Wakefield Press

NOT PART OF THE PUBLIC

Judith Raftery is a history graduate of the University of Adelaide and the Flinders University of South Australia. She is a visiting Senior Lecturer in the Discipline of Public Health at the University of Adelaide and her teaching, research and publications have been in the area of public health history and policy. A major focus of her work has been the impact of colonial and post-colonial history on the health of indigenous people and the current policy implications of this history. In this book she gives a detailed historical account of the impact of non-Aboriginal policies and practices on the health of Aboriginal South Australians, in the light of current public health scholarship about the influence of inequalities on the health of populations.

NOT PART OF THE PUBLIC

Non-indigenous policies and
practices and the health of
indigenous South Australians
1836–1973

JUDITH RAFTERY

Wakefield
Press

Wakefield Press
1 The Parade West
Kent Town
South Australia 5067
www.wakefieldpress.com.au

First published 2006
Copyright © Judith Raftery, 2006

Publication of this book has been assisted by the
Discipline of Public Health, University of Adelaide

Cover designed by Liz Nicholson, designBITE
Text designed by Clinton Ellicott, Wakefield Press
Typeset by Ryan Paine, Wakefield Press
Maps drafted by Christine Crothers
Indexed by Bill Phippard, Seaview Press
Printed and bound by Hyde Park Press

National Library of Australia
Cataloguing-in-publication entry

Raftery, Judith.
Not part of the public: non-indigenous policies and practices
and the health of indigenous South Australians, 1836–1973.

Bibliography.
Includes index.
ISBN-13: 978 1 86254 709 4.
ISBN-10: 1 86254 709 2.

1. Aborigines, Australian – Health and hygiene – South Australia.
2. Medical policy – South Australia – History.
I. Title.
362.1089915

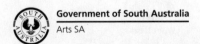

Government of South Australia
Arts SA

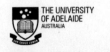

THE UNIVERSITY
OF ADELAIDE
AUSTRALIA

Discipline of Public Health

Contents

This book is dedicated to my children
Simon Peter Raftery and David Jonathon Raftery
and to their children

Acknowledgements

This book had its beginnings in the secure and loving upbringing provided by my parents, Barbara and Lindsay Fitzgerald, and in their unambiguous message that truth, justice and compassion – the hallmarks of a decent society – are things to be fought for. That is the conviction that has energised my career in education, in history and in public health.

I am grateful that throughout my time in the Discipline of Public Health at the University of Adelaide I have been given opportunity to pursue that conviction, on several fronts, but especially in relation to indigenous Australians. When I took up my appointment there were no courses in my discipline, or in the Medical School of which it was a part, dealing with indigenous health. The undergraduate and post-graduate courses on historically-informed indigenous health policy which I developed, and which eventually led to the writing of this book, benefited from three major sources of encouragement and endorsement.

The first was my colleagues' confidence in me, and the provision by the university of opportunities for study leave, which allowed me to learn more about indigenous health issues in New Zealand, North America and in Aboriginal communities beyond Adelaide. The second was the willing cooperation of many South Australian Aboriginal organisations, indigenous units within government departments, and indigenous health professionals, who welcomed me and my students on visits, or participated in classroom sessions. These included Aboriginal Drug and Alcohol Council, Aboriginal Education Unit, Aboriginal Education Development Branch, Aboriginal Health Council of South Australia, Aboriginal Hostels Ltd, Aboriginal Home Care Program, Aboriginal Housing Authority, Aboriginal Legal Rights Service, Aboriginal Services Division of the Department of Human Services, Aboriginal Sobriety Group, Aboriginal and Torres Strait Islander Commission (Adelaide Network Office), Ceduna-Koonibba Aboriginal Health Service, Justice Strategy Unit of the Attorney-General's Department, Nganampa Health Council, Nunkuwarrin Yunti, Nunga Health Team at the Parks Community Health Service, Office of Aboriginal and Torres Strait Islander Health (South Australian Branch), Sacred Site Within Healing Centre, Tauondi College, and the people of Raukkan and Point Pearce. The third source of encouragement and endorsement was the students who elected to enrol in my courses. Their openness to new learning, their willingness to confront uncomfortable truths about the past and the present, and their commitment to building an inclusive and healthier future, were more sustaining of me than they would guess. In all of this, there were some individuals whose strategic support, intellectual companionship, sensitive co-teaching, courageous and imaginative research, or honest sharing of insight and experience was especially significant: Brian Dixon, Neville Hicks, David Raftery, Vicki-Lee Knowles, Jasmine Valadian, Simon Baccanello, Adriana Milazzo, Marguerite Tyson, Major Sumner and Rosemary Wanganeen.

I am grateful for several kinds of practical support. A small grant from the Department of Human Services was invaluable in enabling me to employ Peter Strawhan, who cheerfully did some of the initial, tedious archival searching. Adriana Parrella did final electronic hunting and checking of facts and references with much greater aplomb than I could muster. Brian Fleming, Robert Foster, Neville Hicks and Michelle Renshaw read draft chapters and offered valuable feedback on style and substance. The Discipline of Public Health at the University of Adelaide provided financial support for the publication process.

It has taken much time, energy and self-belief to write this book. There are easier projects I could have pursued, and, along the way, life kept throwing up other challenges and major distractions. That my centre held, and that things did not fall apart, owes much to the wisdom, sensitivity, love and shared commitments of my chief companion on the journey, John Raftery.

Judith Raftery
Adelaide
July 2005

A Note on Language

Finding appropriate and respectful language to refer to the descendants of the original population of Australia presents a challenge, especially when one is writing about an extended period of time. In line with what I understand to be the current preference of many indigenous South Australians I have used specific names of indigenous nations – for example, Ngarrindjeri, Adnyamathanha, Kaurna etc. – where this is possible and appropriate, and 'Aboriginal' as a noun in preference to 'Aborigine', when making more general references. For stylistic purposes I have also used 'indigenous' interchangeably with 'Aboriginal'. Thus I write of Aboriginals, Aboriginal or indigenous South Australians, the Aboriginal or indigenous population etc. When the authorial voice is clearly mine I have adopted this usage regardless of the conventions of period about which I am writing. However, when I am quoting or paraphrasing statements made in earlier times, or referring directly to the details of reports or legislation, I use whatever terms were used then – for example, 'aborigines', 'blacks', 'natives', 'primitives' – even though these are now deemed offensive. While this does not, of course, involve endorsement of such terms it serves to illustrate the attitudes and assumptions prevailing at different times in history. I believe that context, tone and attribution indicate when I am using someone else's language or 'voice' in this way.

The use of the upper case 'A' in 'Aboriginal/s' and 'Aborigine/s' was officially established by the *Aborigines Act, 1962*.

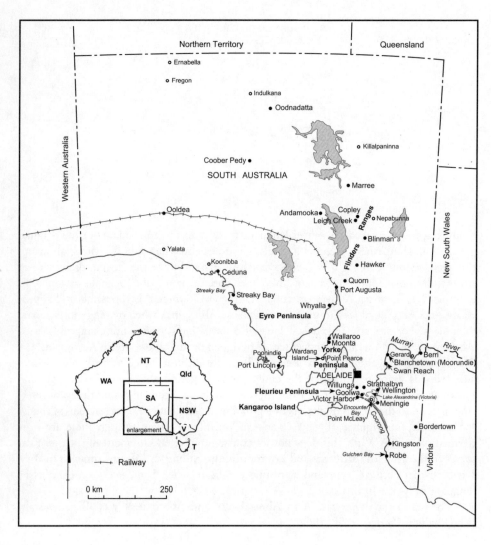

Principal places referred to in the text

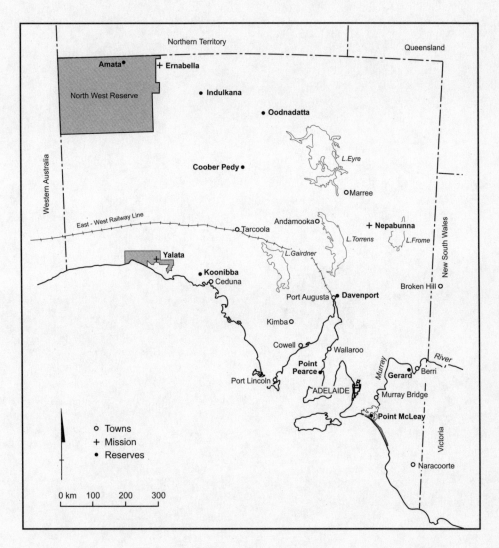

South Australian Main Aboriginal Reserves,
SAPP 23, 1972, page 53.

Chapter 1

History and Health

In announcing to the Colonists of His Majesty's Province of South Australia the establishment of the Government, I hereby call upon them to conduct themselves on all occasions with order and quietness, duly to respect the laws, and by a course of industry and sobriety, by the practice of sound morality, and a strict observance of the ordinances of Religion, to prove themselves worthy to be the founders of a great and free colony.

It is also, at this time, especially my duty to apprize the Colonists of my resolution to take every lawful means for extending the same protection to the Native population as to the rest of His Majesty's subjects, and of my firm determination to punish with exemplary severity all acts of violence or injustice which may in any manner be practised or attempted against the Natives, who are to be considered as much under the safeguard of the law as the Colonists themselves, and equally entitled to the privileges of British subjects. I trust therefore, with confidence, to the exercise of moderation and forbearance by all classes, in their intercourse with the Native Inhabitants, and that they will omit no opportunity of assisting me to fulfil His Majesty's most gracious and benevolent intentions towards them, by promoting their advancement in civilization, and ultimately, under the blessing of Divine Providence their conversion to the Christian faith. **Governor Hindmarsh's Proclamation 28 December 1836**[1]

This much-quoted statement of Governor John Hindmarsh, delivered at Glenelg on 28 December 1836, is solemnly repeated on the anniversary of that day each year in a ceremony attended by the state governor, the premier, the local mayor, other government and community representatives and members of the public. The ceremony is held near the gum tree which provided shade for Hindmarsh and his party, and which is now maintained in its widely recognised curved shape by many tonnes of concrete.

The faithfulness and seriousness of this re-enactment is not matched by public understanding or valuing of the significance of 'Proclamation Day', as 28 December is officially known. Despite the iconic status of the Old Gum Tree and the wrath which is provoked by acts of vandalism against it, most South Australians would not be able to say what was proclaimed on 28 December 1836. The popular significance of the day is that it provides

---

1 *South Australian Gazette and Colonial Register*, 3 June 1837, p.1

an extra public holiday which extends the Christmas break. Indeed the actual date is so unimportant that the holiday is sometimes shifted from the 28 December to whichever nearby day will produce a longer weekend, or a more solid block of 'days off'. And yet in recent years it has become clear that what is annually commemorated at the site of the Old Gum Tree matters greatly to some of the descendants of the indigenous inhabitants whose rights and privileges under British law were proclaimed there in 1836. Aboriginal South Australians have recently used the Proclamation Day ceremony as an opportunity to remind the state's leaders of the ways in which Hindmarsh's promises and admonitions have been ignored.

In the early 1830s there were high hopes for the proposed colony of South Australia. There were persons of humanitarian temper within the British Colonial Office and in British society at large who had a sense of responsibility towards the native population, expressed in a desire to protect their rights to land and to extend to them the benefits of Christianity and civilisation. However, these hopes and desires did not prevail over the more pragmatic concerns of the South Australian Colonisation Commissioners, whose chief concern was the early material success of the colony. In fact, the legislative protection offered indigenous inhabitants by the *South Australia Act* of 1834, especially in relation to land, was vague and in practice easily set aside.[2] It proved to be fragile in the face of the more general context of European beliefs about the relative merits of different 'races' of people and the colonists' day-to-day experiences of 'the natives' in situations that were new and bewildering for both groups.

If the 'lofty motives' of Lord Glenelg, the Secretary of State for the Colonies carried little weight in the Colonial Office in London[3] they carried even less on the Adelaide plains and the surrounding country, where the settlers needed to establish a living and where the inevitable clash between the economic imperatives of the colonial endeavour and the basis of the indigenous population's ancient way of life quickly became apparent. What carried more weight were the widespread beliefs and assumptions, held with varying levels of sophistication and consciousness by scholars, scientists, government officials, missionaries and the general public about various versions of race theory. This was a complex, often contradictory and evolving set of ideas, but whether it invoked Divine Providence, or Enlightenment stage theory, or natural selection of the fittest as its cornerstone, the effect was the same: Aboriginals were at the bottom of the evolutionary scale.[4]

2 For an analysis of views and tensions within the Colonial Office, and between it and the Colonisation Commission and an account of the defeat of humanitarian hopes, see RM Gibbs, 'Humanitarian Theories and the Aboriginal Inhabitants of South Australia to 1860', BA (Hons) thesis, University of Adelaide, 1959. For more general accounts of the settlement of South Australia see Douglas Pike, *Paradise of Dissent: South Australia 1829–1857*, Melbourne University Press, Carlton, Victoria, 1967 [1957], and Dean Jaensch, ed., *The Flinders History of South Australia: political history*, Wakefield Press, Adelaide, 1986.

3 Gibbs, 'Humanitarian Theories and the Aboriginal Inhabitants of South Australia', p.36

4 For a comprehensive and nuanced analysis of the development of this thinking, and the historic shifts in its application to policy and practice in the Australian colonies, see Russell McGregor, *Imagined Destinies: Aboriginal Australians and doomed race theory, 1880–1939*, Melbourne University Press, Carlton, Victoria, 1997.

Some argued that the economic and social 'backwardness' of the natives was the result of isolation and restricted opportunity rather than of racial character, and thus believed in their capacity, given appropriate conditions, for progress. While this Enlightenment view was never completely obliterated and was to resassert itself and increase in authority in the early twentieth century, a less optimistic view quickly gained greater currency in the early colonial period. As the European presence expanded and consolidated, settler and missionary activity produced doubts about indigenous adaptability to western culture or capacity to survive contact with it, and officials and scientists increasingly used evolutionary theory to render 'the difference between savage and civilised as one not merely of attainment, but also of capacity'.[5] McGregor has traced in detail the ebb and flow of these views and their complex relationship to each other and to the intellectual and political currents of the times. He summarises the process whereby, over the course of the nineteenth century, the view of Aboriginals as incapable of civilisation

> rapidly gained ascendancy, as European understandings of other peoples hardened into a science of sharp racial differences. By the end of the century, evolutionary theory had consolidated an image of innately primitive Aboriginals; unable to adapt to the circumstances of civilisation, they would be exterminated by its progress. This view of the Aboriginals as a race irretrievably locked into the Stone Age persisted well into the twentieth century.[6]

It was a view that lent weight to the belief that the Aboriginals were a doomed and dying race, and powerfully shaped policy and practice.

There were other views, of course. Missionaries often saw the fate of the Aboriginals as 'a matter of human responsibility, not the outcome of the inexorable workings of a natural law'.[7] This view was implicit in the objectives and activities of the Aborigines' Friends' Association (AFA), founded in Adelaide in 1858, though it was not always manifest in the missionary work it sponsored. The AFA was established following a public meeting held on 28 July 1857 to consider 'the Condition of the Aborigines'. Those present lamented the general lack of interest displayed by both government and the colonial community in the welfare of 'the natives'. However, they took encouragement from the Anglican experiment at Poonindie[8]: in their view it demonstrated that the Aboriginals were capable of being useful members of society and Christians to boot.[9] Even in the scientific and medical community, where, for the most part, 'evolutionary theory rendered attainment an indicator of capacity'[10], there were differing views. Dr William Ramsay Smith, prominent physician, naturalist, anthropologist and public health official, declared the Aboriginal 'problem' remediable, dependant on the imagination and will of

---

5 McGregor, *Imagined Destinies*, p.24

6 Russell McGregor, 'Protest and progress: Aboriginal activism in the 1930s', *Australian Historical Studies*, vol.25, no.101, October 1993, p.558

7 See McGregor, *Imagined Destinies*, p.60 for some examples.

8 See below, pp.67–9

9 *Observer*, 1 August 1857

10 McGregor, *Imagined Destinies*, p.59

the non-indigenous.[11] Nevertheless, the doomed race theme remained dominant until well into the twentieth century, and all its variants served to underpin the segregationist and protectionist policies and practices, both formal and informal, that were adopted in the Australian colonies from the late nineteenth century.

There was no local academic community of historians to record and analyse this early colonial history. Nor was there such a community for most of the period covered in this book, since, even though modern history was taught at the University of Adelaide from 1900, there was little emphasis on Australian history until much later. However, missionaries, educated colonists and members of the professional and leisured classes in South Australia produced many accounts of the challenges, successes, pleasures, and curiosities of their new lives and the achievements of the South Australian experiment. These, as well as the records of government and administration, which underpin much of the argument of this book, provide insight into the general context of beliefs, values and unexamined assumptions which shaped the colonial experience and, in particular, impinged on the lives of the indigenous inhabitants in complex direct and indirect ways. Edwin Hodder, for example, in his *The History of South Australia From its Foundation to the Year of its Jubilee, with a Chronological Summary of all the Principal Events of Interest up to Date*,[12] noted that in the new colony, 'the welfare of the aborigines' was not 'overlooked'. He claimed that, despite the deficiencies of the 1834 act:

> from the outset of all negotiations for colonizing South Australia, the commissioners made special provision for their welfare, while in the plans of the South Australian company the chairman invariably set the claims of the natives, and the duty of the servants of the Company in regard to them, in the forefront.[13]

The first volume of Hodder's history contains several accounts of newsworthy events involving the original inhabitants. These included massacres, punitive expeditions, missionary activity, and the inexplicable behaviour of the native girl, 'Nancy', who, despite instruction at the Native School, regular church attendance and employment as a domestic servant at Government House, 'suddenly, without any apparent or sufficient reason, left her situation, returned to her tribe, and, to a great extent, to her primitive mode of life'.[14] On occasion, Hodder reported on the views of government regarding the natives, but made no attempt to provide a complete account of these views. He recorded, for

---

11 WR Smith, 'The Aborigines of Australia', *Official Year Book of the Commonwealth of Australia*, no.3, 1901–1909, p.175. For a summary of Smith's career, see Ronald G Elmslie and Susan Nance, 'Smith, William Ramsay (1859–1937)', in Geoffrey Serle, (ed.), *Australian Dictionary of Biography, vol.11, 1891–1939*, Melbourne University Press, Carlton, Victoria, 1988, pp.674–5.

12 Edwin Hodder, *The history of South Australia from its Foundation to the Year of its Jubilee, with a Chronological Summary of all the Principal Events of Interest up to date* (two volumes), Sampson Low, Marston and Company, London, 1893. Hodder was the biographer of Colonization Commissioner and prominent South Australian pioneer, George Fife Angas, and had access to the records Angas had collected with the aim of writing a history of the colony.

13 Hodder, *The History of South Australia from its Foundation to the Year of its Jubilee*, vol 1, p.85

14 ibid., p.168

example, that in 1844 Governor Grey commended to the Legislative Council a bill for the care of Aboriginal orphans, maintaining that 'the care of such orphans afforded the best chance of civilizing the race, by educating the children and attaching them to our customs'.[15] However, it is clear that, to Hodder, the real history of South Australia was the history of its European settlers. The indigenous people appear in his narrative only sporadically, and by the second volume, which deals with the years from 1868, they have disappeared entirely. At the end of that volume he summarised the situation which presented itself to Lord Kintore when he arrived in April of 1889 to take up the governorship of the colony: whereas 'a little more than fifty years before the site was a nameless wilderness', he 'found in Adelaide a model city, beautiful for situation, and marvelously developed'. Hodder concluded:

> There can be little doubt that the future of South Australia will be one of wealth and usefulness ... all the vast extent of the land which is not under settlement has a prospective value ... this enormous extent of unalienated land, hundreds of thousands of square miles ... sources of wealth practically illimitable.[16]

The original owners of this 'unalienated land' and of its potential wealth had simply disappeared, unremarked, from his story.

Another prominent commentator, the Rev. John Blacket, Methodist minister and author of eight books of philosophy and history[17], saw the early history of South Australia as 'a most romantic one', which revealed 'the grit, the energy, the perseverance, and the determination which are such potent factors in the mental and moral make-up of the British race'. The colonists, were, in his view:

> men and women who could 'replenish the earth and subdue it' ... Their motto was 'conquer or die' ... and they made 'the wilderness and the solitary place glad' and 'the desert blossom as the rose'.[18]

The indigenous population he described as treacherous, warlike, dangerous and 'barbarous in the extreme', pursuing 'peculiar customs' and 'strange ways'. They 'gave the early settlers much trouble'.[19] However, he acknowledged that they 'suffered much from contact with some unprincipled and lecherous whites', and were soon reduced to 'a weak, degraded, decimated race, doomed to speedy extinction'.[20]

The writings of Hodder and Blacket belong to a genre which flourished from the late

---

15 ibid., p.192

16 ibid., vol 11, pp.124, 141

17 For a summary of Blacket's life, see Arnold D Hunt, 'Blacket, John (1856–1935)', in Bede Nairn and Geoffrey Serle, (eds), *Australian Dictionary of Biography*, vol. 7, 1891–1939, Melbourne University Press, Carlton, Victoria, 1979, pp.312–13.

18 Blacket, Rev. John. *History of South Australia: a romantic and successful experiment in colonization*, second edition, Hussey and Gillingham, Adelaide, 1911, p.xvii

19 ibid., pp.161–63

20 ibid., p.46

nineteenth century, that is, personal memoirs and chronological histories detailing local events and developments. Such writing, which was often associated with memorialising on the occasions of significant anniversaries, cemented a legend of noble pioneers securing the colony's future in the face of the depredations of the primitive, treacherous and ultimately doomed natives. It sustained its appeal over a considerable period, sometimes bolstered by scholarly and institutional support, as seen, for example, in the 1936 centenary publication of the Royal Geographical Society of Australasia, South Australian Branch.[21] In their examination of instances of frontier violence in the colony's early history, Foster, Hosking and Nettelbeck have demonstrated how such writing effectively silenced alternative voices, and normalised a sanitised and heroic account of European settlement. This account, which largely denies the violence done to the indigenous population and reveals scant sympathy with their reaction to it, became accepted as fact and formed the basis of public attitudes and policy.[22]

Another category of writers, who travelled extensively in the Australian colonies and produced promotional material of a popular kind describing many aspects of the natural, social and economic environment, also contributed to this process. May Vivienne was one such commentator. Her assessment of the initial contact between colonists and natives matched that of Blacket: she wrote of a 'noble band of pioneers' who at first needed protection from the 'savage attacks' and 'artful ways' of the natives.[23] However, the natives soon became 'poor creatures, who are grateful for any kindness they receive'. Her journeying took her to the mission at Point McLeay, where it was

> quite a novelty to go ashore and see these civilized natives at work. They look very happy and contented ... and the government is certainly doing all it can for 'our black brudders', who are so swiftly but surely dying out.[24]

These 'civilized', easily pleased but doomed natives at Point McLeay were the Ngarrindjeri people to whom the AFA had been sending missionaries since 1859. The first and most distinguished of these was the Rev. George Taplin, whose experience led him to conclude that:

> it has now been proved the Aborigines of Australia are not altogether a hopeless case. We may hope that the Gospel of Christ will be the means of saving a remnant from extinction.[25]

---

21 See below, pp.18–19

22 Robert Foster, Rick Hosking and Amanda Nettelbeck, *Fatal Collisions: the South Australian frontier and the violence of memory*, Wakefield Press, Adelaide, 2001

23 May Vivienne, *Sunny South Australia: its city-towns, seaports, beauty-spots, fruit, vineyards and flowers; its wheat, wool, wine, sheep, dairying, copper, iron, phosphates, and other progressive industries from 1837 to 1908 with map. 4000 miles of travel*, Hussey and Gillingham, Adelaide, 1908, pp.15–23

24 ibid., p.169

25 Rev. George Taplin, *The Narrinyeri; an account of the tribes of South Australian Aborigines inhabiting the country around the Lakes Alexandrina, Albert, and Coorong, and the lower part of the River Murray: their manners and customs. Also, An Account of the Mission at Point McLeay*, JT Shaw, Adelaide, 1874, p.iv

Taplin was an educated and reflective man. He made careful study of the language of the Ngarrindjeri and tried to discern the meanings and values underlying their beliefs and customs. And although he did not foster their independence and was adamant that much of their culture was injurious and needed to be proscribed, he showed concern for their welfare, and was energetic in arguing their cause with the government:

> In common justice, we are bound to see that the Aborigines do not suffer from our occupation of the soil. We are under moral obligation to see that they are no worse off than before.[26]

The influence of nineteenth-century evolutionary thinking was evidenced in his belief that the culture of the Ngarrindjeri was indicative of a previous 'higher state of social life', but at the time of contact they were sunk in barbarism, and barbarism led inevitably to extinction. As fellow human beings they deserved whatever protection the state and the missions could provide, but they had no choices and not much hope of a future:

> It is not wise to attempt to civilize these people too fast. Judgment has to be exercised and the treatment to be adapted to their condition. We are not to suppose that they are capable of taking upon them the duties of a state of society which we have been trained for by ages of civilisation.[27]

Thus the natives whom Governor Hindmarsh and the colonists were enjoined to consider as much under the safeguard of the law as themselves and equally entitled to the privileges of British subjects, soon either disappeared from view and thought, or became a problem sub-population, imagined and dealt with as a group quite apart from the rest of his majesty's subjects. As a group apart, they were perceived as either dangerous and troublesome, or as pathetic, simple and easily pleased, or as needing to be controlled, protected, civilised and enlightened. In any case, their demise seemed inevitable. From the beginning, their economic and social needs for such fundamental provisions as land, shelter and food were assumed to be different from and less than those of the colonists, and their loyalties, affections and values to be lacking in evidence of civilisation. In the context of such views and beliefs, it was easy to read the decline in Aboriginal numbers, the escalation of illness and despair, the growth of dependence and the breakdown of traditional life as evidence of cultural inferiority, rather than as a result of European intrusion. From there it needed only a short conceptual step for the colonists to convince themselves that they and their government had exhausted their responsibility to the native population, and were doing 'all that could be done'. In this context, a doctrine of minimal provision could as readily be accommodated by those whose attitudes were sympathetic as by those who were more hostile and unashamedly racist.

---

26 ibid., p.100

27 ibid., pp.75–6, 100–1

This book traces the impact of non-indigenous views, policies and practices in South Australia on the health of indigenous South Australians. It offers a critical synthesis and overview that has not been attempted before. There is a growing body of historical and other work that focuses on the impact of European settlement, and of the entrenchment of European culture, values, political and economic structures and priorities on the original inhabitants of South Australia. This material includes the prolific pioneering anthropological work of Catherine and Ronald Berndt, beginning with *From Black to White in South Australia* (1951); Graham Jenkin's sympathetic study of the Ngarrindjeri people of the lower Murray area, *The Conquest of the Ngarrindjeri* (1979); Peggy Brock's *Outback Ghettos: a history of Aboriginal institutionalization and survival* (1993), which questions blanket judgements about institutionalisation and demonstrates indigenous resilience and ingenuity in the face of social and economic encroachment; sections on South Australia within studies of missionary enterprise, such as John Harris's *One Blood— 200 years of Aboriginal encounter with Christianity: a story of hope*, (1990) and Tony Swain's and Deborah Bird Rose's, *Aboriginal Christians and Christian Missions* (1988); and Foster, Hosking and Nettelbeck's analysis – already mentioned – of the ways in which frontier conflict has been portrayed and used to shape policy and practice. In addition to these studies by non-indigenous writers, there are South Australian indigenous publications, often making use of oral history and very local sources, which focus on the direct impact of non-indigenous policies on indigenous communities, families and individuals. Most substantial and influential among these is Christobel Mattingley's and Ken Hampton's *Survival in Our Own Land: 'Aboriginal' experiences in 'South Australia'* (1988). The submissions of indigenous South Australians to the National Inquiry into the Separation of Aboriginal and Torres Strait Islander Children from their Families, *Bringing Them Home* (1997), add another dimension to this history. A brief but valuable summary account of South Australian 'Aboriginal histories' – histories by and about indigenous people – is Victoria Haskins' essay in *The Wakefield Companion to South Australian History*.[28]

These South Australian accounts can be read against a national context of historical and anthropological scholarship on the impact of European colonisation on indigenous Australians. Among the significant markers in this wider field are WEH Stanner's 1968 Boyer lectures, *After the Dreaming: black and white Australia – an anthropologist's view* (1969), which draws attention to 'the great Australian silence' which had prevailed in historical literature to that time in relation to the continuing presence of Aboriginal people in Australia; CD Rowley's three pioneering volumes on Aboriginal policy and practice across the nation, *The Destruction of Aboriginal Society* (1970), *Outcasts in White Australia* (1971), and *The Remote Aborigines* (1971); the journal *Aboriginal History*, which since 1978 has promoted a multi-disciplinary approach to the study of 'Aboriginal history' and encouraged indigenous authors and co-authors; Henry Reynolds' *The Other Side of the Frontier* (1981), which questions the received wisdom about frontier conflict and

---

28 Victoria Haskins, 'Aboriginal Histories' in Wilfrid Prest (ed.), *The Wakefield Companion to South Australian History*, Wakefield Press, Adelaide, 2001, pp.3–6. *The Wakefield Companion*, reflecting the enlarged awareness of recent years, contains entries on various aspects of indigenous history and culture.

initial indigenous responses to European invasion; Richard Broome's *Aboriginal Australians: black response to white dominance, 1788–1980* (1982), which details a variety of indigenous responses to the establishment of European political, economic and cultural hegemony; Anne McGrath's *'Born in the Cattle': Aborigines in the cattle industry* (1987) which makes use of 'new' methodologies and categories of analysis to show that Aborigines could 'inhabit both sides of the frontier' and incorporate work 'for the coloniser' into 'their own cultural frameworks'; Bain Atwood's *The Making of the Aborigines* (1989), which presents an argument about the 'construction' of Aboriginality by the experience of colonisation; McGrath's (ed.) *Contested Ground: Australian Aboriginals under the British Crown* (1995), an anthology which provides, along with historical overviews from each colony/state, an analysis of the 'contested ground' of 'Aboriginal history' and historiography; Anna Haebich's *For Their Own Good: Aborigines and government in the south west of Western Australia, 1900–1940* (1998) and Rosalind Kidd's, *The Way We Civilise: Aboriginal affairs – the untold story* (1997) which expose the institutionalised racism and ongoing production of indigenous marginalisation in Western Australia and Queensland; Tim Rowse's *White Flour, White Power: from rations to citizenship in Central Australia* (1998), which offers a complex analysis of the meanings attached to rationing and the program and policy goals which it served; and Attwood's and SG Foster's *Frontier Conflict: the Australian experience* (2003) which, as well as canvassing current scholarship about the frontier, analyses the state of 'Aboriginal history' and the political and intellectual debates it has raised.[29]

My project acknowledges and makes use of this earlier scholarship but also attempts something new. My focus is health. None of the works mentioned above focuses specifically on health, although many have much to say about health. What they say is implicit rather than explicit, and may not even be recognised as health-related. Often when they make specific mention of health, it is in the restricted context of disease, medical services and other forms of health care. In fact, their focus is on illness and how it is dealt with, rather than on health and how it might be produced and safeguarded.

When I write about health I am referring to well-being, that is, a state of being which enables individuals and populations to live a life that is good, according to their values and aspirations, and which, for individuals, extends as long and is marked by as much opportunity for human flourishing, as is experienced by others who share their time and place in history. Health has physical aspects, most clearly manifested in freedom from and control over illness and injury, and in longevity. It also has psychological aspects, for example, a reasonably robust sense of self-worth and of control over one's circumstances, and spiritual aspects, such as a sense of at-one-ness with one's community and with those things which are deemed to give life its deepest meaning. Thus health is relative and

---

29 This selective and non-exhaustive list indicates some of the important dimensions of the now extensive body of scholarship which has broken Stanner's 'great Australian silence'. For detailed and insightful discussion of 'Aboriginal history' and historiography see Anne McGrath (ed.), *Contested Ground: Australian Aborigines under the British Crown*, Allen and Unwin, Sydney, 1995, chapter 10: Contested ground: what is 'Aboriginal history', pp.359–97, and Bain Attwood and SG Foster (eds), *Frontier Conflict: the Australian experience*, National Museum of Australia, Canberra, 2003, especially 'Introduction', pp.1–30 and chapter 13: Historiography on the Australian frontier, pp.169–84.

culturally and historically determined. It is also politically determined, in that it can be withheld from or undermined in some groups within populations, according to how power and opportunity are divided and shared, and according to which values and aspirations are legitimated and valued, and which are not.

We need to be clear at this point that the current health status of Aboriginal people, now well documented and often referred to as a national disgrace, is of recent origin.[30] It is a product of colonisation. We need to be clear also that late in the eighteenth century, when non-Aboriginal people first settled permanently in Australia, the health of the indigenous population compared favourably with that of the European populations from which the settlers came. Those European populations experienced high levels of mortality, especially infant mortality, as a result of infectious diseases. They needed to work very long hours in order to feed themselves, often in environments that were unsafe or disease-producing. As urbanisation and industrialisation advanced, they were exposed to the manifold health threats associated with overcrowded and insanitary housing, polluted water supplies, unsafe food production and gross inequalities in access to material comforts and opportunities of all kinds. Medical care, like other social goods, was much less available to the poorer groups than to the well-off, and in any case was very limited in its efficacy.

Without falling prey to a modern tendency to romanticise the traditional, we can say that, by comparison, indigenous Australians were at that stage a relatively healthy lot. Certainly the harshness of much of their physical environment, their hunter-gatherer economy and the absence of agricultural development meant that they lacked the capacity to produce surpluses, to sustain a large population or to protect the weak at either end of the life span. And certainly traditional Aboriginal culture legitimated forms of violence and gender-based inequalities that were both distinctly unhealthy and unacceptable to modern sensibilities – as did the culture of the colonisers.[31] However, indigenous Australians enjoyed near-complete freedom from infectious disease, and had a nutritionally sound diet based on food procured without exposure to unhealthy or unsafe working conditions. Their controlled, semi-nomadic lifestyle meant the gross inequalities and health threats associated with urbanisation and industrialisation in the context of an unregulated market economy were unknown among them. Ancient law and ceremonial life, which made individuals aware of their place within the group, their obligations to it, and what they could expect of others, provided the means to maintain communal harmony and well-being, or restore it when disrupted. Within that system, health was seen as evidence and outcome of proper group functioning and the maintenance of right relationships. When illness or injury occurred, there were recognised healers whose skills

---

30 For an historically informed account see Milton J Lewis, *The People's Health: public health in Australia, 1788–1950* (vol.1) and *1950 to the present* (vol.2), Praeger, Connecticut, 2003, pp.20–7, vol.1, pp.234–58, vol.2. See also Edith Cowan University's comprehensive indigenous health website: <www.healthinfonet.ecu.edu.au>. See also below, Appendix 1 for a summary of current indigenous health status.

31 For discussion about the contribution of traditional culture, especially when distorted by the unresolved disruption caused by colonisation, to the recent and current poor health of indigenous people, see Peter Sutton, 'The Politics of Suffering: indigenous policy in Australia since the 1970s', *Anthropological Forum*, vol.11, no.2, 2001, pp.125–73.

and therapeutic advice, although undoubtedly not always efficacious, were available to all and focused on the psychological and spiritual, in the sense described above, as well as the physical aspects of health.[32]

At the time of colonisation, therefore, the health of the indigenous population compared favourably with that of the settlers. Subsequent history has reversed that situation. As already argued, health is politically determined and can be withheld from or undermined in some groups within populations. Since European colonisation the population from whom the experience of health has been most consistently and comprehensively withheld or undermined is the indigenous population. Of course there is evidence of good health among indigenous Australians and there are other groups of Australians whose health suffers because of Australia's social and political arrangements. It is clear that there are, within the Australian population as in other populations, gradations of health that reflect social gradations and inequalities. It is also clear that, when non-indigenous researchers and policy-makers measure health, they do not usually include all those things that indigenous people take as markers of health or its absence. Nevertheless, on the basis of a range of factors that have been clearly demonstrated to have a bearing on health in Australian society and in others like it – income, education, employment, housing, nutrition, rate of incarceration, social connectedness and access to health services – Aboriginal people do worse than any other sub-population. This book asks, 'Why is this so?' It seeks answers in a history of policies and practices which have not merely disadvantaged indigenous Australians but constructed them as not part of the public.

There is an existing literature on the health of indigenous Australians and some of it understands health in broad terms and explores it within historical contexts. This includes, for example, Janice Reid and Peggy Trompf's *The Health of Aboriginal Australia* (1991), Ernest Hunter's *Aboriginal Health and History* (1993), Stephen Kunitz's, *Disease and Social Diversity: the European impact on the health of non-Europeans* (1994) and Tim Rowse's *Traditions for Health* (1996). However, none of these sets out to survey the impact of non-indigenous interventions on indigenous health over a long historical period in the light of current understandings of what contributes to the health of populations, and none concentrates on South Australia. That is what this book does.

In South Australia, as in the rest of Australia, there were no Aboriginal health policies as such for most of the period since European settlement, although there were some health

---

32 For further insight into indigenous health prior to European settlement, see Geoffrey Blainey, *The Triumph of the Nomads: a history of ancient Australia*, Sun Books, Melbourne, 1976; Jenny Burden, 'Health: an holistic approach', in Colin Bourke, Eleanor Bourke and Bill Edwards (eds), *Aboriginal Australia: an introductory reader in Aboriginal studies*, 2nd edn, University of Queensland Press, St Lucia, 1998, pp.189–93; Margaret-Ann Franklin and Isobel White, 'The History and Politics of Aboriginal Health', in Janice Reid and Peggy Trompf (eds), *The Health of Aboriginal Australia*, Harcourt Brace Jovanovich, Sydney, 1991, pp.1–3. For a brief summary of traditional indigenous approaches to healing see Report of the House of Representatives Standing Committee on Aboriginal Affairs: 'Aboriginal Health', *Commonwealth Parliamentary Paper*, no.60, 1979, pp.67–9, 124.

services and practices designed especially for the indigenous population. However, there were other policies and practices directed at Aboriginals which had a profound impact on their health. These included, for example, educational and economic policies which were designed to provide them with just enough education to fit them for a narrow range of low-paid and low-status jobs. Aboriginal health was also shaped by social attitudes which construed Aboriginals as inferior and, in complex ways, provided them with negative views of themselves. Such constructions frequently became self-fulfilling prophecies leading to underachievement, constrained choices and poor health. My intention is to link what we now know, from the burgeoning and multi-disciplinary area of public health research – and especially recent research into the links between social inequalities and health – with the history of policies, practices and social views relating to Aboriginal people. The purpose of this is to demonstrate that this history was a recipe for poor health and constitutes a substantial explanation for ongoing poor health.

At a time when politicians, pundits and historians are turning black and white arm-bands into heavy artillery, it is worth insisting that my project is not about 'reading backwards', or about blaming or reprimanding previous generations for what they did or did not do. Rather it is about using the new insights delivered by recent and ongoing public health scholarship to illuminate the past, explain why things are as they are now, and allow that understanding to radically challenge our current prescriptions for improving health and to suggest alternative futures. This critical historical analysis recognises that 'the truth' is never arrived at, and that understandings are always partial and contingent, but nevertheless engages seriously with the question of how things could be different. Thus I claim for the discipline of history a complex, fundamentally social and moral role. This is not new in health history. Charles Rosenberg has written of the potential of social and historical analysis to drive social action by focusing our attention on 'the perceived gap between the "is" and the "ought to be"'.[33] Paul Starr has argued that 'analyses of roads not taken remind us that the past had other opportunities and so do we today'.[34] And Michel Foucault has argued powerfully for history unashamedly linked to social and moral purpose. According to Thacker, Foucault's final and most mature understanding of writing history is that it

> is one way we can bring to prominence those restrictions upon our present subjectivities that perhaps should be transgressed, the points where change in values and action is possible. The past then does not merely help us understand the present, it also helps us have the courage to imagine that the present could be different from the form it manifests at the moment.[35]

While there were no specific or targeted *Aboriginal* health policies prior to the devel-

---

33 Charles E Rosenberg, 'Framing Disease: illness, society and history', in Charles E Rosenberg and Janet Golden (eds), *Framing disease: studies in cultural history*, Rutgers University Press, Rutgers NJ, 1992, p.xxii

34 Paul Starr, *The Social Transformation of American Medicine*, Basic Books, New York, 1982, p.xi

35 Andrew Thacker, 'Foucault and the writing of history', in Moya Lloyd and Andrew Thacker (eds), *The Impact of Michel Foucault on the Social Sciences and Humanities*, Macmillan, Basingstoke, 1997, p.39

opment of the National Aboriginal Health Strategy in 1989[36], there have been general health policies in South Australia since the early days of colonisation. The earliest of these reflected the immediate health concerns of a young population seeking to establish itself in a raw environment at a time when the therapeutic capacity of medicine was limited. These concerns were the control of infectious disease, quarantine regulations and vaccination against smallpox. The *Public Health Acts* of 1873 and 1898 reflected growing understandings of the conditions that contributed to the health of individuals and populations and also greater intervention by government to ensure that those conditions were provided and protected. They were modelled on similar legislation enacted to meet the health crises of rapidly industrialising Great Britain. By offering protection against some of the most obvious and far-reaching dangers to health which, although not new, became more apparent in urban settings (for example, unsafe water supplies and lack of sewerage and public sanitation), they acted as a force for social order and economic progress as well as for better health. Two further acts in 1935 and 1987, as well as frequent amendments between these dates, responded to emerging health issues and needs and involved governments in a growing range of responsibilities for protecting the health of the public in their homes, at school, at work and in the community at large. These acts also committed the government to the provision of increasingly complex infrastructure and a panoply of regulations and regimes of monitoring and surveillance.

This public health legislation purported to maintain and protect the health of the public, that is, the people of South Australia. None of it specifically stated who belonged to this 'public', and it is clear that the earlier legislation left untouched many threats to the well-being of the least powerful groups. It is worth noting that the earliest nineteenth-century public health reforms, and the easiest to achieve, were those that dealt with conditions directly affecting the rich as well as the poor. Conditions affecting mainly the poor, and from which, in many cases, the rich profited were much more resistant to reform. This reflects the limited political franchise and limited notions of citizenship operating in the nineteenth century.[37] However, the public health acts did not indicate that any groups of the population were excluded from or not covered by their provisions. In the

---

36 National Aboriginal Health Strategy Working Party, *A National Aboriginal Health Strategy*, AGPS, Canberra, 1989. The working party arose out of the perception of Commonwealth, state and territory ministers that, despite the Commonwealth takeover of responsibility for indigenous affairs in 1973 and subsequent increases in funding and effort, there had been little or no improvement in indigenous health. The working party, which consulted widely throughout Australia and received many written submissions, was set up by the Keating Labor Government in 1987. It had 19 members, two, including the chair, appointed by the Commonwealth Government, eight appointed by state governments and nine appointed by the Aboriginal community. South Australian members were Barbara Wingard, Aboriginal Health Worker, Aboriginal Health Organisation, Murray Bridge, and Clare Coulthard, Chairperson, Pika Wiya Health Service, Port Augusta. For details of the working party's membership and its consultation process, see *A National Aboriginal Health Strategy*, chapter one, pp.1–6.

37 For further insight into the political forces and fears that shaped the reform agenda, and accorded some groups only a limited membership of the 'public', see Gareth Stedman Jones, *Outcast London: a study in the relationship between classes in Victorian society*, Peregrine, Harmondsworth, 1984. For a detailed account of threats to the health of the public and how these were understood and responded to, see Anthony S Wohl, *Endangered Lives: public health in Victorian Britain*, Methuen, London, 1983.

absence of any specific exclusions, the common-sense reading of the term 'public' must therefore be an inclusive one. Indeed, the 1987 act stated explicitly that it was the duty of the South Australian Health Commission, the body responsible for the administration and enforcement of the act, 'to promote proper standards of public and environmental health in the state generally'. However, there was in fact a radical exclusion. The historical record makes it clear that Aboriginal South Australians were not regarded as part of the general public. They were seen as a separate 'public', with different needs which could be satisfied by different and lesser provision of services and opportunities than were deemed suitable or necessary for the rest of the population. And that is what they received.

Throughout most of the period covered by this book, the health of indigenous South Australians, and many other aspects of their lives, were dealt with through laws, regulations and mechanisms different from those which applied to the rest of the population. Of course they were a different population. Their lives had been governed for tens of thousands of years prior to the coming of the colonists by political, social, economic and spiritual values and patterns of life that set them apart from the newcomers. The newcomers, by intention and default and with varying degrees of hostility and good will, blindness and insight, undermined those ancient values and patterns and deprived them of their capacity to support healthy and vigorous lives. The newcomers simultaneously denied the indigenous population any genuine opportunity to take its place as part of the new public whose aspirations and way of life quickly became dominant. As we have seen, this denial was despite official instructions to extend to the Aboriginals the rights of British subjects and the protection of British law. In other words, the colonists had been enjoined to recognise the indigenous population as part of the public, and they failed to do so. In a system replete with contradictions, the Aboriginals were instead to be a separate group, governed and provided for separately. At some stages this distinctive treatment and provision was based on segregation and on a perceived need for protection; at other times it was based on a goal of assimilation which was understood in a variety of ways. But whatever the theoretical underpinnings, Aboriginals were, to all intents and purposes, deemed to be not part of the public. It is the central argument of this book that the poor health and restricted life chances of Aboriginal people today stem inexorably from this negative and exclusionary construction. There is little chance of indigenous Australians enjoying better health until this history is understood, and until as a nation we respond to it by building the more equal, inclusive and 'civic' society that research now tells us is the basis of good health for all.

While policies and mechanisms of protection and assimilation readily accommodated the construction of indigenous Australians as not part of the public during the time span covered by this book, in the ensuing decades there have been significant changes. It might be expected that the recognition of Aboriginals as citizens, the abolition of restrictive, special legislation and the adoption of the policy of self-determination represent a rejection of that earlier construction. I argue that the situation is more complicated than that, and complicated in a way that is deeply ironical. Aboriginals have certainly been officially and legally constructed as part of the public by those changes and they have declared themselves so in word and deed. But some of them have also insisted that their membership of the Australian public must be on their terms – and that involves recognising that they are different, that they subscribe to different cultural values, and that they have distinctive ideas about what their needs are and how they can best be provided for. Despite a considerable degree of assimilation to dominant values and goals, they maintain a sense of themselves as culturally distinctive. They ask that their separate identity be respected and given opportunity to flourish, and argue their right to do some things differently and separately. This has occasioned disquiet and resentment within the wider community. Ironically, Aboriginals are now told *to be part of the public* by other Australians who believe that the public cannot, with safety, be plural and heterogeneous. It seems that it was acceptable for Aboriginals not to be part of the public when this meant being seen and provided for as *less than the public*. But there is fear now, in some quarters, that indigenous freedom to choose to be different and separate might amount to preferential treatment, in effect to being *more than the public*. Such fear and the political stances it spawns is a significant obstacle to indigenous well-being. We can help to exorcise it by honestly confronting our history and being willing to take on the radical implications of what we now understand contributes to the health of populations.

My experience, since 1989, of teaching graduate and undergraduate public health students, almost all of them non-indigenous, suggests that this book is needed. Students emerging from school frequently have little appreciation of world views different from their own, or knowledge of what has happened to indigenous Australia and Australians since the arrival of the settlers. Older students, including those working in public health, often have little understanding of why indigenous health is as it is. This is hardly surprising and should not be taken as a simplistic criticism of what happens in schools. Several tendencies cohere to militate against the development of richly textured understandings of the impact of historical processes on health. Firstly, people focus more readily on immediate situations, which are the end result of complex processes, and read these as causes rather than results. Secondly, complex political and structural explanations are hard to sell and often not taken seriously, because biomedical views of health and individual behavioural explanations for illness are so pervasive in Australia, as elsewhere. Thirdly, the power and appeal of the social and economic *status quo* for those who are favoured by it means that there is a reluctance to 'own' problems as the problems of the social order: it is more convenient to blame the victims. Thus 'Aboriginals' and 'Aboriginal health' appear as discrete problems for the rest of the community to solve, and as areas for special targeting within health policies.[38] Thoughtful students of public health may be less likely to do this than many others, or may be more aware of the inadequacies of such an analysis. Even so, they often lack the historical knowledge and insight that would allow them to make an alternative case, or to encourage the building of the alternative policy responses and commitments essential to producing better health across the whole population. My experience is that they want to know more of this history once it is introduced to them. Hence this book.

I am aware that some people will dispute my right to be writing this history, arguing

---

38 I suggest that the Report of the Generational Health Review, 2003, commissioned by the South Australian Government, is not entirely free of this limited and limiting analysis. See below, pp.41

that as a non-Aboriginal, I am fundamentally disqualified from doing so. They will see it as further evidence of ongoing colonisation and of appropriation of roles that rightfully belong to indigenous people. And they will have read into my argument thus far yet another protectionist or assimilationist prescription. Some, who accept my legitimacy as an historian, may nevertheless have other concerns. For example, they may think that the division of the book into chapters delineated by time periods which relate to non-Aboriginal developments and historical markers indicates an approach that is both too western and too chronological to properly illuminate what has happened to the health of Aboriginal South Australians since non-Aboriginals settled in their country. Still others may question the wisdom of exposing a history which once more reveals the indigenous people as victims and losers. These are important considerations, and I think it important to indicate how I react to them.

I acknowledge that the way I undertake research, what I understand from it, what and how I write, the conclusions I come to and the positions I endorse are inevitably informed by who I am, that is, a non-Aboriginal academic historian. However, I do not see this as a disqualification or even a serious limitation. This work is what I can do, as a non-Aboriginal and an historian. I am claiming for history a social role that is endorsed from within the discipline: 'writing history is about trying to think and act differently towards oneself, towards others, and towards the present more than the past'.[39] More importantly, given the current political and social context in Australia, and given a past marked by paternalism at best and racism at worst, my work has been endorsed, personally and in a more general fashion, by indigenous Australians.

On the personal level I have consciously sought this endorsement. My teaching about Aboriginal health policy has been done in partnership with Aboriginal colleagues from the health field. This has involved joint planning of teaching sessions, the presentation of differing and sometimes opposing views, not only about health and ways of providing health care, but also about the sources and authority of different kinds of knowledge. It has involved the juxtaposition of archival, research-based, academic history with the personal, lived histories of Aboriginal people. In addition, my teaching has provided scheduled opportunities for my students to reflect on such partnerships and on the limits to non-indigenous roles that are imposed by a genuine embrace of the principles of self-determination. Aboriginal colleagues involved in this teaching have endorsed it through repeated involvement, and by welcoming further contact with my students. They have frequently cited the emphasis which I place on learning about and confronting our colonial history as of central importance in my teaching.[40]

In a more general way, my work has also been endorsed by those Aboriginals who call

---

39 Thacker, 'Foucault and the writing of history', p.51, and see above, pp.12

40 I have taken this issue seriously and written about it. See Judith Raftery, 'Aboriginal Health and "Black Armband History"', in Suzanne Parry (ed.), *Migration to Mining: medicine and health in Australian history: collected papers of the fifth biennial conference of the Australian Society of the History of Medicine, Darwin 1997*, Australian Society of the History of Medicine, Casuarina, Northern Territory, 1998, pp.106–15; Judith Raftery, 'Non-indigenous Teaching and Learning about Indigenous Health Issues', unpublished paper prepared for a teaching/learning course, Advisory Centre for University Education, University of Adelaide, 1997.

for cooperation among indigenous and non-indigenous people of good will in the process of reconciliation. I have taken encouragement, for example, from the public statements of Lowitja O'Donoghue. In her 1999 'Sorry Day' address she named as the key elements in the reconciliation process, the recognition and acknowledgement of the past and its continuing legacy, commitment to practical action, and working towards unity for a better future for us all. She acknowledged that this is a collective effort, and in particular stressed the need for truth-telling about our history.[41] She advanced the same views in her 2003 Duguid Memorial Lecture, and in addition argued the need for white Australians to study the political meanings of 'whiteness' and the impact of white privilege on black Australians.[42] As an historian, this is work that I am equipped to do. As an historian working in the field of public health it is work that I have felt compelled to do as a matter of fundamental justice. This book continues and extends what I have already done in the classroom and in the area of curriculum development.

The way the book is organised provides a means of understanding the non-Aboriginal history that, I argue, has determined the current health status of Aboriginals. It does this by paying attention to what seem to me to be significant changes in thinking, policy and practice over time. In addition, it provides a clarifying framework through which to view the experiences and understand the perceptions of both Aboriginal and non-Aboriginal South Australians whose stories make up the historical record, regarding those things which have determined the health of the public. This historical record is not a neatly organised given. It has to be searched for and discovered in many places and is often hidden under other guises. A chronological ordering and dividing is a valuable guide in this search, providing some elements of context and explanation. However, what has become clear to me in my searching, and what I hope will be clear to the reader, is that neither policies, nor experiences, nor perceptions of those experiences are respecters of the historian's chronology of convenience. For example, all policy views and positions may be present at any one time, regardless of what the official line is. Assimilationist views and practices, and Aboriginal experiences of being assimilated, abound during the period officially designated protectionist, as well as during the period designated assimilationist. And indeed, both assimilationist and protectionist views and behaviour thrive today when both are officially things of the past. Even so, changes over time in the dominant policy thrust, reflected in legislative changes, did occur, and occurred at specific times. Noting these changes and using them to create 'periods' and 'eras' is thus more than a chronological convenience: it provides a theoretical context against which to understand and measure what happens to people.

However, the chronological chapter division and the focus on policy changes should not be taken to suggest that I have employed no other mechanisms of explanation. Running through all the chapters are several strands of argument. These all relate to well-established political theory: they also emerge vividly from the historical record as lively and material issues in the relations between Aboriginal and non-Aboriginal South Australians.

---

41 Lowitja O'Donoghue, Address to the foreign correspondents' press conference, Canberra, 25 May 1999, broadcast on ABC Radio National

42 Lowitja O'Donoghue, Duguid Memorial Lecture, University of South Australia, Adelaide, 13 August 2003

The first of these strands relates to the complex relationship between policy and its implementation. Clearly, it is the way that policy is implemented, rather than the intentions or ideological positions underlying its development, which determines how it is experienced by those to whom it refers. And there are many ways in which implementation can modify policy. At the centre, policy implementation occurs through the frail and volatile mechanisms of meetings and discussions among people possessed of varying degrees of insight and good will, and often far-removed from the situations and people about whom they are making decisions. In the field, far from the centre, policy may well appear to those charged with its implementation to be vague, peripheral or irrelevant to the urgent concerns of day-to-day survival. It may even be unknown or invisible. This may allow other views and values to prevail, and these will not necessarily be consonant with those which inform official policy. This can account for time lags between official policy and actual practice, local variants on the central theme, or, in some cases, practices which are clearly at odds with it. This phenomenon is common in situations where policy is made by a central body but carried out by a constituency which is organisationally, geographically and culturally disparate. We see something similar in the relations between education departments and schools, and between church synods and local congregations. In the sphere of 'indigenous affairs' this tension between policy and its implementation is made particularly problematic by a history of oppression and distrust and by an ongoing debate, linked to differences in values and world views, about how Aboriginals are to relate to and be part of the rest of the Australian public.

A second strand of argument relates to whether Aboriginals were – or were seen as – active agents in their own history, or merely passive recipients of non-Aboriginal decisions and actions. Passive recipients, who do not act on their own initiative and who are handed a script rather being free to develop their own, are not, in any meaningful sense, part of the public. A denial of indigenous agency pervades some of the earlier non-indigenous accounts of dealings with the indigenous population. In these accounts there are 'natives' and, interacting with them are missions and government and commercial enterprises, but there are rarely any actual, delineated indigenous people with a sense of themselves, their descent, their identity or their future. For example, in 1936, JB Cleland, the prominent medical scientist and anthropologist who spent much of his professional life 'understanding' the native population concluded, in his contribution to *The Centenary History of South Australia*, that:

> taking them altogether ... they are a lovable race, good-humoured and kind, but they are incapable of mixing successfully with the European population, and so require guidance and care, like grown-up children.[43]

He presents them as a shadowy group, with individuals and sub-groups largely indistinguishable from one another, and certainly not as actors in their own destiny. This is powerfully reinforced, albeit without Cleland's hope that some might be assimilated

---

43 JB Cleland, 'The Natives of South Australia', in Royal Geographical Society of Australasia, South Australian Branch, *The Centenary History of South Australia, Supplementary to vol. xxxvi of the Proceedings of the Society*, Adelaide, 1936, p.29

into the broader community, in the final, summary chapter of *The Centenary History*, which concludes:

> The story of the aborigines leaves us with little cause for satisfaction. We have read of these happy, cheerful, simple folk at their hunting and fishing in the early days. We have noted the efforts made by Church and State to ameliorate their lot, and we have seen the fatal margin of contact between the whites and the blacks slowly and inevitably moving towards those remote districts where the remnants of the aborigines survive.
>
> Today, a few earnest missionaries still preach Christianity to the blacks; bands of eager scientists confer with them to snatch some further records of the habits and customs of Stone Age men; and thoughtless tourists visit camps to purchase uncertain souvenirs.
>
> Meanwhile, almost unnoticed, the everyday contacts between blacks and out-back settlers and prospectors hasten these primitive people towards extinction.[44]

The game is all but up. 'The blacks' have played no active or independent part in it, and have no future role.

This lack of agency is implicit in much missionary literature as well, especially that designed to inform the 'home' churches of progress in evangelism and to encourage a continual flow of funds. Until well into the twentieth century, Aboriginal people are much more likely to appear in mission records as nameless and de-contextualised success stories than as people with a distinctive culture and identity, making active and strategic choices about their lives, or as partners and co-workers with the missionaries in the interests of their own people. Even as late as the 1960s and 1970s a sense of Aboriginals as active citizens is largely missing from government deliberations about them as well. Instead, there is evidence of the notion, deeply ingrained in the thinking of even well-intentioned and sympathetic non-Aboriginals that Aboriginals are a problem group within the population, who need non-Aboriginals to 'do something about them'. It may be imagined that the public health scholarship which I invoke will tend towards a continuing denial of agency. Certainly much past public health practice would feed this concern. However, I argue that the implications of research into the social determinants of health, and in particular into the impact of inequalities on the health of populations, constitute a significant challenge to the structures and power imbalances which have been so damaging to Aboriginal self-determination and have excluded them from genuine membership of the public.

A third strand of argument which runs through the book is the notion that, throughout the period covered by this study, all policies and most practices, whatever they were called, were essentially assimilationist. They all proceeded from the position, sometimes crudely spelled out and on other occasions presented in more sophisticated guise, that the best hope for Aboriginal people was for them to become more like the rest of the community. Only then could they eventually become part of the 'public'. This assumption is still present in the age of self-determination. In fact the policy of self-determination, established by the 1972–75 Whitlam Government, was soon modified by subsequent

---

44 Charles Fenner, 'Retrospect and Prospect', in *The Centenary History of South Australia*, pp.379–80. Fenner was a leading South Australian geographer, and a member of the editorial board of the *Centenary History*.

governments to become a policy of self-management and trimmed of whatever might have delivered genuine autonomy. However, as has been argued by field workers and scholars who have investigated the mechanisms, structures and organisations set up under the rubric of 'self-management', governments have claimed to give Aboriginal people the freedom to determine and manage their own affairs while denying them the power and opportunity to do so.[45] This may represent unwillingness to relinquish control, fear of division or separate development, or a means, perhaps only superficially different from the older, more explicit assimilation, of 'drawing them inexorably into the corporate State'.[46] The persistent preference among non-Aboriginals for Aboriginals to be assimilated in one way or another reflects Australia's historical concerns about being 'white', but it is also evidence of humankind's generally limited capacity to cope with difference and our high level of fear of and discomfort with it. In race relations, as in other areas where this fear of difference is manifested and becomes the basis of policy and practice, injustice abounds.

The time frame of the book perhaps needs some explanation. The reason for the starting date, 1836, is obvious. It is the year of the arrival of the first official European settlers and the formal establishment of British rule in the colony of South Australia. As such, it marks the beginning of sustained, formally sanctioned, non-indigenous encroachment on the land and life of the original inhabitants and the consequent tragic impact on their health. The reason for adopting 1973 as the cut-off date may be less obvious. It can be argued, however, that this date signifies a significant break with the historical period this book explores and indicates the beginning of a new era. It is the year in which the Commonwealth took over responsibility for Aboriginal affairs from the states, and in which a reformist Labor government, led by Gough Whitlam, established the new policy of self-determination and greatly expanded the government's financial commitment to Aboriginal well-being. From this time, indigenous organisations proliferated in health and other spheres. They attempted to make self-determination a reality, suggesting revised roles for non-indigenous people. From 1973, then, the story becomes a different one, perhaps needing someone else to tell it. In addition, in 1973 South Australia was on the eve of instituting major new arrangements in its system of health care administration[47], providing a pragmatic reason, as well as the more important philosophical one, already mentioned, to stop there.

Seven chapters follow this introductory one. Chapter Two outlines the public health

---

45 For insightful examples of this scholarship, see Robert Tonkinson and Michael Howard (eds), *Going It Alone? Prospects for Aboriginal autonomy: Essays in honour of Ronald and Catherine Berndt*, Aboriginal Studies Press, Canberra, 1990. See especially Hans Dagmar, 'Development and Politics in an Interethnic Field: Aboriginal interest associations', pp.99–123, and Kingsley Palmer, 'Government Policy and Aboriginal aspirations: self-management at Yalata', pp.165–83.

46 This point is made by JR von Sturmer, one of the discussants in Christopher Anderson, Ian Keen, Tim Rowse et al. in 'On the Notion of Aboriginality: a discussion', *Mankind*, vol.15, no.1, 1985, pp.41–55.

47 See the 'Bright Report': CH Bright (Chairman), Report of the Committee of Enquiry into Health Services in South Australia, Government Printer, Adelaide, 1973. The report's only reference to indigenous health was to note the need for a health service in the remote north-west of the state.

research to which I have alluded in this chapter and summarises the case that can now be made about the determinants of health in individuals and populations and the impact of social inequalities on health. It indicates the capacity of this research to generate egalitarian social and economic policy and to suggest inclusive and compassionate models for democratic and pluralist societies. Subsequent chapters develop a detailed historical analysis of non-indigenous policies and practices in South Australia in relation to indigenous people, and, in the light of the theory presented in Chapter Two, trace the impact, both short-term and long term, on their health. Chapter Three deals with the period 1836–58, when the colony could be said to have been in search of a policy towards its indigenous population. Chapters Four and Five deal with the periods 1858–1911 and 1911–39 respectively. This was the era of protection, when separate legislative and administrative arrangements were established to govern the lives of Aboriginal people, who for much of this time were considered to be doomed to extinction. It was also the era in which two waves of missionary activity and an expanding and diversifying non-Aboriginal economy impinged in direct ways on the lives of some Aboriginal communities. Also during this time scientific and anthropological developments exerted a significant influence on government and community thinking about the 'native question'. Chapter Six focuses on the period 1939–62, when the survival of indigenous people and of some aspects of their culture, the increase of the 'half-caste' population, and the failure of protection to deal with their ongoing material needs led to the dismantling of the segregationist structures of protection and the adoption of a complex and evolving policy of assimilation. Chapter Seven deals with the period 1963–73, when changed government and community attitudes and a growing indigenous consciousness were undermining the foundations, always shaky and incomplete, of assimilation and suggesting alternative futures. Chapter Eight revisits the theoretical arguments of the first two chapters and considers their application to the ongoing challenges of the self-determination era. In particular it raises questions about how the unhealthy historical legacy of indigenous dispossession, marginalisation and cultural denigration can be replaced by a healthy, inclusive and equitable future without sacrificing respect for indigenous identity and choice.

Chapter 2

Health and Inequalities: Evidence and Implications

In the developed world, it is not the richest countries which have the best health, but the most egalitarian.   **Richard Wilkinson 1996**[1]

Societies that enable all their citizens to play a full and useful role in the social, economic and cultural life of their society will be healthier than those where people face insecurity, exclusion and deprivation.   **Richard Wilkinson and Michael Marmot 1998**[2]

The lesson of history is that it is only through the awkward and complex processes of political conflict and ideological negotiation over the allocation of resources between differently empowered social groups that rapid economic growth can be harnessed to yield beneficial outcomes.
                                                                      Simon Szreter 1999[3]

It has long been apparent that the determinants of health and illness in populations are largely social and economic. This understanding grew from the middle of the nineteenth century and helped to fuel the sanitary and environmental reforms that, in Britain and in other parts of the western world, including the Australian colonies, made significant inroads into the morbidity and mortality associated particularly with infectious disease. The analysis that underlay these reforms, however, was limited and did not constitute a fundamental challenge to the structures and ideologies that allowed class-based inequalities and associated health inequalities to remain. These inequalities have persisted, despite a sustained overall rise in standards of living during the last century. Advances in science and medicine have done little to alter this. In fact, health inequalities were entrenched when, from the end of the nineteenth century, the growth of scientific medicine encouraged a retreat to

1 Richard Wilkinson, *Unhealthy Societies: the afflictions of inequality*, Routledge, London, 1996, p.2

2 Richard Wilkinson and Michael Marmot, *Social Determinants of Health: the solid facts*, World Health Organization, WHO Regional Office for Europe, 1998

3 Simon Szreter, 'Rapid Economic Growth and 'the four Ds' of disruption, deprivation, disease and death: public health lessons from nineteenth century Britain for twenty-first century China?', *Tropical Medicine and International Health*, vol.4, issue 2, February 1999, pp.146–52

23

individualist and behaviourist explanations of health and illness. There have been significant late-twentieth-century challenges to this approach, arising from epidemiology and
from the social sciences. These challenges have been resisted by those who hold the bio-
medical high ground, by policy-makers and health professionals who prefer 'life-style', that
is individual behavioural explanations of health and illness, and, most recently, by those
who are dazzled by the extravagant promises of the gene-mappers. However, it is becoming
ever more difficult to ignore the growing body of scholarship that points to the complex
impact of socioeconomic inequalities and relative deprivation on health and illness.

Much of this scholarship rests on foundations laid by the *Black Report*, the report of
the Working Group on Inequalities in Health, commissioned by the British Government
in 1977 to investigate national and international evidence on health inequalities and
suggest policy implications arising from this.[4] To illuminate the unequal health experiences
of people of different social class or socioeconomic status, the *Black Report* made use of the
system of stratification by occupation used by the Registrar General.[5] This had the
advantage of being already widely used and understood within government and research
circles, as well as being regarded as more able than alternative measures to provide an accurate guide, not just to level of income but to other aspects of life for which occupation may
act as a proxy measure:

> Occupation not simply designates type of work but tends also to show broadly how strenuous
> or unhealthy it is, what are the likely working conditions – for example whether it is indoors or
> outdoors and whether there is exposure to noise, dust or vibration – and what amenities and
> facilities are available, as well as level of remuneration and likely access to various fringe ben-
> efits. Pay will also determine family living standards, and while members of a family will not
> be exposed to some features of the working conditions experienced, there are others which may
> affect them indirectly, like the risk of intermittent employment, or the stress of disablement and
> of shift work.[6]

The authors of the *Black Report* were aware of the weaknesses as well as the strengths of
this system of stratification by occupation. They encouraged the development of more
refined indicators that would take into account the occupations of married women,
groups such as the elderly and the unemployed who are not economically engaged, and
the access of family units to wealth and resources not captured by a focus on occupation.
It is worth noting, in the light of subsequent research into the impact of inequalities
on health, that such resources might be regarded as social and cultural, and might influence health and maintain health inequalities through mechanisms other than physical
ones.

---

4 In this section I have relied on the interpretative comments found in Peter Townsend, Nick Davidson and Margaret
  Whitehead, 'Introduction to *Inequalities in Health*', in Peter Townsend, Nick Davidson and Margaret Whitehead, (eds).
  Inequalities in Health: the Black Report *and* The Health Divide, Penguin Books, London, 1988, pp.1–28. The versions of
  the *Black Report* and *The Health Divide* to which I refer are the ones included in this volume.

5 See below, Appendix 2

6 Townsend, Davidson, and Whitehead, *Inequalities in Health*, pp.39–40.

At the time when the *Black Report* was commissioned, within the British Department of Health and Social Security there was an acknowledgement of 'Britain's failure to match the improvement in health observed in some other countries' and of 'the relationship of this to persistent internal inequalities of health'.[7] The *Black Report* concluded that the poorer health experiences of the lower occupational groups applied at all stages of life, and that, in the twenty years prior to the period covered in the report, mortality rates in the lowest occupational groups had remained constant or deteriorated, while in the highest groups they had steadily diminished. In other words, health inequalities, at least insofar as these can be measured by mortality rates, had been increasing. The report put human flesh on these statistical bones by indicating that the lives of 74,000 people aged under 75, including nearly 10,000 children, would have been saved if the mortality rates that applied in the highest occupational class had applied across the whole population.[8]

Recognising that the roots of the problem lay largely outside the areas normally considered to be within the purview of health policy and health services, the report's recommendations reflected two major policy thrusts: 'a total and not merely a service-oriented approach to the problems of health', and 'a radical overhaul of the balance of activity and proportionate distribution of resources within the health and associated services'. This whole-of-government approach, which recognised the importance of good health care but avoided the common mistake of equating improvements in health with improvements in health care, included in its recommendations:

> giving effect to improvements in information, research and organization so that better plans might be drawn up, redressing the balance of the health care system so that more emphasis was given to prevention, primary care and community health, and, most important of all, radically improving the material condition of life of poorer groups, especially children and people with disabilities, by increasing or introducing cash benefits, like child benefit, maternity grant and infant care allowance, and a comprehensive disablement allowance, and developing new schemes for day nurseries, ante-natal clinics, sheltered housing, home improvements, improved conditions at work and community services.[9]

The *Black Report*, commissioned by a Labour government, was submitted in April 1980 to a Conservative administration, and was summarily dismissed. Apart from being too costly to implement, its explanations of the causes of health inequalities were deemed inadequate and thus its recommendations for remedial action could not be endorsed. The Secretary of State for Social Security, Patrick Jenkin, in opposing the report, showed the extent to which he had not understood it, by focusing on health service usage, quoting other evidence which demonstrated that 'the poor' did indeed have 'a proper crack of the whip when it comes to using the National Health Service' and arguing that there was no point in spending more money on services since 'we have been spending money in ever-increasing amounts on the NHS for thirty years and it has not actually had much effect

---

7 ibid., p.1

8 ibid., p.2

9 ibid., pp.2–3

on increasing people's health'.[10] The government declared itself in support of the *Black Report's* recommendations on prevention of illness, but interpreted this narrowly as 'encouraging health education, personal responsibility for health, and encouraging voluntary organisations to help in the personal social services and helping to complement the NHS'.[11] This again was missing the point, and confirmed the individualist approach to health which ensures that the structural problems identified by the *Black Report* persist.

Despite the failure of the British Government to take the *Black Report* seriously as a basis for national health policy development, the report itself stimulated much interest and research activity among academics and health professionals and within health and social services, local government bodies and voluntary organisations.[12] One outcome of this was the commissioning, in 1986, of another inquiry, to update the evidence on inequalities and report on progress with the *Black Report* recommendations. This resulted in the publication of *The Health Divide* in 1987. This took as the central question to be addressed:

> Are there groups in the population who are disadvantaged to such an extent that it affects their opportunity to achieve good health? For instance, do a person's financial resources, social position, ethnic origin or gender affect their chances of good health? Are certain areas of the country or certain neighbourhoods unduly disadvantaged in health terms? Are the unemployed disadvantaged compared with those in work? Does the health care system treat some people more favourably than others? Are the resources available to the NHS fairly distributed around the country? These are the sorts of issues which arise when trying to answer the question of whether the social justice in health has been achieved.[13]

In answering this question, *The Health Divide* noted that two different research thrusts had emerged: one which identified the central issue as inequality and therefore focused on the health gradient across whole populations, and one which was more concerned with deprivation and therefore focused on the most disadvantaged groups. These two

---

10   Rodney Deitch, 'The Debate on the *Black Report*', *Lancet*, 18 July 1981, pp.158–9, cited in Townsend, Davidson and Whitehead, *Inequalities in health*, pp.4–5

11   Sir George Young, under-Secretary of State for Health and Social Security, *British Medical Journal*, 22 August 1981, p.567, cited in Townsend, Davidson and Whitehead, *Inequalities in Health*, p.5

12   This 'grass roots' interest in and positive response the *Black Report*, despite, or perhaps partly because of, lack of government endorsement of its findings, was not limited to Great Britain. It was very apparent to me in my work (from 1989 to 2002) as a public health academic, teaching Australian graduate students who, in most cases, worked either as clinicians or in government or non-government public health agencies. The *Black Report* was quoted or referred to in many quarters as an inspiration or foundation for health initiatives. This informal and difficult-to-quantify impact of the *Black Report* on thinking, research and action about health inequalities is in many ways analogous to the impact of the report on the Royal Commission into Aboriginal Deaths in Custody on thinking, research and action about Aboriginal health. While critics maintain that Australian governments have failed to take this report seriously or to act on its many recommendations, it has encouraged initiatives within many indigenous organisations, and is regularly quoted as the source and inspiration of ideas, programs and services.

13   Townsend, Davidson and Whitehead. *Inequalities in Health*, p.222

approaches clearly had different policy implications. They had not been equally embraced at the time of the publication of *The Health Divide*, and they have not been equally embraced subsequently. This is an issue which has implications for current Australian health policy and practice and for the health of Aboriginals, and I shall return to it later. Perhaps the most important interpretive work of *The Health Divide* was its canvassing of the main ways in which researchers tried to explain health inequalities. It found no reason to support the notion that these inequalities were largely artefactual, and only sketchy evidence that they might in some cases be the result of natural and social selection. It rejected the simplistic 'lifestyle' arguments, which, maintaining that individual behaviour and lifestyle determine health, wave a judgemental finger at the dangerous and damaging choices of the lower social groups and their apparent lack of interest in long-term health protection. Instead, *The Health Divide* endorsed materialist/structuralist explanations of health inequalities. That is, it argued that health is determined by the external environment, by the conditions of life and work, and the pressures and risks to which people are subjected. While such explanations do not discount the impact, both positive and negative, of behaviour on health, they recognise that behaviour is constrained by material circumstances, and thus 'the whole structure of society is implicated' in the production and maintenance of health inequalities.[14] *The Health Divide* was unequivocal in arguing that the determinants of health inequalities are social and economic. Its conclusions are worth quoting at length, since they neatly summarise an understanding which, although regarded as commonplace within public health circles, is frequently not known or understood beyond them:

> The weight of evidence continues to point to explanations which suggest that socio-economic circumstances play the major part in subsequent health differences. For example, the evidence that health-damaging behaviour is more common in lower social groups continues to accumulate, especially concerning smoking and diet. But can such life-style factors account for all the observed differential in health between different social groups? The short answer is: no. When studies are able to control for factors like smoking and drinking, a sizeable proportion of the health gap remains and factors related to the general living conditions and environment of the poor are indicated. In this context there is also a growing body of evidence that material and structural factors, such as housing and income, can affect health. Most importantly, several studies have shown how adverse social conditions can limit the choice of life-style and it is this set of studies which illustrates most clearly that behaviour cannot be separated from its social context. Certain living and working conditions appear to impose severe restrictions on an individual's ability to choose a healthy lifestyle.
>
> The evidence suggests that policies to reduce inequalities which focused entirely on the individual would be misguided. The importance of social and material factors highlighted by the research suggests that broader policies incorporating structural improvements in living and working conditions would be required in addition.[15]

---

14 ibid., pp.286–9
15 ibid., pp.304–5

Reaction to *The Health Divide* was, predictably, mixed. Some people read the evidence on inequalities with alarm, accepted the structural explanation, and called for wide-ranging reform which recognised the links between poverty and poor health. Others sought to discredit the report, by calling it biased, unscientific or Marxist, labels guaranteed to unnerve those already wary of calls for structural reform. A common government reaction was to discount the report's findings by focusing on overall improvements to health as measured by particular indicators such as infant mortality and population life expectancy, or by re-running the familiar and more comfortable line that health inequalities are the result of individual choices and behaviour.[16] However, as had happened with the *Black Report*, the health professional and research communities responded more warmly to *The Health Divide* than the government did. Its publication ensured that 'inequalities in health were once again put firmly on the agenda', and professionals and academics made sure that they stayed there by making them the topic of conferences, seminars, journal articles and position papers.[17]

This is a familiar scenario. I have written elsewhere about how reformist, even radical ideas about the health of the public, when endorsed by key groups of health professionals, public servants and health academics, can be kept alive in an increasingly unsupportive and hostile political climate.[18] There is an instructive story to be told about how this occurred in South Australia in the 1970s and 1980s. The social and economic priorities of the federal Labor Government elected in December 1972, and its willingness to fund initiatives designed to enhance social justice and encourage community participation in social planning resonated with the aspirations of a reforming South Australian Labor Government enjoying office after many years of non-Labor rule. The national Community Health Program, established in 1973, and designed to provide health services that were accessible, coordinated, multi-disciplinary, tailored to community needs and focused on prevention, and which would attempt to improve 'the habits, conditions and environment that may precede disorders in health',[19] was embraced with greater enthusiasm in South Australia than elsewhere. At first glance it appeared to offer an answer to the inadequacies of the traditional health system and the increasing mismatch between what it could offer and the health needs of the Australian community. However, closer inspection revealed it as:

> unquestioning about certain bio-medical assumptions that were central to the shortcomings of the existing arrangements; its analysis of the origins of ill-health and of ways in which good health is achieved was shallow; it was lacking in ideas about strategies to achieve its objectives; and it was vague and naïve about the prevention of illness. It revealed little understanding of the connection between public policies and health, and despite some mention of the impact of social environments on health, its orientation was largely individualist.[20]

---

16 ibid., *Inequalities in Health*, pp.9–11

17 ibid., *Inequalities in Health*, p.16

18 See Judith Raftery, 'The Social and Historical Context' and 'Health Policy Development in the 1980s and 1990s', in Fran Baum (ed.), *Health for All: the South Australian experience*, Wakefield Press, Adelaide, 1995, pp.19–37, 51–64

19 Hospitals and Health Services Commission, *A Community Health Program for Australia*, AGPS, Canberra, 1973, p.4

20 Raftery, 'The Social and Historical Context', p.23

A 1976 national review of the Community Health Program commended its principles and objectives, and pointed to specific successes and 'some smaller inroads' into 'special needs areas', including Aboriginal health. However it also acknowledged a lack of support for its principles among health professionals, many of whom saw it as 'basically a health centre building program'.[21] Two years later, a study of South Australian use of community health funds reported on the proliferation of health-related community groups and activities, the establishment of women's community health centres, and an occupational health centre, which not only provided treatment and rehabilitation services, but worked with employers to promote healthy work environments.[22] None of this amounted to a major reorientation of health services or of thinking about health, but it did indicate that, in some quarters at least, there was a broadening definition of health and of those things which contribute to a healthy community. From that time, other forces combined to lend support to this emerging view.

After the election of the Hawke federal Labor Government in 1983, new federal funding for community health became available, and the South Australian Labor Government, willing to take on the federal government's philosophy as well as its money, used this to match local government initiatives in community health. At the same time it boosted its spending on education, housing, job creation, opportunities for women, and Aboriginal affairs.[23] Influential in maintaining and extending this commitment to community health, was the energetic and reformist John Cornwall, Minister of Health, 1982–85 and of Health and Community Welfare, 1985–88, and some imaginative bureaucrats supported by and supportive of him within the South Australian Health Commission. These bureaucrats staffed the Social Health Office established by Cornwall in 1986 to promote an inter-sectoral, public policy approach to improving the health of the public. Cornwall argued that such an approach involved 'a redistribution of power ... a redistribution of important goods, services and conditions of life so that all Australians have an equal opportunity to enjoy good health'.[24] The Social Health Office was clearly influenced by the Declaration of Alma Ata and the Ottawa Charter, whose principles and vision it frequently invoked.[25] It also reflected the more radical readings of

---

21 Hospitals and Health Services Commission, *Review of the Community Health Program*, AGPS, Canberra, 1976, pp.29, 37

22 South Australian Health Commission & South Australian Association of Community Health Centres, *Community Health Centres in South Australia: a study of the use of community health funds to develop community health centres, in South Australia, to June 1978*, Adelaide, 1978

23 The impact of the particular economic and political climate that existed in South Australia at this time on the fate of the Community Health Program was noted by Nancy Milio, a visiting American academic who undertook substantial analysis of Australia's community health policy and programs. See Nancy Milio, 'Keeping the Promise of Community Health Policy Revival under Hawke 1983–85', in F Baum, D Fry and I Lennie (eds), *Community Health: policy and practice in Australia*, Pluto Press, Sydney, 1992, pp.28–47, and also, Raftery, 'The Social and Historical Context', pp.27–30.

24 John Cornwall, *Just For the Record: the political recollections of John Cornwall*, Wakefield Press, Adelaide, 1989, p.157

25 The Declaration of Alma Ata, emerging from a World Health Organization conference in 1978, marked the beginning of the 'Health for All' campaign based on primary health care principles. The Ottawa Charter for Health Promotion, 1986, built on Alma Ata and developed strategies for health promotion that affirm that the determinants of the health of populations are social, economic and political. World Health Organization, *Primary Health Care: report of the international conference on primary health care, Alma Ata*, World Health Organization, Geneva, 1978; World Health Organization,

the *Black Report* and *The Health Divide*, that is, as indicated above, 'the whole structure of society is implicated' in the production and maintenance of health, and of health inequalities.[26]

What did this thinking achieve? I have argued that it encouraged commitment among some health professionals, bureaucrats, academics and researchers to the public policy approach to producing and sustaining a healthy community, that it constituted a minor challenge to bio-medical orthodoxy, and that it supported a network of community health services and programs.[27] However, we should be careful not to make too much of this. It is one thing for ideas to enjoy intellectual currency and even, through some strategic bureaucratic support, to remain on the policy agenda; it is quite another for them to exert a strong influence on policy. Standing agenda items can too easily be postponed, dealt with superficially or in a variety of ways accorded a low priority. They may continue to have some effect, but often not in the most influential places, and often not sufficiently to influence big initiatives. And bureaucratic structures which endorse particular ideas can be dismantled as easily as they can be established.

In assessing the impact of the *Black Report* and *The Health Divide*, Townsend, Davidson and Whitehead concluded that, 'Above all, the prospects for doing something about inequalities in health have been affected by the government's ideology in favour of a private market and cutting public expenditure'.[28] This was as true in Australia and in other parts of the western world as it was in Britain. During the 1980s, governments and political parties of various stamps became captive to philosophies that produced and maintained inequalities. Their embrace of the values inherent in the private market, the principle of 'the user pays', and a fundamental commitment to containment or reduction of government expenditure, amounted to a significant threat to social reform agenda. The effects of this could be seen in South Australia by the late 1980s. In 1989, John Cornwall, reflecting on his achievements in South Australia, suggested that the public policy approach to improving health did not flourish because, among other reasons, it implied 'a consensus on equity of distribution of important health-producing goods and services which we have not yet achieved'.[29] The downgrading of the Social Health Office, the loss of its high-level staff and its direct access to the minister by 1989 provided tangible evidence of this lack of consensus and of how difficult it is for complex, radical views to make inroads into entrenched positions.

Indeed, at the very time that the *Black Report* and *The Health Divide* were demonstrating the connections between social inequalities and health inequalities, those inequalities were becoming more marked. In the early 1950s, Britain had experienced the smallest mortality differentials on record, and been at its most egalitarian in terms of income distribution, as result of the government seeking legitimacy and cohesion through the redis-

---

'Ottawa 1986: report of an international conference on health promotion, 17–21 November 1986, Ottawa, Ontario, Canada', *Health Promotion: An International Journal*, vol.1, no.4, pp.i–v, 405–60.

26 See above, pp.27

27 Raftery, 'The Social and Historical Context', pp.30–1

28 Townsend, Davidson and Whitehead, *Inequalities in Health*, p.24

29 Raftery, 'The Social and Historical Context', p.35

tributive mechanism of rationing.[30] Since then, despite overall gains in prosperity, the proportion of the population living in relative poverty (that is, on less than half the average income) had been increasing, rising from eight per cent in the early 1950s, to 30 per cent in the early 1980s. During the same period, death rates were reduced, but the differential in death rates between the highest socioeconomic groups and the lowest increased significantly.[31] Reporting a few years later, the Acheson inquiry indicated a continuation of these trends: from the early 1970s to the early 1990s, mortality rates fell by 40 per cent in social classes one and two, by 30 per cent in classes three and four, but by only 10 per cent in class five, with the inequalities more marked among men than among women.[32] Similar trends have been reported in Australia. Here, as in other advanced economies, 'mortality differentials are finely stratified from top to bottom of the socioeconomic hierarchy', and have persisted, and in some cases increased, despite marked improvements in health across the whole population. For example, in 1985–87, male mortality rates among the most disadvantaged were 55 per cent higher for coronary heart disease, 60 per cent higher for lung cancer and 73 per cent higher for motor vehicle accidents than among the least disadvantaged. By the period 1995–97, these differentials had risen to 87, 98 and 133 per cent respectively.[33]

While governments were embracing the economic ideologies that produced and maintained these inequalities, research and debate continued among academics, policy analysts and health professionals committed to understanding more fully the impact of inequalities on the health of the public. This has resulted in the establishment of a significant and burgeoning school of health research and produced a substantial body of evidence that links inequalities in health within populations with underlying social and economic inequalities.[34] This research endeavour has engaged both the epidemiology and

---

30 JM Winter, Public Health and the Extension of Life Expectancy in England and Wales, 1901–1960, in M Keynes, DA Coleman and NH Dimsale, (eds), *The Political Economy of Health and Welfare: twenty-second annual symposium of the Eugenics Society 1985, Studies in Biology, Economy and Society*, Macmillan, London, 1988, pp.184–203

31 Alison Quick and Richard Wilkinson, *Income and health*, Socialist Health Association, London, 1991, pp.15–16. Quick and Wilkinson claimed that death rate differentials doubled or tripled, and suggested that there was some evidence that 'mortality rates rise increasingly rapidly as you move down the income scale'.

32 Sir Donald Acheson, *Independent Inquiry into Inequalities in Health Report*, the Stationery Office, London, 1999 [1998]. pp.11–17. The report indicated that, in the 1970s, mortality for men in classes four and five was 53 per cent higher than for those in classes one and two, but by the late 1990s it was 68 per cent higher. For women, the corresponding figures were 50 per cent and 55 per cent.

33 Gavin Turrell and Colin D Mathers, 'Socioeconomic Status and Health in Australia', *Medical Journal of Australia*, vol.172, 1 May 2000, pp.434–8. See also, G. Turrell, 'Social Class and Health: a summary of the overseas and Australian evidence', in GM Lupton and JM Najman (eds), *Sociology of Health and Illness: Australian readings*, Macmillan, Melbourne, 1995, pp.113–42.

34 It is impossible here to provide more than a brief summary of some of the major foci, findings and implications for policy of this major area of research. Those wishing to pursue it further may find useful starting points in Richard Wilkinson, *Unhealthy Societies: the afflictions of inequality*, Routledge, London, 1996; Michael Marmot and Richard Wilkinson, (eds), *Social Determinants of health: the solid facts*, World Health Organization, Geneva, 1998; Ichiro Kawachi, Bruce P. Kennedy and Richard G Wilkinson, *The Society and Population Health Reader, vol.1: income inequality and health*, The New York Press, New York, 1999; Michael Marmot and Richard G Wilkinson, *Social Determinants of Health*, Oxford University Press, Oxford, 1999; Michael Marmot, 'Social Determinants of Health: from observation to policy', *Medical*

social science wings of public health, employed a range of methodologies, drawn its evidence from a variety of sources and demonstrated its findings in different social and political settings. It has broadened the concept of risk factors for morbidity and mortality beyond the individual and behavioural to include the material and structural, and from the physiological to include the psychological and the emotional. Its aim has been to interrogate the conventional modern wisdom that rising prosperity is the main source of rising health standards and that the only remaining relationship between income and health is the relationship between absolute poverty and health, and that this will disappear as affluence spreads. Further, it has challenged the economic rationalists' argument that inequalities are the engine of productivity, by demonstrating that egalitarian societies too are characterised by economic growth and vibrancy.[35]

To see this conventional wisdom as not merely simplistic but actually erroneous is not to deny the importance of living standards to health. One has only to compare the health experience of the people of a rich country such as Australia with that of the people of a very poor country such as Bangladesh, or the health experience of nineteenth century Australians with that of twenty-first-century Australians, to know that living standards matter. It is more difficult, however, to explain why, among a group of countries which can all be categorised as rich, it is not always those with the highest standards of living that have the lowest mortality rates or the highest life expectancy. Prosperity and health appear to be linked, but not in straightforward way. Something else is going on which should make us wary of assuming that economic growth will guarantee better health. Richard Wilkinson, a prominent and prolific contributor to the inequalities debate has explained this succinctly:

> There is an important paradox at the heart of the relationship between health and living standards. Among the richer countries it looks as if economic growth and further improvements in living standards have little effect on health. They have advanced beyond a crucial stage in economic development when living standards reached a threshold level adequate to ensure basic material standards for all. This point is marked by the epidemiological transition when infectious diseases give way to the cancers and degenerative disease as the main causes of death. During the same period the so-called 'diseases of affluence' become the diseases of the poor in affluent societies.[36]

Comparisons over time and contemporary observation show us how important to our health and indeed to all aspects of our lives is the attainment of this living standards threshold. However, as Wilkinson goes on to say:

Journal of Australia, vol.172, 17 April 2000, pp.379–82; Vicente Navarro and Leiyu Shi, 'The Political Context of Social Inequalities and Health'. *Social Science and Medicine*, vol.52, 2001, pp.481–91. Also useful, especially for demonstrating the application of inequalities research to conventional policy areas, as well as its capacity to suggest new policy foci, is a series of eight articles published in the Education and Debate section, under the general heading of 'Socio-economic Determinants of Health', *British Medical Journal*, vol. 314, 22 February 1997–vol.314, 24 May 1997.

35 Quick and Wilkinson, *Income and Health*, p.9

36 Richard Wilkinson, *Unhealthy Societies: the afflictions of inequality*, Routledge, London, 1996, pp.2–3

the other side of the paradox is that differences in the standard of living remain closely related to health *within* [emphasis in original] societies. That is to say, poorer people in developed countries may have annual death rates anywhere between twice and four times as high as richer people in the same society.

These differentials persist and may even widen despite overall rises in standard of living.[37]

At first glance this may seem unremarkable and scarcely new. After all, detailed information about significant class-based, occupational and regional differences in mortality within populations has been increasingly available from the mid-nineteenth century in Britain and somewhat later in Australia through the establishment of national censuses and centralised government registers of national vital statistics. Any student of the history of public health knows that within any society it is the poorest who are sickest and die earliest. However, this history has been best documented in situations in which the epidemiological transition has not occurred, in which the minimum living standards threshold has not been met, in which governments have not accepted the role of providing what we now call safety nets to protect the most vulnerable, and in which medicine and health services can offer little. This history, with its graphic tales of human misery and suffering, is frequently shocking to modern readers, who, perhaps out of a need to protect their values and interests, can read it as a commentary on the effects of ignorance, absolute poverty and lack of political and scientific 'progress', and miss what it is saying about the effects of structured inequality. Or, if they do focus on inequality, they may well understand this as simply a division between 'the rich' and 'the poor'. Such readings of history support some extensions of the role of governments to maintain the welfare of the population, and suggest economic growth to combat poverty and scientific advance to enhance our capacity to deal with illness. They also frequently lead to behavioural prescriptions whereby 'the poor' can improve their lot. What they miss or downplay or avoid is the more radical implication of the effects of inequality, effects which persist even when other factors which undermine health have been attended to. What is new and powerful about the recent and current public health research which is the focus of this chapter is that it focuses directly on the effects of these inequalities. And its findings are unequivocal: 'In the developed world, it is not the richest countries which have the best health, but the most egalitarian'.[38] Furthermore, this research has demonstrated that it is not just the poorest and the most marginal whose health suffers as a result of inequalities:

> the message is not simply that inequality kills [or makes sicker] the poorest, but that it reaches well beyond the poor to become the major determinant of health standards among the population as a whole.[39]

There is, in fact, a social gradient in health which reaches across the whole population and disadvantages progressively those furthest down the social scale.

---

37 ibid., p.3

38 ibid., p.2

39 Quick and Wilkinson, *Income and Health*, p.10

The link between social and economic inequalities and health inequalities is robust and persistent. Its existence has been established through careful epidemiological studies, through analyses of census data and official records of life expectancy and mortality for various occupational groups, and through studies that compare the experience of different countries, or the experience within a country over time. For example, it is clearly illustrated by comparative studies of recent developments in Japan and the United Kingdom. At the beginning of the 1970s, life expectancy and income distribution in these two countries were very similar and close to the average of the OECD countries for which data are available. Subsequently, Japan achieved the most egalitarian income distribution in the world and also the highest life expectancy. During the same period, the United Kingdom became much less egalitarian in terms of income distribution, death rates for men and women rose significantly and life expectancy lagged behind that of Japan. In addition, it is demonstrable that, within the United Kingdom, life expectancy was at its highest and increased most rapidly not during periods of greatest overall national prosperity, but during periods when governments made deliberate attempts to reduce social stratification by policies of income redistribution.[40]

The discovery of the continuing link between social and economic inequalities and health within developed countries, where absolute poverty is not the issue and where increases in standard of living do not nullify the impact of inequalities, has prompted further research into the mechanisms by which this link operates. The nature of the link makes it seem likely that other factors beyond the physical must be involved and thus the research agenda has been broadened to scrutinise the possible impact of other factors connected to social stratification and inequality, especially as mediated by income. This has involved moving into new and challenging territory where new research questions and measurement tools are needed in order to produce new kinds of evidence. Some of these challenges were hinted at in Quick and Wilkinson's summary of the emerging project:

> If the issue is not absolute income levels, this suggests that health is no longer determined primarily by the directly physiological effects of the material circumstances in which people live. The importance of relative income implies that the crucial issue is *what a person's income or standard of living means in the social context of their society* [My emphasis]. The problem lies less in the physical consequences of the material conditions of life than with their psychological and emotional consequences ... for most people it is hard to live on a low income without financial worries and stress, without it cramping your style or limiting your social contacts and confidence, and without a sense of diminishing self-esteem and worthlessness ... in societies where appearances count for so much, few will have the emotional resources or the alternative sources of self-esteem to avoid the demeaning effects of a low income.[41]

---

40 ibid., pp.14–15. Here Quick and Wilkinson draw on the work of a distinguished earlier contributor to the field: Richard Titmuss, 'War and Social Policy', in *Essays on the Welfare State*, Unwin, London, 1958. See also Winter, above, footnote 30, 31.

41 Quick and Wilkinson, *Income and Health*, pp.28–9. The debate is ongoing. A comprehensive recent overview and analysis is found in Brian J Fleming, 'The Social Gradient in Health: trends in twentieth century ideas, Australian health policy 1970–1998, and a health equality evaluation of Australian aged care policy', PhD thesis, University of Adelaide, 2003.

Thus researchers interested in elucidating the links between social inequalities and health inequalities have increasingly turned their attention to such non-physical factors as the levels of stress that people experience, their sense of control over their circumstances, the degree to which they are isolated or socially connected, and the quality of the social environment in which they live. This research has gone beyond a focus on individuals and attempted to show, for example, that income inequality, which is often accompanied by residential segregation and reduced levels of social cohesion has significant 'spillover effects on society at large, including increased rates of crime and violence, impeded productivity and economic growth, and the impaired functioning of representative democracy'. The development and use of the notion of 'social capital' is an attempt to capture and measure the effects on population health of this lack of social cohesion.[42]

Evidence of interest in this research and its implications for policy can be seen in the commissioning, by a new British Labour Government in 1997, of the Independent Inquiry into Inequalities in Health. This inquiry was chaired by Sir Donald Acheson, chair of the International Centre for Health and Society at University College, London, and included in its scientific advisory group eminent members of the inequalities research school.[43] The inquiry's remit was to moderate a Department of Health review of the latest available information on health inequalities, to summarise the evidence and identify trends, and to identify priority areas for policy development likely 'to offer opportunities for government to develop beneficial, cost-effective and affordable interventions to reduce health inequalities'.

In the preface to the report, Acheson identifies the health differentials existing between social groups in Britain, despite increased overall prosperity and reduced mortality rates, as 'fundamentally a matter of social justice'.[44] While acknowledging the primary importance of the *Black Report* to an understanding of the impact of social inequalities on health, the *Acheson report* traces the historic development of this understanding from Farr and the work of the General Register Office, through Chadwick, Rowntree and Titmuss to the *Beveridge Report*, which focused on social inequalities and inadequate access to health care, and led to the development of social services to combat 'the five giants of Want, Disease, Ignorance, Squalor and Idleness'.[45] He noted that it was the perception that Britain was falling behind in the march to better health, despite this history, that led to the commissioning of the inquiry that resulted in the publication of the *Black Report*.

---

42 Ichiro Kawachi and Bruce P Kennedy, 'Health and Social Cohesion: why care about income equality?', *British Medical Journal*, vol.314, 5 April 1997, pp.1037–40. Insight into the scope of this research and into what it claims to demonstrate can be gained from Wilkinson, *Unhealthy Societies* and Kawachi, Kennedy and Wilkinson, *The Society and Population Health Reader, vol.1*. See above, footnote 34, pp.31–2.

43 These were Professor David Barker, Director of the Medical Research Council's Environmental Epidemiology Unit, University of Southampton; Dr Jacky Chambers, Director of Public Health, Birmingham Health Authority; Professor Hilary Graham, Director of the Economic and Social Research Council's Health Variations Programme, Lancaster University; Professor Michael Marmot, Director of the International Centre for Health and Society, University College, London; Dr Margaret Whitehead, Visiting Fellow, the King's Fund, London.

44 Acheson, *Independent Inquiry into Health Inequalities*, p.v

45 ibid., pp.4–5

The *Black Report*, as discussed above, fell on largely deaf government ears in 1980. The *Acheson Report* represented the next opportunity to present formally to government the inequalities evidence, which was by then much enhanced and refined. The Acheson Inquiry judged that the commissioning of the new report reflected genuine government support for tackling the 'root causes of health' (sic) and a conviction about the link between income, inequality and poor health, and about the need for policies to deal with this that went far beyond the more equitable provision of health services.[46] The report was forthright in its endorsement of this view, claiming that:

> socio-economic inequalities in health reflect differential exposure – from before birth and across the life-span – to risks associated with socio-economic position. These differential exposures are also important in explaining health inequalities which exist by ethnicity and gender.

Furthermore, it argued that '... health inequalities are the outcome of causal chains which run back into and from the basic structure of society'.[47]

While this might be seen as the *Black Report* revisited, the *Acheson Report* pushed the boundaries further. It invoked the most recent research on the capacity of social inequalities within populations to produce health inequalities, despite overall gains in prosperity, stressing the importance of non-impoverished social environments and social connectedness to the health of individuals. It concluded that:

> policies to reduce social inequalities and to promote social networks are part of a strategy to reduce inequalities in health in just the same way as action on economic inequalities or improvements in the material environment of disadvantaged communities.[48]

The bulk of the report consists of recommendations, supported by specific evidence and detailed argument and strongly linked to the reformist principles expounded in the Introduction, for policies aimed at reducing inequalities in health. While these policies have the capacity to bring about general improvements in health, they are specifically designed to have a greater impact on those who are less well off in terms of income, education, employment and material environments. There is a recognition that 'well-intentioned', classic illness prevention and health promotion policies will not do, as they are usually taken up by those who are better off, and can actually lead to an increase in inequalities. The areas identified for policy development include poverty, income, taxation and benefits, education, employment, housing, mobility and transport, nutrition, and inequalities in access and resource allocation within the health care system. The report notes that policies designed to reduce inequalities in all these areas need to focus specifically on the particular needs related to ethnicity, gender and age.

At about the same time as the British Government commissioned the *Acheson Report*, the World Health Organization's Regional Office for Europe commissioned the

---

46 ibid., p.7

47 ibid., pp.6–7

48 ibid., pp.8–9

publication of a booklet that would 'present the evidence on social determinants in a clear and understandable form', as part of its campaign 'to broaden awareness, stimulate debate and promote action'. This resulted in the publication in 1998 of *Social Determinants of Health: the solid facts*, edited by Professors Richard Wilkinson and Michael Marmot.[49] This presents key evidence in a summary and accessible fashion, naming health inequalities within countries as 'an important social injustice' and arguing that 'people's lifestyles and the conditions in which they live and work strongly influence their health and longevity'. It begins by explaining the phenomenon of the social gradient in health and then discusses ten interrelated aspects of the social determinants of health which explain:

> the need for policies to prevent people from falling into long-term disadvantage; how the social and psychological environment affects health; the importance of ensuring a good environment in early childhood; the impact of work on health; the problems of unemployment and job insecurity; the role of friendship and social cohesion; the dangers of social exclusion; the effects of alcohol and other drugs; the need to ensure access to supplies of healthy food for everyone; and the need for healthier transport systems.[50]

The conclusion is unequivocal:

> Societies that enable all their citizens to play a full and useful role in the social, economic and cultural life of their society will be healthier than those where people face insecurity, exclusion and deprivation.[51]

The bold title and the forthright tone of *The Solid Facts* reflect its provenance as a booklet commissioned for popular consumption. However, while research findings reported in other more scholarly settings usually employ less emphatic language and hedge their arguments carefully to preempt criticism, it is apparent that there is increasing assurance in the conclusions that have been drawn from health inequalities research. While some aspects of the research, especially those dealing with such difficult concepts as social cohesion and social capital, remain somewhat contentious, the inequalities debate has been advanced through creative links between researchers operating within different research paradigms and the use of classic epidemiological methods to explore the effects on health of factors suggested by social science perspectives.

Perhaps most widely accepted and influential in this process has been the work of the epidemiologist Professor Michael Marmot. His much-cited 'Whitehall studies', begun in the 1960s, have identified the existence of a steep gradient in coronary heart disease incidence between the top and bottom ranks of the British civil service and demonstrated that the degree of control which workers have in their work situation, especially in

---

49 Richard Wilkinson and Michael Marmot, *Social Determinants of Health: the solid facts*, World Health Organization, WHO Regional Office for Europe, 1998

50 ibid., Introduction

51 ibid., Section 1, 'The social gradient'

relation to experiences of stress, is an important factor in explaining this gradient.[52] Since then, other researchers, using a variety of research methods, have explored further both the phenomenon of the social gradient and the mechanisms by which it operates. In addition, they have been willing to articulate the implications of this research for public policy and to promote the public policy approach to reducing health inequalities. Marmot himself has been involved in this. For example in 2000 in an article entitled 'Social Determinants of Health: from observation to policy', he reiterated the by-then-familiar arguments about the relative unimportance of medical care and 'lifestyle' in establishing and maintaining the social gradient in health and the absence of known biological or genetic reasons for its existence, and concluded that 'rather, the causes are social, economic and political'. Further, he argued that since variations in the steepness of the gradient both across countries and within countries over time indicate that it is not fixed, it must potentially be susceptible to change: 'if inequalities in health increase as an unintended consequence of socio-economic forces, then perhaps they may be reversed to varying degrees by instituting deliberate social and economic measures'. Such measures would go beyond those designed to deal with poverty *per se* and focus on a range of psychosocial factors.[53]

This frankly political response to a persistent health problem does not go far enough for some, including the noted sociologist and policy analyst, Vicente Navarro. In 2001, Navarro and Leiyi Shi claimed that the health and social inequalities literature 'rarely touches on the importance of political forces in influencing inequalities'. They set out

> to show the importance of political parties, and the policies they implement when in govern-
> ment, in determining the level of equalities or inequalities in a society and in explaining the
> level of health of its population.

Their study of advanced OECD governments from a range of political traditions in the period 1945–80 indicated that those traditions had a significant impact in four areas: income distribution, and other mechanisms affecting income inequalities, such as levels and types of government benefits; levels of public expenditure on health care and health insurance coverage; public support of services to families, such as child care; and level of population health as measured by rates of infant mortality. They concluded that those political traditions more committed to redistributive policies and full employment have generally been more successful in improving the health of populations.[54] A related point is made by Kawachi and Kennedy in an article which probes the links between income inequality and social cohesion. They point out that 'the extent of inequality within a

---

52 M Marmot, H Bosma, H Hemingway, E Brunner and S Stansfield, 'Contributions of Job Control and Other Risk Factors
    to Social Variations in Coronary Heart Disease Incidence', *Lancet*, vol.350, 1997, pp.235–9

53 Michael Marmot, 'Social Determinants of Health: from observation to policy', *Medical Journal of Australia*, vol.172,
    17 April 2000, pp.379–82

54 Vicente Navarro and Leiyu Shi, 'The Political Context of Social Inequalities and Health', *Social Science and Medicine*,
    vol.52, 2001, pp.481–91. See also Vicente Navarro, 'A Historical Review (1965–97) of Studies on Class, Health, and
    Quality of Life: a personal account' in *International Journal of Health Services*, vol.28, no.3, 1998, pp.389–406

society is often a consequence of explicit policies and public choice'.[55] Thus, reducing inequality and realising the promise that such reduction offers of creating greater social cohesion and better population health rests on the political will to make different choices. This is supported from within the discipline of public health history by Simon Szreter's work, in particular his 'four Ds' argument. Szreter argues that the 'disruption' that is caused by periods of rapid economic growth within populations – such as industrial revolutions – is inevitably associated with 'deprivation, disease and death', unless the disruption is resolved through specific social and political negotiations about how the wealth resulting from economic growth is to be used and distributed.[56] While Szreter's focus is not on colonial settings, his argument appears to offer a useful model for analysing the immediate and long-term effects of colonial and post-colonial 'disruption' on the well-being of indigenous populations.

Although there has been some scholarly interest in and contribution to the inequalities debate in Australia, its epicentre and major impacts have been elsewhere, as the above discussion indicates. There has been no equivalent in Australia of the Black or Acheson reports. However, an innovative South Australian project, reflecting the 'social health' focus of the 1980s, has contributed to an ongoing and growing understanding of the impact of relative deprivation on health. This is the social health atlas project. The first social health atlas, *A Social Health Atlas of South Australia*, was published in 1990 by the South Australian Health Commission and was followed by a national version in 1992, a second edition of the South Australian atlas in 1996 and a much expanded national version, consisting of one volume for the whole nation and volumes for each of the states and territories in 1999.[57] The 1999 publication provides a summary of how the atlas project has refined its methodology and strengthened its statistical analysis over time. The initial aims of the project were to illustrate the spatial distribution of socioeconomic disadvantage within the population and to compare this with the patterns of distribution of major causes of morbidity and mortality and with the use of health services. To do this, the atlas uses a summary measure of relative disadvantage – the Index of Relative Socioeconomic Disadvantage (IRSD). The IRSD, produced by the Australian Bureau of Statistics on the basis of census data, summarises information regarding education, occupation, unemployment, income, family structure, race, ethnicity and housing. The atlas has used this information to calculate an IRSD score for all Statistical Local Areas (SLAs), which measures the relative socioeconomic disadvantage of an area in comparison with the average

55 Kawachi and Kennedy, 'Health and Social Cohesion', p.1037

56 Szreter, 'Rapid Economic Growth and 'the Four Ds' of Disruption, Deprivation, Disease and Death: public health lessons from nineteenth century Britain for twenty-first century China?', *Tropical Medicine and International Health*, vol.4, no.2, February 1999, pp.146–52; Simon Szreter, 'The Population Health Approach in Historical Perspective', in *American Journal of Public Health*, vol.93, no.3, March 2003, pp.421–31

57 South Australian Health Commission, *A Social Health Atlas of South Australia*, South Australian Health Commission, Adelaide, 1990; John Glover and Tony Wollacott, *A Social Health Atlas of Australia*, vols 1 and 2, Commonwealth Department of Health and South Australian Health Commission, Adelaide, 1992; John Glover, et al. *A Social Health Atlas of South Australia*, 2nd edn, South Australian Health Commission, Adelaide, 1996; John Glover and Sarah Tennant, *A Social Health Atlas of Australia*, 2nd edn, Public Health Information Development Unit, University of Adelaide, 1999

socioeconomic status of Australia as a whole.[58] On the basis of this analysis the authors conclude:

> The information in this atlas adds to a convincing body of evidence built up over a number of years in Australia as to the striking disparities in health that exist between groups in the population. People of low socioeconomic status (those who are relatively socially or economically deprived) experience worse health than those of higher socioeconomic status for almost every major cause of mortality and morbidity.[59]

In addition, by grouping SLAs into quintiles based on their IRSD score, the authors are able to demonstrate that significant health inequalities exist, not just between the most and least advantaged groups, but also at each of the intervening levels of socioeconomic status.[60] In other words, a social gradient of health exists in Australia, as it does elsewhere in the world. The unique contribution of *A Social Health Atlas of Australia* to this understanding is that it demonstrates the existence of this gradient graphically, in relation to a large number of socioeconomic status variables and measures of health and illness, and maps it at the local level across the whole nation.

  The social health atlas project is an impressive achievement and constitutes a 'challenge for policy makers, health practitioners and governments ... to find ways to address [the] inequities' which it has identified.[61] It seems however, that there has been no rush to take up this challenge or even to take very seriously the evidence underlying it. Milton Lewis and Stephen Leeder, in a paper entitled, *Where To From Here? The need to construct a comprehensive national health policy*, argue that 'the impetus for change must come from a government with capacity extensively to mobilise authority, and with the will to institute major reform'. Such opportunities for major change, they say, come only rarely, and, to be fruitful, need not only 'the strong commitment of governments of the time for change, but a large political and economic context favourable to change'.[62] I have argued above that the want of such a context limited the chances of the *Black Report*, *The Health Divide* and reformist ideas within the South Australian Health Commission to effect major change. Such a context still does not exist in Australia, and despite mounting evidence of the extent to which health and health inequalities are socially and politically determined, governments continue to avoid the implications of this evidence and to reduce concerns about health to concerns about health care. As Lewis and Leeder conclude:

---

58 For more detailed discussion of the background to the project, and issues related to methodology, analysis, data, selection of indicators etc., see Glover and Tennant, *A Social Health Atlas of Australia*, 2nd edn, *vol.5: South Australia*, Executive summary, pp.v–vii, and Introduction, pp.1–18.

59 ibid., p.v

60 ibid., pp.vi–vii

61 ibid., p.v

62 Milton J. Lewis and Stephen R. Leeder, *Where To From Here? The need to construct a comprehensive national health policy*, Australian Health Policy Institute, University of Sydney, 2001, pp.46–7

Since the population health approach (including amelioration of health inequalities) demands a major change in policy championed by a national government, it is difficult to see a window of opportunity opening in the near future in Australia. Much more likely is further conflict between the major parties over the long-established issue of health care funding ... The population health approach may be of increasing significance to health researchers and practitioners, but the window of opportunity to translate it into a major policy change has not even begun to open in Australia.[63]

The Generational Health Review, a review of the South Australian health system commissioned by the South Australian Government in 2002 and reporting in 2003, supports this contention.[64] Despite the fact that its aim was to deliver 'a plan ... that provides effective strategies for health system reform, which ensures that all South Australians enjoy the best possible health and have access to high standards of health care', the Generational Health Review failed to take seriously the social determinants and health inequalities research, the *Acheson Report*, or even, except in a token fashion, the information yielded by the social health atlas. It did attempt to come up with approaches that would ensure greater equity in provision of and access to health services, and in expending most energy on this, attested to the continuing hegemony of bio-medical explanations of health and illness, despite compelling evidence that suggests alternative explanations. These alternative ideas, with their disturbing insistence that 'the whole structure of society is implicated' and their critique of prevailing orthodoxies, remain as an irritant to those charged with the responsibility of crafting government policy.

The decades in which the *Black Report* and *The Health Divide* appeared, in which research into health inequalities burgeoned and produced robust findings – even 'solid facts' – and in which the *Acheson Report* translated these findings into a substantial policy reform agenda coincided with the period in which non-Aboriginal Australia officially recognised Aboriginals as part of the public. At the broadest level this recognition involved the extension of full citizenship rights to Aboriginals, the dismantling of old structures and policies of protection and assimilation, and the declaration of a new policy to guide 'Aboriginal affairs', that is, the policy of self-determination. Old arguments about an appropriate place, or indeed any place for Aboriginals within the nation, were officially declared to be over: Aboriginals would henceforth participate on an equal basis with all other Australians in the affairs of the nation, exercise their rights and responsibilities as citizens, and make decisions about their own affairs, being free to preserve whatever they wished of their own identity. In the light of these new commitments and grand hopes, the material deprivation experienced by many Aboriginal people, their continuing lack of educational attainment, social inclusion or productive incorporation into the economic

---

63 ibid., p.47

64 I was member of one of the five task groups which were established to carry out the Generational Health Review and recommend a plan for reform the South Australian Minister of Health. My comments in this section are based on my experience as a member of that task group and on my analysis of the final report of the Generational Health Review.

structures of Australian society, and their poor health status appeared as major policy challenges and an affront to democratic ideals.[65]

There is a deep irony and much capacity for distortion in the fact that the policy of self-determination was devised and imposed on Aboriginals by non-Aboriginals. In any case, within a very short time of its establishment, governments became uncomfortable with its potentially radical implications and set about repackaging it as self-management. Despite these limitations, the adoption of the policy of self-determination from 1973 was a significant development. It coincided with a time in which indigenous confidence and aspirations were flourishing and being reflected in the positive reclaiming of a separate identity and the establishment of indigenous organisations of many kinds. Among these were Aboriginal community-controlled health services.

These services, which proliferated after the establishment of the prototype in Redfern, Sydney in 1971, combined a community development function with the provision of health services. They understood the health of Aboriginal people to be powerfully influenced by historical circumstances and by ongoing social, economic and political forces, and in their attempts to improve health, adopted a community focus as well as an individual one. These services were not simply more culturally appropriate alternatives than 'mainstream' services. Fundamental to their philosophy and their organisational structures was the principle of community control. The community-controlled health services and similar organisations which emerged around the same time, such as legal rights services and community and housing associations, were supported by government funding of various kinds but run by and for the benefit of Aboriginal communities through representative boards of management. This of course is problematic, and many 'community-controlled' organisations are faced with ongoing argument about who 'the community' is, how it is to be represented and whose interests the organisations are serving. Nevertheless, these organisations, through the employment and training of indigenous staff, are able to provide services that are acceptable to many Aboriginal people. In addition, they contribute to growth of confidence among their staff and clients, imparting a sense of being in control, of being actively involved in restoring well-being to their communities, and of having their own priorities and ways of doing things valued.

The philosophy of 'community control', as both evidence of and a means to self-determination, has been promoted nationally through the umbrella body, the National Aboriginal Community Controlled Health Organisation (NACCHO) since 1993 and is fundamental to the National Aboriginal Health Strategy of 1989. This strategy was developed by a working party set up in 1987 in response to ministerial concern about the apparent lack of improvement in the health of indigenous Australians, despite the commitment of 'significant resources' since the Commonwealth assumed responsibility for Aboriginal affairs in 1973. The concern was not just that health might not be improving, but that resources might not be being well-used:

Ministers are continually being assailed with allegations of duplication, competition and

---

65 See below, Appendix 1 for a summary of Aboriginal health status. The historical origins of this health status will
    be traced in subsequent chapters.

waste in the health service area. There is also a growing belief amongst politicians and particularly Ministers, that sufficient resources are currently available to make significant improvements in Aboriginal health and that the task is to redirect and focus those resources.[66]

There is an implicit assumption here that the issue is one of health services and the
efficient use of resources directed to these services. By restricting their focus to discussion of
services and strategies for dealing with particular health issues, much of the introductory
section of the strategy, and most of its executive summary and its specific recommendations support this assumption. They constitute a strong endorsement of community-
controlled services and of providing opportunities, through better education and training,
for greater participation by Aboriginal health professionals in these services. However, this
serves to elide the distinctions between health and health services and reinforces the argument that the former is secured through improvements to the latter. This is strangely at odds
with the highly polemical opening section of the strategy which constructs the problems
faced by Aboriginal Australia as the result of colonisation, dispossession and marginalisation.[67] This construction is not reflected strongly in the rest of the document, although
it is hinted at in section headed 'Political Realities'. This section expresses doubts about the
existence of the political will to do what needs to be done to improve Aboriginal health.
It reads the current context as one in which there are 'increasing demands for smaller and
leaner government' and a 'hardening of general community attitudes to assisting Aborigines'.[68]
In 1994 *The National Aboriginal Health Strategy: an evaluation* was published.[69] It
concluded that the strategy had never been effectively implemented, and reported
'minimal gains in the appalling state of Aboriginal health'. This 'appalling state' could not

> by any accurate reading of the factors influencing health and life expectancy, be attributed to
> anything other than the impact of dispossession and its effects on the lives of Aboriginal and
> Torres Strait Islander peoples.

However, the document does not, on balance, reflect this reading. Rather it focuses on 'the
health hazards of a hostile physical environment', and inequity in access to the 'health-
promoting knowledge' and the medical and other services that are needed to 'equip individuals to achieve a lifestyle and level of economic stability which permits healthy choices'.
The major recommendations offer little insight into what might be involved in addressing
dispossession and reduce the notion of 'equity' to 'equal access to equal care appropriate
to need'.[70] In the world of policy-making, this phenomenon of a radical mismatch
between a broad construction of the problem and the much narrower recommendations

---

66 National Aboriginal Health Strategy Working Party, *A National Aboriginal Health Strategy*, p.xii. For further information
    about the Working Party, see above, footnote 36, p.13.

67 ibid., pp.i-viii. This section is entitled 'Aboriginal Australia – the reality and not the myth', and is attributed to John Newfong.

68 ibid., p.xi

69 National Aboriginal Health Strategy Evaluation Committee, *The National Aboriginal Health Strategy: an evaluation*,
    AGPS, Canberra, 1994

70 ibid., pp.1–5

which are then made to address it is a common one. It is apparent in both *A National Aboriginal Health Strategy*, and in the evaluation of that strategy, and in subsequent Aboriginal health policy initiatives in South Australia, for example, *Dreaming Beyond 2000* and *The First Step*.[71] It is still there in the *National Strategic Framework for Aboriginal and Torres Strait Islander Health* produced by the National Aboriginal and Torres Strait Islander Health Council in 2003. This document endorses the 1989 strategy as the 'key document' for indigenous health and advocates a program for health improvement based on more comprehensive, better-funded and more accountable primary health care services, in which indigenous control over priority setting and service delivery and partnerships between government and indigenous communities are the hallmarks. While the National Strategic Framework acknowledges that the health of Aboriginal Australians is linked to underlying poverty and multi-faceted disadvantage, its 'key action areas' do not address this. Its only nod in the direction of the public health research discussed in this chapter relates to community control as a means of building the capacity to allow individuals and communities to make healthy choices.[72]

What does the research and the evidence on inequalities, the chief focus of this chapter, have to say to this situation? Very little of the inequalities research alludes to or draws its evidence from Australia. Certainly, it neither makes reference to the health of indigenous Australians, nor focusses on other analogous situations. However, the implications of this research for the health of indigenous Australians are far-reaching and complex. It is abundantly clear from the available data that indigenous Australians have the worst health of all groups within the Australian population. Since, as has now been demonstrated, health is largely socially and economically determined, and since social and economic inequalities are reflected in health inequalities across populations, with those groups who suffer the greatest deprivation also suffering the worst health, we are able to conclude that the complex social and economic marginalisation of Aboriginal Australians is linked to their poor health. In the light of current evidence, previously advanced alternative explanations which posit racial inheritance, evolutionary stage, behaviour or culture as the source of health status are no longer tenable. This being the case, the prerequisites for improved indigenous health become clear. They are not merely more and better services of various kinds, or greater and more sustained funding, or the training of more indigenous health professionals, or better coordinated administrative arrangements, or improved accountability and governance, although all of these things are important. What is needed are the more fundamental shifts required to minimise social inequalities

---

71 Aboriginal Health Council of South Australia Inc. and South Australian Health Commission, *Dreaming beyond 2000: our future is in our history. South Australian Aboriginal health policy and strategic framework*, Aboriginal Health Council of South Australia Inc.; South Australian Health Commission, Adelaide, 1994; South Australian Aboriginal Health Partnership, *The First Step: South Australian Aboriginal health regional plans*, South Australian Aboriginal Health Partnership, Adelaide, 1998. The phenomenon of problem/solution or cause/remedy mismatch is not confined to Aboriginal health. It is a persistent *motif* in the history of public health and relates to the reluctance of governments and those benefiting from the *status quo* to embrace structural solutions that involve changes to existing power balances.

72 National Aboriginal and Torres Strait Islander Health Council, *National Strategic Framework for Aboriginal and Torres Strait Islander Health: framework for action by governments*, Canberra, 2003,

among the Australian population, to build civic environments that include and engage rather than exclude and alienate, and, in particular, that allow Aboriginal Australians, dispossessed and marginalised as a result of non-indigenous policies and practices, to become part of the public.

There are dangers, however, in imagining that the health inequalities argument, developed from information gathered in different circumstances, can be applied to the situation of indigenous Australians without some modification. One danger is that superficial readings of the evidence, which focus most attention on the deprivation and ill-health of the most disadvantaged, have the capacity to be counter-productive. They frequently take too narrow a view of what impinges on health and encourage victim-blaming and individualist, behavioural responses to structural problems. More considered readings which recognise that the social gradient in health persists across whole populations are more likely to suggest radical, whole-of-government, structural reform. If this understanding were to be taken seriously by governments and policy-makers, then it would offer hope for improvements in the health of Aboriginal people.

Even so, the fit between the problem and the solution implied by the health inequalities argument is far from neat. The situation of indigenous people in post-colonial societies is unique. There is no obvious place for them in the stratification by occupation used by the Black Inquiry and, with some refinements, found useful by many other inequalities researchers. Aboriginal Australians should not be seen as occupying the lowest levels of occupational class five or constituting some kind of class six. They are a population group whose place in the social order was, until the early 1970s, decided for them in a way that did not apply to any other group within the Australian population. It is not that the policies and practices of protection and assimilation which governed the lives of indigenous Australians until then left them as merely the most disadvantaged section of the population, scrambling to get onto the lowest rungs of the socioeconomic ladder, and therefore in need of a leg-up. Rather, it situated them differently, as 'inmates against the management' within 'the politics of the asylum, hospital, camp, or other authoritarian institution'.[73] The legacy of this distinctive history continues to be reflected in many aspects of the lives of Aboriginal Australians. It is clearly seen, for example, in the nature of some remote indigenous communities, which, in terms of mainstream understandings, have no rational or natural economic base, and where ways have yet to be found to guarantee the rights and well-being of those who choose to live there. It is seen also in the dependence, lack of autonomy and lack of opportunity of the kind enjoyed by other sections of the population that continues to characterise many Aboriginal lives and communities. This historical legacy, then, is not merely about disadvantage and inequality: it is about – even yet – not being part of the public.[74]

There is another aspect to the imperfect fit of the inequalities research with the problem of Aboriginal health. The *Black Report* recommended 'radically improving the

---

73 CD Rowley, *Outcasts in White Australia: Aboriginal policy and practice – vol.11*, Australian National University Press, Canberra, 1971, p.190. See below, pp.272–3

74 Here Szreter's argument about unresolved disruption, associated with deprivation, disease and death seems apt. See above, pp.39

material conditions of life of poorer groups ... by increasing or introducing certain cash benefits'. Subsequent researchers, including the authors of the *Acheson Report*, have stressed the primary importance of income guarantees via increased government benefits as a means to reducing inequalities.[75] While such a response to community need is fundamental in any society making claims to decency and inclusivity, in cases of grave social dysfunction and entrenched, inter-generational dependence it may also be problematic. Such dysfunction and dependence is an historical burden borne by some Aboriginal communities, families and individuals. In these situations the routine provision of benefits or welfare payments, according to unimaginative and restrictive formulae and at levels bound to keep recipients in or near poverty, may be the very antithesis of beneficial and may actually undermine their welfare. In recent years, the view has been growing among some Aboriginal people that 'welfare' or 'sit down money' does not contribute to equality, that it exacerbates some serious social problems, inhibits the growth of autonomy, militates against social inclusion and is at odds with the notion of self-determination.[76] This view may generate creative thinking that will lead to the adoption of healthier policies and greater independence, or it may encourage a regression to something more paternalistic and ultimately inimical to health. In any case, it is clear that, while the inequalities research has much to offer to indigenous Australians, it would be foolish to imagine that there can be one policy agenda arising from it that will fit all situations.

Viewed in the light of the scholarship and major inquiries discussed in this chapter, the history of non-Aboriginal policies and practices in relation to Aboriginal Australians appears as a neat and fail-safe recipe for the production of poor Aboriginal health. Aboriginals have suffered not only from the individualist, genetic, biological, and behavioural analyses of health which frequently limit our understanding of what determines the health of populations and lead to inappropriate interventions; they have suffered also from the unhelpful and hostile victim-blaming that public health history demonstrates is the lot of all deprived and marginalised groups. Their poor living conditions, damaging or destructive behaviour and attitudes, low levels of educational achievement and exclusion from roles and functions associated with social acceptance and physical and psychological well-being are seen as uncomplicated individual choices, rather than as the end point of complex processes of deprivation and lack of choice. Perhaps even more significantly, Aboriginal people have also been subjected to an overtly racist construction of themselves as different and 'other', with different and lesser needs than the rest of the population, and different and lesser claims on the resources and opportunities which Australia has had to offer. The inequalities research tells us clearly that there will not be improvement in the health of the indigenous population until the Australian community addresses the profound, complex, and entrenched inequality and alienation that is the result of this history.

The political will needed to effect such a transformation does not currently exist. In

---

75   Townsend, Davidson and Whitehead, *Inequalities in Health*, pp.2–3; Acheson, *Independent Inquiry into Health Inequalities*, p.30

76   Noel Pearson has been a prominent exponent of this view. See, for example, Noel Pearson, 'On the Human Right to Misery, Incarceration and Early Death', *Quadrant*, December 2001, pp.9–20

fact, in recent times, an insecure global climate and conservative domestic political philosophies which laud individual responsibility, maintain fictions about equal opportunity and level playing fields and legitimise the retreat of government from social provision have allowed old fears, prejudices, hostilities and social divisions to resurface. This situation is inimical to the extension to indigenous Australians of the resources and the opportunities to make choices about their future that will overturn the effects of their dispossession and allow them to be part of a plural and heterogeneous Australian public. My contention is that it is only by knowing and confronting our history, and by embracing the radical implications of what research now tells us determines the health of populations, that we can transcend these insecurities. It is only when we acknowledge that 'the appalling state of Aboriginal health' is a result of non-indigenous policies and practices that we will be in a position to respond appropriately. The rest of this book is about uncovering and confronting that history.

Chapter 3

1836–1858:
In Search of a Policy

Black men, we wish to make you happy. But you cannot be happy unless you imitate white men. Build huts, wear clothes and be useful.

Above all things, you cannot be happy unless you love God who made heaven and earth and men and all things.

Love white men. Love other tribes of black men. Do not quarrel together. Tell other tribes to love white men and to build good huts and wear clothes. Learn to speak English.

If any white man injure you, tell the Protector and he will do you justice.

Governor George Gawler 1838[1]

Resplendent in full dress uniform, George Gawler, newly arrived governor of the colony of South Australia, addressed these words to a crowd of about 200 indigenous inhabitants assembled in the park near Government House, Adelaide, on 1 November 1838. The 'natives' were 'highly delighted' with the occasion, at which they not only enjoyed a 'plenteous supply' of roast beef, tea, sugar, rice and biscuit, but also received gifts of rugs, blankets, woollen frocks, caps, tin dishes and cups. When the speech-making and the distribution of food and gifts were over, the governor and the ladies and gentlemen of the colony retired to a marquee for refreshments, and the 'natives departed to their usual haunts'. The whole occasion was taken to be 'gratifying evidence' of the friendly relations that had been established between the colonists and the indigenous inhabitants, and of the latter's gratitude for the forbearance and consideration with which they had been treated.[2]

Governor Gawler's words were no doubt taken by the colonists as confirmation that the official message of protection, justice and advancement through conformity to white ways, which had been consistently preached since Governor John Hindmarsh proclaimed the establishment of the government and the rule of British law at Glenelg on 28 December 1836, remained unchanged.[3] Gawler's speech was an endorsement of their belief in the

---

1 Governor Gawler's speech, 1 November 1838, *South Australian Gazette and Colonial Register*, 3 November 1838, p.4

2 *South Australian Gazette and Colonial Register*, 3 November 1838, p.4

3 Governor Hindmarsh's Proclamation, 28 December 1836, *South Australian Gazette and Colonial Register*, 3 June 1837

superiority of their own culture and of their right, indeed their duty, to extend its insights and benefits to 'these poor people ... our friendly natives'.[4] It is now clear that it was also a poignant foreshadowing of future policies, practices and attitudes which, far from protecting the indigenous inhabitants, making them happy and guaranteeing them justice, came close to destroying them. In addition, before the long-term destructive potential of these apparently benign beliefs became clear, the immediate failure of practice to conform to the official pronouncements brought misery, injustice and degradation to the indigenous inhabitants of South Australia rather than the promised boons. This lack of congruence between what governments proclaim as their policy, or less grandly, their hopes, and what actually happens, is a recurring phenomenon and underscores the need to be wary of mistaking prescription for description.

Governor Gawler's words, and the events at Government House on 1 November 1838 exemplify three other important themes which were repeatedly played out in the subsequent history of South Australia. Firstly, they are clear evidence of the view that the original inhabitants were not seen as part of the public. The 'poor natives' provided a spectacle for the European guests to observe; they were fed and entertained separately and differently from them, and they then disappeared to 'their usual haunts', which were not part of the fledgling colonial settlement. Secondly, these events indicate a failure on the part of the governor and his guests to apprehend among the assembled 'natives' any existing economic and cultural life of any value or any aspirations for the future independent of non-indigenous plans for the colony. Thirdly, the provision of food to a crowd of Aboriginals gathered at official behest constituted an early act of rationing. This had obvious political purposes and was to become the basis of the government's attempts to order relations between settlers and 'natives' for some time to come. This chapter traces those attempts to order indigenous/non-indigenous relations in the early years of the colony's development. It demonstrates that the entrenchment of colonial authority and the growth of the settler economy severely undermined indigenous cultural and economic independence, and that the government failed to adequately protect or provide for the indigenous population, confirming them as a problem to be dealt with, rather than as part of the public whose interests it existed to serve.

The locus of responsibility for providing the indigenous inhabitants with the protection of British law, of 'promoting their advancement in civilization, and ultimately, under the blessing of Divine Providence, their conversion to the Christian Faith'[5], was the office of Protector of Aborigines. However, no permanent appointment was made to the office until June 1839 and in the meantime three Protectors were appointed on an *ad interim* basis. The first of these was George Stevenson, who came to the colony on the *Buffalo* as Governor Hindmarsh's Private Secretary. In the first months of 1837 Stevenson collected many additional roles, as well as attracting the disapproval of those at odds with Hindmarsh, who considered Stevenson self-serving and not fit for the offices he held.

---

4 *South Australian Gazette and Colonial Register*, 3 November 1838, p.4

5 ibid, p.4

Appointed as Protector on 3 February, he resigned on 1 April in response to public agitation against him, leaving behind not 'a single reference to any act of administration on his part while holding the office of Protector'.[6]

On the surface of it, Captain Walter Bromley, who was appointed to succeed Stevenson on 7 April 1837, was better equipped for the job. He had previously worked among indigenous people in Canada and had been conducting a school for Aboriginal children in Kingscote, Kangaroo Island, since his arrival in South Australia in October 1836. In Adelaide he was given no official instructions, but set out to establish good relations with and provide protection and education for the local Kaurna people at the Aborigines Location, an area on the north bank of the Torrens set aside by the government for that purpose. He supervised initial building activity there, and, on 25 May 1837, in a letter to the Colonial Secretary, outlined his aims and hopes. He wanted to 'teach the natives to regard us as neighbours and brethren', and to 'lead them to assimilate their habits and feelings to ours'. They would 'be gradually initiated into the great doctrines of Christianity' and through that experience would be 'led to consider themselves as allied to us through our common parent'. He expected the natives to embrace all of these opportunities and believed that they would quickly come to 'look upon their former habits and situation with abhorrence'. He intended to learn their language 'as a preliminary step to every improvement in their moral and religious condition'. He asked for a plot of land on which the natives could grow food while learning practical skills. This land was to be for the local natives only, and while they would be free to come and go on it, the more distant tribes were not to be invited for fear of causing trouble. Whites were not to be on the reservation without official permission.[7]

However, Bromley soon proved to be unequal to the job, lacking the physical and mental stamina and the personal presence it required. All events seemed to conspire against him. A badly scalded leg incapacitated him physically; the Aboriginals scorned the oatmeal he offered them when the biscuit ration ran out and refused to cooperate with him; and his assistant, Cooper, whose official role was interpreter, was 'usually drunk and frequently an absentee'.[8] On 24 July 1837 Bromley was interviewed by the Legislative Council and was counselled to resign, which he did on 26 July.[9]

The colonial government's next appointment as *ad interim* Protector was Dr William Wyatt who took up his duties on 1 August 1837. Wyatt was a surgeon who was also appointed as colonial coroner and magistrate. Unlike his predecessors, he had government instructions to guide him.[10] This proved to be a two-edged sword and he was later accused of not fulfilling his duties as specified in the instructions. From the start Wyatt set about inculcating in the minds of the Aboriginals a connection between work and material reward. In his first report he wrote:

---

6 AA Lendon, Short Biographical Sketches, typescript, no date [c. 1933], pp.179–84, PRG 128/2/11

7 Walter Bromley, to the Colonial Secretary of South Australia, 25 May 1837, GRG24/1/1837/117

8 Lendon, *Short Biographical Sketches*, p.188

9 ibid., p.194

10 *South Australian Gazette and Colonial Register*, 11–12 August 1837

A general rule has been adopted of not giving anything to them except for some trifling service done, so that by thus teaching them to look upon what they receive as equivalents for what they do, they may gradually be brought into habits of industry and may eventually become more profitable members of society.[11]

By the end of 1837, a group of concerned citizens, 'perceiving how essential it is to conciliate the natives, and by kind treatment to entice them into social and industrious habits' had formed a committee to support the Protector.[12] Although this committee shared Wyatt's frankly assimilationist aims and declared it 'extremely desirable to lead the natives to habits of industry by adequate remuneration', they also believed that providing them with food, work and accommodation was 'only an act of common justice to those whose land we have occupied and whose game we have destroyed'.[13] This notion of the provision of benefits as compensation for dispossession had been present, although not predominant, in negotiations in Britain prior to the foundation of the colony, and reappeared frequently in early South Australia. Although somewhat at odds with the more prevalent position, which saw benefits as a reward for and inducement to work, the two views seemed to sit easily together. In fact, they were often espoused by the same person, with no apparent awareness of contradiction.[14]

Wyatt set about erecting sheds and establishing a school at the Aborigines Location, and reported on 1 April 1838 that it would be ready for occupation by the end of the following month.[15] In July he reported positively about progress: the Location was appreciated by the Aboriginals; James Cronk, who had replaced Cooper as interpreter when the latter was dismissed for misconduct in March, had settled in well; and a biscuit ration was being issued twice daily. However, he also described the natives as 'indolent' and attributed this to the 'salubrious climate' which fairly readily supported subsistence. This indolence was 'the grand obstacle to their civilization', and he had come to the conclusion that the solution was 'first to teach them the simple and divine doctrine of Christianity and that to begin by any other method is truly to commence at the wrong end'. Therefore, he recommended the appointment of a missionary, adding rather cryptically that this would please those 'who look upon the aborigines of South Australia as fellow members of the same great human family'.[16] Whether Wyatt included himself in this company is not entirely clear. However, it is clear that he was aware that this inclusive view was by no means universally held.

Meanwhile, outside the Location, and despite the official policy, relations between natives and colonists were sufficiently punctuated by violence and unrest for dissatisfaction to mount

---

11 Report of Protector of Aborigines, 1 October1837, GRG 24/1/1837/389

12 Report of Protector of Aborigines, 1 January 1838, GRG 24//1/1838/3

13 Resolutions of meeting of Aborigines' Committee, 10 January 1838, GRG24/1/1838/8

14 See RM Gibbs, 'Humanitarian Theories and the Aboriginal Inhabitants of South Australia to 1860', BA (Hons) thesis, University of Adelaide, 1959, for a discussion of Colonial Office ideas about the responsibility of the South Australian Government for the indigenous inhabitants.

15 Report of Protector of Aborigines, 1 April 1838, GRG24/1/1838/69

16 Report of Protector of Aborigines, 1 July 1838, GRG24/1/1838/142

over the Protector's inability to control matters. A public meeting to discuss the situation was held on 7 May 1839. It resolved that colonists and Aboriginals alike had a right to security of life and property and attributed current threats to this security to the inefficiency of the Protector and his failure to comply with his instructions, especially those pertaining to his living among the Aboriginals.[17] Wyatt insisted that this had never been an expectation of his office. Governor Gawler came to his defence by reminding the public that no formal complaints had ever been brought against Wyatt, and that since his appointment was *ad interim* and expected to finish in the near future when a permanent appointment was made, there were limits to what could be expected of him.[18] The situation was resolved when the crown appointed Dr Matthew Moorhouse to the position of Protector. Moorhouse arrived in Adelaide in June 1839, and was to prove much more durable and effective than the *ad interim* appointees whom he followed. But Gawler was not leaving things to chance or to Moorhouse's unguided judgement: he drew up and gazetted rules for the guidance of the Protector of Aborigines in the carrying out of his duties, to which Moorhouse assented on 26 June 1839.[19] These guidelines provide us with a template by which to assess the achievements of Moorhouse's long term of office and also to gauge developments in the concerns and activities of subsequent Protectors and of the South Australian public.

In the first place, the Protector was to be wholly devoted to the office, and was to pursue no other occupation. He was expected to spend 'a great part of his time among the natives in such a manner that he may acquire their friendship and confidence' and to acquaint himself with their language, customs and prejudices and with their numbers and the localities of the various tribes. He was not to spend all his time in Adelaide and was expected to visit all the tribes frequently. He was to keep a detailed journal of his journeys and his dealings with the Aboriginals and report any extraordinary events to the Governor without delay. He was to protect his charges from exploitation by ensuring that all agreements made with them were honoured and that people who were paid to provide services to them, performed these 'actively and faithfully'. The aim was to promote mutual understanding and justice between the races and this required that the Protector bring offenders, whether Aboriginal or non-Aboriginal, to justice. While he was to leave the Aboriginals as far as possible to their own means of subsistence, ensuring only that they did not fall into destitution, he was to see to it that they were instructed in reading, writing, building houses, making clothes, cultivating land and in 'all the other ordinary arts of civilization'. Above all, he was to bring them to a knowledge of God and of the fundamental truths of Christianity.[20]

It seems reasonable to assume that these demanding guidelines reflected the dissatisfaction of the authorities with the achievements of the earlier Protectors and also that they amounted to a good deal of pressure on Moorhouse to perform. They probably also encouraged his meticulous reporting of his activities, which provides us with a rich

---

17 *South Australian Gazette and Colonial Register,* 11 May 1839

18 *South Australian Gazette and Colonial Register,* 18 May 1839

19 *South Australian Government Gazette (SAGG),* 4 July 1839, pp.5–6

20 *SAGG,* 4 July 1839, pp.5–6

record of his and his Sub-Protectors' views of relations between settlers and indigenous inhabitants in the earliest years of the colony.[21]

The guidelines provided for Moorhouse are also a clear reflection of the values and assumptions of early colonial society in South Australia and of the contradictions and seeds of conflict inherent in them. There is no mistaking the good will and the hope for peace and harmony that lay behind them. Here was a government wanting to engage the friendship and trust of the indigenous inhabitants, to protect them from exploitation and injustice, and to relate to them on the basis of knowledge rather than ignorance. But nor is there any mistaking the blindness of the colonisers to the fact that by their very presence and by the erection of their own institutions and the pursuit of their own economic and social ends, at the expense of those of the indigenous inhabitants, they were perpetrating a fundamental and comprehensive act of subjugation and dispossession. They were confident in the assumption that the natives were in need of civilising and learning to live according to the material habits, spiritual beliefs and moral standards of the colonisers. However, they saw no need for the natives to develop skills beyond the menial, or to aspire to comforts beyond those which kept them out of destitution. The Aboriginals were no longer in charge of their own land or their own affairs, and while they were being offered entry into some aspects of the world of the newly arrived authorities, they were clearly not being invited to become an integral part of it.

Thus, unwittingly, the early colonial governments set the pattern for all subsequent policies regarding the original inhabitants of South Australia. These policies were either an expression of the assumption of the superiority of European culture and the primacy of European aspirations and of the unquestioned value of indigenous assimilation to them, or they were a reaction to the effects of these assumptions. They impacted profoundly on Aboriginal health and well-being and, in a deeply ironical way, given the assimilationist thread that ran through them all, ensured that Aboriginals were always seen as a race apart and not as part of the public whose interests the laws and provisions of the state were supposed to serve.

———————————

When Moorhouse took up his position as Protector of Aborigines he found the Adelaide natives 'in a state of perfect quietude'. This was induced in part, he thought, by a plentiful supply of shirts and blankets, although the judgement of history focuses more on the Kaurna being 'simply overwhelmed by the sheer weight and concentration of European settlement'.[22] Early census data collected in the colony indicate the extent to which the indigenous population was outnumbered.[23] Through his own recording of population

21 For discussion of this context of dissatisfaction and expectation see Robert Foster (ed.), 'Two Early Reports on the Aborigines of South Australia', in *Aboriginal Adelaide:* special issue of the *Journal of the Anthropological Society of South Australia*, vol.28, nos 1 and 2, December 1990, pp.38–63.

22 Robert Foster, Rick Hosking and Amanda Nettelbeck, *Fatal Collisions: the South Australian frontier and the violence of memory*, Wakefield Press, Adelaide, 2001, p.3.

23 The first official census, taken in 1840, indicated that there were 14 160 Europeans in South Australia, that 7000 hectares of land had been enclosed, of which 1200 were under crop, and that there were 200 000 sheep and 15 000 cattle in the

numbers, Moorhouse's reports hint at the inevitable impact of European settlement and occupation of land on indigenous patterns of life. He estimated in his second report that there were 540 natives currently living between the Para River and Encounter Bay, with only 80 in Adelaide. A year later he was reporting 271 men, 178 women and 183 children in or close to Adelaide, and 650 in an area that extended 80 miles to the north of Adelaide, 60 miles to the south and 20 miles eastwards from the coast. He believed he had 'met everyone' in this area.[24] While the precise numbers are likely to be inaccurate, and the patterns subject to seasonal and periodic change, the lure and disruptive effect of Adelaide is apparent. In the city there was little chance of the Aboriginals being other than dependent on and marginal to the social and economic priorities of the colonists, or of being protected from its various corrupting influences.

From the start, Moorhouse tried to provide such protection. For example, he was quick to make clear one of the guiding principles that directed his efforts, namely that there should be no handouts or rations without work. He regretted that the 'characteristic indolence of the natives' had already been reinforced by the unthinking behaviour of many colonists. As a way of addressing this situation, he suggested two alternative approaches. The first was for the government to issue instructions against the colonists giving anything to the Aboriginals, so that all rationing could occur at the Aborigines Location and be seen to be linked to the work of building houses and developing productive gardens. The second approach was to abandon plans for 'locating and civilizing' adult Aboriginals and focus instead on the children, leaving the adults to fend for themselves. Moorhouse clearly favoured the first of these alternatives, but despite pursuing it energetically, was soon forced to opt for something closer to the second, which, as subsequent history has shown, was uncannily prophetic of much future policy and practice.[25]

Moorhouse fulfilled Gawler's faith in him as a man of energy and commitment. Assiduous in his attention to the issues that confronted him in Adelaide, he also quickly acquainted himself with the country and population beyond, where, as the survey of rural land enabled the spread of settlement, 'a state of perfect quietude' was frequently not to be found. He travelled to Encounter Bay, the Fleurieu Peninsula, the River Murray and the area of the Para 'tribe', north of Adelaide, and investigated reports of 'aggressions', sheep stealing by the Aboriginals, and 'disproportionate retaliation' on the part of the settlers. He was aware of the likelihood that, through contact with Europeans, the indigenous population would decrease as it had done in New South Wales and Van Diemen's

---

colony. By 1851 the European population had grown to 63 700, the area under cultivation to 26 150 hectares, and the livestock to one million sheep and 100 000 cattle. The number of Aboriginals recorded in that census was 3730. See Trevor Griffin and Murray McGaskill, (eds), *Atlas of South Australia*, South Australian Government Printing Division/Wakefield Press, Adelaide, 1986, pp.11–12. This publication provides an accessible and graphic summary of Aboriginal patterns of settlement and trade in South Australia prior to 1836, and of the spread of European settlement and economic activity into Aboriginal land since 1836.

24 Report of Protector of Aborigines, 14 Jan 1840, 20 February 1841, published in the *Fifth Annual Report of the Colonization Commissioners for South Australia* (29 July 1842), and reproduced in *British Parliamentary Papers: Papers relating to Australia, 1842–1844: Colonies Australia 7*, Irish University Press, Shannon, Ireland, 1969, pp.352–4, 356–8

25 Report of Protector of Aborigines, 9 October 1839, *Fifth Annual Report of the Colonization Commissioners*, pp.350–2

Land, and expressed particular concern about the spread of venereal disease among the natives as a result of their contact with sealers and whalers.[26] By 1841, his authority had been formally extended to areas isolated from Adelaide. In that year he appointed the German missionary, Clamor Schurmann, Deputy Protector at Port Lincoln, where there were considerable numbers of Aboriginals and only a few Europeans. He also responded, although only on a short-term and limited basis, to the request of Dr Richard Penny, surgeon at the whaling station at Encounter Bay, for medicines to treat the large numbers of Aboriginals in that area suffering from introduced diseases, particularly venereal disease.[27] These early reports of Moorhouse's attention to issues beyond Adelaide indicate his commitment to some aspects of indigenous health and welfare, especially where these constituted a threat to the health of the wider community. They also illustrate his concern to maintain peace and order and encourage 'sufficient forbearance' among the settlers who, with their stock, were extending European influence further into Aboriginal territory.[28] However, the task was beyond him. The formal extension of authority did not always afford protection to either indigenous or settler populations, and was often ineffective against frontier violence.

The spread of European settlement and economic activity brought more colonists and Aboriginals into contact with each other, albeit in unequal numbers, and sometimes at a considerable distance from Adelaide and the influence of the protectorate. This spread of settlement had the potential to provide some employment opportunities for the indigenous population, but before this potential could be realised there was usually a period of what Moorhouse called 'collisions' to be weathered. These 'collisions', which others were more inclined to label as Aboriginal treachery and count as evidence of their savage and uncivilised nature, bred fear and insecurity among many settlers. This often led to disproportionate retaliation in the face of actual or perceived threats and a tendency to confuse and conflate retaliation with self-defence. Moorhouse suggested that in the rural areas peaceful relations between Aboriginals and colonists were usually established only after two to three years of occupation, and that before that there was often a marked absence of 'good feeling and mutual forbearance'.[29]

This was moderate language to describe a situation which recent historians have described in more forthright terms. Robert Clyne, for example, suggests that a 'sense of

---

26 Reports of Protector of Aborigines, 9 October 1939, 14 Jan 1840, *Fifth Annual Report of the Colonization Commissioners*, pp.350–2, 352–4

27 Report of Protector of Aborigines, *SAGG*, 22 April 1841, p.6. See also Graham Jenkin, *Conquest of the Ngarrindjeri*, Rigby, Adelaide, 1979, pp 46–8. Dr Richard Penny's name sometimes appears in records as Penney. He arrived in South Australia from England in 1840 and was employed at Encounter Bay by the United Fishing Company. See AA Lendon, 'Dr Richard Penney (*sic*), 1840–1844', *Proceedings of the Royal Geographical Society of Australasia, South Australian Branch*, vol.xxxi, 1929–30, pp.20–33. He is not to be confused with Dr Robert Banks Penny (see below, pp.104–5), who arrived in the colony c. 1850 and worked first at Robe and then Bordertown.

28 Report of Protector of Aborigines, 14 January 1840, *Fifth Annual Report of the Colonization Commissioners*, pp.352–4

29 Moorhouse frequently reflected on these matters in his reports. See for example, Reports of Protector of Aborigines, 14 January 1840, *Fifth Annual Report of the Colonization Commissioners*, pp.352–4; 10 February 1842, GRG 24/6/1842/32; *SAGG*, 17 July 1845, pp.173–4.

war was prevalent in the colony during 1840–1842'.[30] Foster, Hosking and Nettelbeck describe a 'climate of crisis' brought about by 'a series of dramatic events' and 'bloody clashes' in 1841.[31] They, and others, in investigating some of the more serious 'collisions' of 1840–42 have shown how theft of Aboriginal land and livelihood, settler fears and insecurities, abuse, and dishonoured promises and contracts, encouraged resistance and retaliation from the Aboriginals. This in turn fuelled settler demands for punitive police action, in order to 'pacify' the Aboriginals.[32]

Governor George Grey, who replaced Gawler early in 1841, responded to demands for government action to protect settlers and maintain the safety of the overland stock routes, by asserting the rights of the indigenous inhabitants as British subjects, rights which made being in a state of war with them improper.[33] Moorhouse was always inclined to judge European rather than indigenous behaviour as the real source of the troubles and exhibited considerable understanding of Aboriginal reactions to the usurpation of their land. He judged their theft of sheep to be predictable and rational. They were, after all, hunters, and must have been 'astonished' to see, on their land, 'a flock of sheep, tame, and tractable', and apparently for the taking. In his view, 'it appear[ed] a difficult matter to suggest any plan that would prevent them from doing so'.[34] But such attitudes were not the prevailing ones, and even though emanating from high places, were not able to avert violence. Settlers and overlanders, relying on the support of public opinion, the strength of economic arguments about protecting stock and other property, and the protection often afforded by time, distance and lack of witnesses were prepared to ignore the government and take the law into their own hands. The resulting conflicts impelled the government to act, thus establishing a violent cycle of aggression, retaliation and retribution, in which the government played a punitive role at odds with its responsibility to protect the rights and safety of the Aboriginals. The historical record shows that across the continent, colonial governments, in response to the 'condition of incipient clash' created by the presence and activities of the settlers, were frequently willing to be involved in this way.[35] Punitive expeditions, while

---

30 Robert Clyne, 'At War with the Natives: from the Coorong to the Rufus, 1841', *Journal of the Historical Society of South Australia*, no.9, 1981, pp.91–110

31 Foster, Hosking and Nettelbeck, *Fatal Collisions*, pp.3–4

32 The events which were most unsettling at the time and have subsequently attracted most historical investigation include the murder of the survivors of the shipwrecked *Maria* on the Coorong in 1840, clashes between Aboriginals, overlanders droving stock from the eastern colonies, and police on the upper River Murray in 1841 (often referred to as the Rufus River conflicts), and attacks on pastoral stations in the Port Lincoln district in 1842. TA Coghlan in his monumental *Labour and industry in Australia from the First Settlement in 1788 to the establishment of the Commonwealth in 1901*, Oxford University Press, Melbourne, 1918, had almost nothing to say about the indigenous inhabitants, but he did note that in South Australia in 1840, 'there had been some trouble with the aborigines', and provided some details of the *Maria* murders, 'outrages by the blacks upon white travellers' and clashes with 'offending blacks' and 'disaffected aborigines'. Coghlan, *Labour and industry*, vol.1, part iii, chapter i, pp.310–11

33 Clyne, 'At War with the Natives', p.100; Foster, Hosking and Nettelbeck, *Fatal Collisions*, pp.31–2

34 Report of Protector of Aborigines, *SAGG*, 17 July 1845, pp.173–4

35 A nuanced account of this history and of the historiography of frontier conflict in Australia is found in Bain Attwood and SG Foster (eds), *Frontier Conflict: the Australian experience*, National Museum of Australia, Canberra, 2003

worrying Grey and Moorhouse, were widely accepted as an effective means of showing that 'the intruders' power is paramount', and that resisting it 'means defeat and death'.[36] The greater toll of death and injury experienced by the indigenous population in these conflicts and the government's failure, in most cases, to bring the Europeans involved to justice were indeed a powerful lesson to the indigenous about who was now in charge of their country and about the price of their survival.

Moorhouse travelled extensively, often in the company of police officers and Aboriginal interpreters, to investigate reports of 'collisions' and to attempt to control reactions to them. In addition, from 1841 the government appointed Sub-Protectors to provide a continuous official presence in those country areas where significant numbers of Aboriginals lived and congregated and where 'collisions' between them and settlers were likely. In most cases, the Sub-Protectors relied on the distribution of rations and the demands of employment to pacify the Aboriginals and bring them into the European sphere of influence. However, from 1853, in response to vice-regal directions, some appointed Aboriginal constables to aid them in their work of pacification, and by the end of March 1855 the Native Police force numbered 22, with ten stationed at Moorundie on the Murray, nine at Venus Bay on Eyre Peninsula and three at Port Augusta.[37] Such initiatives were deemed necessary because the process of 'settlement' in fact continued to be unsettling, and violence between the indigenous population and the colonists, although not on the scale of 1840–42, continued to occur. Indeed, it seemed to be an expected and unremarkable aspect of colonial life and was officially reported in resigned and fatalistic tones. For example, in January of 1850, Moorhouse wrote of the usual mix of 'quietude' and upheaval: five Aboriginals were alleged to have been poisoned by a shepherd, six had been shot by Europeans, and four Europeans had been murdered by natives. There had been Aboriginal convictions: six for murder, four for assault, three for larceny, one for petty theft and one for possessing stolen property.[38] A year later, the Protector reported theft, and 'outrages', but 'nothing of serious moment'. In fact:

> The natives have generally been at peace with the Europeans, if the unfortunate case of the murder of Mr Baird is excepted, and but one death has been caused by the Europeans amongst them, which occurred at the recovery of upwards of seven hundred sheep stolen from the late Mr Baird.[39]

One of the earliest Sub-Protectors to be appointed was the celebrated explorer Edward John Eyre. Vested with the powers of a police magistrate, in late 1841 he took up his post at

---

36 AP Elkin, 'Reaction and Interaction; a food gathering people and European settlement in Australia', *American Anthropologist*, vol.53, no.2, 1951, pp.164–86, 167. This article, well known for its description of the phenomenon of 'intelligent parasitism', provides an insightful summary of stages of government policy and indigenous reactions to them from the time of earliest settlement.

37 Cameron Raynes, '*A Little Flour and a Few Blankets': an administrative history of Aboriginal Affairs in South Australia, 1834–2000*, State Records of South Australia, Adelaide, 2002, p.16

38 Report of Protector of Aborigines, *SAGG*, 17 January 1850, pp.46–8

39 Report of Protector of Aborigines, *SAGG*, 30 January 1851, p.79

Moorundie, the territory of large numbers of River Murray Aboriginals.[40] Reporting in 1842, Eyre indicated his fidelity to Moorhouse's principle of linking provisioning with work. He suggested that the monthly muster of Aboriginals and the distribution of flour was 'admirably adapted to bring about a friendly intercourse in the first instance, and subsequently to establish a controlling influence over them of the most salutary kind'. He said that he

> invariably made it a rule never to give anything to a native (except at the monthly issue of flour) unless he has first earned it by work, or brings some equivalent for it in barter.[41]

Other Sub-Protectors appointed during Moorhouse's term of office included the missionary Schurmann and the Government Resident, Driver, at Port Lincoln; Mason at Wellington, on Lake Alexandrina near the mouth of the Murray; Minchin in the Northern Districts, in the vicinity of Mt Remarkable and Mt Brown in the southern Flinders Ranges; Scott, who followed Eyre at Moorundie; and Brewer at Guichen Bay, later known as Robe, in the South-Eastern Districts. These Sub-Protectors, appointed to areas of expanding European influence, economic activity and settlement, often filled some other official role as well, for example police officer or Government Resident. Living at some distance from Adelaide, they were faced with many differing and often difficult circumstances and exercised some independence in the carrying out of their duties. Their reports indicate a range of approaches, for example, to the question of rationing, and incorporated differing diagnoses of problems and of prospects for the future.

By 1853, Brewer, at Guichen Bay, was proposing the discontinuation of the monthly flour ration to the men, 'it being only an inducement to some of them to remain idle and unsettled', which was particularly problematic in 'these times of scarcity of labour' when 'their services are so important'.[42] At the more recently established ration depot at Mt Brown, however, Sub-Protector Minchin saw rations as a means

> to induce the wild natives from the hills to live at [the feeding] station, and by keeping them some time in contact with himself and the police, so far civilize them, as to render them not only harmless but useful to the settlers.

In mid-1853 he was feeding 130 Aboriginals on a weekly basis, but was asking Moorhouse for an extra allowance so that he could feed them every third day. This, he predicted, would 'ensure peace and quietness for the settlers, and have the natives content'. In the same report he noted some of the complexities of the situation: the natives' capacity to feed themselves had been diminished by the loss of game in the neighbourhood, they led indolent lives, and they found little in the way of employment or welcome at the cattle stations of the settlers. Later in the year, Minchin reported, rather plaintively, that while

---

40 Moorundie, also spelt Moorunde and Moorundi, is on the River Murray, near the present site of Blanchetown.

41 Report, Sub-Protector EJ Eyre, Moorundie, 10 January 1842, *Fifth Annual Report of Colonization Commissioners*, pp.335–6

42 Report, Government Resident Captain Brewer, Guichen Bay and South-Eastern Districts, *SAGG*, 28 July 1853, p.499

most of the northern settlers are as kind as possible to the blacks, if deserving ... this has not
the desired effect ... It is indeed a sad pity that [the blacks] do not understand the whites better.
I spoke much to them upon the advantages of acting a friendly part towards the whites, and
also led them to understand that the latter would protect themselves as well as their property
from injury. I must confess that I felt some little difficulty in explaining to them why the white
man should take possession of the best part of their country[43]

Scott, at Moorundie, was often expansive and philosophical in his reporting. He was
very clear about the inadequacies of government attempts to control the Aboriginals
and at the same time to ensure they were useful to the settlers. He regretted that Adelaide
exerted such a pull on the natives that they regularly left their work in the Murray area
during the winter and travelled to the city, 'notwithstanding that their numbers are
thinned yearly by their migration'. He wanted the government to take action to stop their
wanderings, since 'year after year they return more squalid and miserable than ever, and
possessed of greater vices, and consequently much more difficult to manage'. He admitted
that part of the problem was that the work offered them by the settlers was insecure and
poorly paid, but his response to this was merely to ask for more rations and 'extras' as a
means of rewarding good behaviour. He had already formed a gloomy view of the future
of the Aboriginals: 'It is melancholy ... to observe that as civilization advances, and as the
country of the aborigines becomes more thickly populated by Europeans, the number of
the former decrease'.[44]

Moorhouse's involvement in crises and developments outside Adelaide did not detract
from his work in Adelaide. His reports in the early 1840s revealed close attention to the
matter of the education of indigenous children and meticulous accounting of what was
being achieved in that area. This reflected the reality of the situation: efforts to educate and
'civilise' the children might draw only lukewarm and inconsistent responses, even when
food and blankets were held out as inducements, but this was a much greater reward than
was to be had from working directly with the adults. The indifference of the Aboriginals
to the settled life and the agricultural and horticultural pursuits promoted at the
Aborigines' Location and their continuing commitment to their seasonal journeyings
and ceremonial obligations were a source of frustration to the Protector and the other
colonists. Not only did they militate against the development of industrious habits
among the adults, but they hindered the children's regular attendance at school and
stood in the way of efforts to wean them from traditional cultural values and practices. In
fact, in his very first quarterly report, Moorhouse expressed doubts about the value of
working with the adults[45], and in December of 1839 confided in the German missionary
Schurmann that he had given up any hope of civilising and Christianising the adults at the

---

43 Report, Sub-Protector Minchin, Northern Districts, SAGG, 2 June 1853, p.362; 28 July 1853, p.498; 15 December
    1853, p.816

44 Report, Sub-Protector Scott, Moorundie, SAGG, 28 July 1853, p.499; 25 May 1854, p.413

45 Report of Protector of Aborigines, 9 October 1839, Fifth Annual Report of the Colonization Commissioners, pp.350–2

Location.[46] Several years later nothing had happened to modify these feelings, and in 1842 he reported in unequivocal terms:

> The adults are become more confirmed in habits of mendicity ... We find it difficult to make them believe that begging lessens them in the estimation of Europeans, and that their supplies would be much more certain and more creditable if produced by cultivation from their own ground. The parents are great hindrances to the improvement of the children, and will continue to be so for several generations unless some decisive measures are adopted, to separate in a degree the one from the other.[47]

In addition, the behaviour of the colonists in Adelaide exacerbated the difficulties of the situation. The instructions issued to *ad interim* Protector Wyatt in 1837 had noted the deleterious effects of handouts not associated with work, and complaints about this matter became a constant refrain in Protectors' reports.[48] The Aboriginals were quick to learn how to optimise the benefits for themselves, and every new boatload of colonists reinforced the situation. At the beginning of 1844 Moorhouse acknowledged that the Aboriginals had 'kept themselves from outrage' and were generally in a more 'satisfactory condition' than at any time in the previous three years. However, he bemoaned the fact that while in the country 'settlers adopt the plan of having an equivalent in labor for all they give to the natives', in Adelaide food was too often given for nothing, and hence idleness and begging were encouraged.[49] This had brought to nought his efforts to turn the Aboriginals into settled cultivators of the land. They saw no need to live permanently at the Location, with all that this implied in relation to their traditional social and ceremonial practices. Hunting and gathering supplemented by handouts remained a viable and much more attractive option. Thus from the earliest contact, they were exhibiting those attitudes of independence and that power of discrimination that much later came to be referred to as 'intelligent parasitism'.[50] In short:

> During the early years of its operation, the Location was a convenience: the Aborigines could camp there, receive rations and use the huts, but they did so at their own discretion. Europeans undoubtedly exerted an influence over the Aborigines at the Location, but very little control.[51]

This was not what the government or the colonists had bargained on, and it irked them. They wanted control, or at least responses which fitted their own notions of what it meant

---

46 CW Schurmann, Diary, 16 December 1839, cited in Robert Foster, 'The Aborigines' Location in Adelaide: South Australia's first 'mission' to the Aborigines', *Journal of the Anthropological Society of South Australia*, vol. 28, nos.1–2, December 1990, p.21

47 Report of Protector of Aborigines, 10 February 1842, GRG, 24/6/1842/32

48 *South Australian Gazette and Colonial Register*, 12 August 1837, p.1. See also, Report of Protector of Aborigines, 9 October 1939, 20 February 1841, 10 February 1842 etc.

49 Report of Protector of Aborigines, *SAGG*, 11 January 1844, pp.14–15

50 Elkin, 'Reaction and Interaction, pp.164–86, and especially pp.168–74

51 Foster, 'The Aborigines' Location in Adelaide', p.18

to be a responsible member of the community, that is, working for rewards, and leading a settled, industrious and orderly existence. When this did not happen, there were some, probably many, who, although slow to see how settler behaviour might contribute to Aboriginal responses, were quick to judge the Aboriginals as non-civilised and non-civilisable, at least not by the methods currently being used.

The local press was active in promoting such views. In 1840 for example, both the *South Australian Register* and the *Southern Australian* were politely sceptical about Governor Grey's views on 'civilizing the natives'. They judged Grey to be only 'partially informed' and were not dissuaded from their 'known opinion of the *impracticability* (original emphasis) of the Natives of South Australia being civilized'.[52] Grey believed that, although the Aboriginals were 'naturally perfectly capable of being civilized', no schemes had worked thus far because they had all made the mistake of allowing them to continue with their own customs, which were barbarous and kept them in a state of savagery. The only hope of civilising and making Christians of them lay in outlawing their customs and making them subject to British law, not just in their relations to Europeans but in their dealings with each other.

The continuing resistance of the indigenous population to attempts to assimilate it served to harden public attitudes. Criticism frequently focused on the Protectorate and the missionaries, who were deemed to be ineffective in dealing with such offences as the natives washing themselves in the River Torrens, which was the colonists' water supply, or scandalising the 'Christian inhabitants' by walking through the streets of Adelaide 'in a state of almost complete nudity'.[53] The solutions that were suggested, editorially and by correspondents to the press, were sometimes extreme. The *Adelaide Examiner* declared the efforts of the missionaries and Protector a 'woeful failure' and a 'waste of public money'. It stopped short of recommending the exclusion of the natives from the town altogether, since some of them were useful to the colonists, but insisted that they should be clothed and be required to carry around their necks 'a tin or brass ticket with [their] name on it, which might be given by the Protector to all those who were the most industrious and respectable'. A correspondent to the same paper went so far as to suggest that if the country were 'invaded' by anyone other than these 'protégés of Mr Moorhouse' there would be no difficulty in raising a militia force to deal with them.[54]

There were of course some colonists whose approach to civilising the native inhabitants was more respectful. The Adelaide Literary and Scientific Association and Mechanics Institute, and the Statistical Society of South Australia were keen to learn about Aboriginal language, culture, practices and belief systems from Moorhouse and the missionaries, so that appropriate policy could be built on a firm foundation of accurate knowledge.[55] However, the more common view was that such concerns were of little practical value. What mattered was to get the natives into regular employment. This was the sure path to civilisation, and those Aboriginals who were already treading it were the only ones who

---

52 *South Australian Register*, 18 April 1840, pp.5–6; *Southern Australian*, 23 April 1840, p.5

53 *Adelaide Examiner*, 10 March 1842, p.2; 17 December 1842, p.2; 25 January 1843, p.1

54 ibid., 10 March 1842, p.2; 28 January 1843, p.2

55 ibid., 20 January 1842, pp.3–4; 25 February 1843, p.3; *South Australian Register*, 25 February 1843, p.2

earned commendation. The implications were clear: South Australia now belonged not to its original inhabitants, but to the recently arrived British settlers whose intention was to govern and develop it according to their own values and aspirations. Unless the original inhabitants were prepared to conform to this intention, as grateful subordinates, their fate would be that of savages, nuisances and vagrants.

In this context of considerable community contention and negativity, and despite his own ambivalence and disappointments, Moorhouse continued to carry out his duties as Protector with energy and positive spirit. He earned high praise from Governor Gawler who believed that Moorhouse underestimated the positive effects of his work. Gawler found the Protector 'unremitting' in his efforts, 'always to be found with the natives, in their Location, instructing them and encouraging them to work', and noted that he had visited 'almost all the distant tribes of the district'.[56] In addition, he had given serious attention to the education of Aboriginal children.

In 1843 Moorhouse provided a summary report on the state of education among the Aboriginals since the beginning of schooling at the government Aborigines' Location in Adelaide on 23 December 1839.[57] The first teacher employed during his protectorship was William Oldham. After Oldham's resignation in January 1840, Moorhouse secured the services of Christian Teichelmann and Clamor Schurmann, two Dresden Mission Society missionaries who had arrived in the colony in October 1838 and had been living at the Location, building gardens and houses and gaining knowledge of the Kaurna language. Average daily attendances at the Location school of between 10 and 13.5 children from December 1839 until the end of 1842 masked considerable seasonal fluctuations and give little idea of the total number of children influenced by the school. This is clarified somewhat by Moorhouse's claim that, by the end of 1842, 41 children knew the alphabet, 25 could read monosyllables, 18 could read polysyllables, 15 could write on slate and on paper, 14 were acquainted with addition, 11 with subtraction, nine with multiplication and five with division, while one could perform compound addition. Furthermore, 17 had been

> most regular in their attendance, [were] able to repeat the commandments, and narrate the history of the creation, fall of our first parents, and other portions of the old and new testaments.

Meanwhile, the Wesleyan ladies were imparting the skills of one of the female arts of civilisation: needlework.[58] While the detail of Moorhouse's reports refers to activities and achievements at the Location school in Adelaide, the influence of education extended beyond the Location fence. In fact, in his report for the second quarter of 1843 he claimed:

---

56 Gawler, Annual Finance Minute, *SAGG*, 21 April 1841, p.5

57 This report deals only with education during Moorhouse's Protectorship and disregards earlier shortlived attempts at schooling undertaken during the Protectorships of Bromley and Wyatt.

58 Report of Protector of Aborigines, *SAGG*, 23 March 1843, pp.85–6

There is not a child between the age of five and ten years, sixty miles to the North or sixty miles to the South, with an average breadth from East to West of ten miles, that does not know the alphabet, and some are advanced in reading, writing and arithmetic.[59]

However, the influence of the parents continued to be a constant challenge to the authority and impact of the school and to the maintenance of regular attendance. In an attempt to combat this, 'a kind of boarding school' was established in June 1843. Fifteen of the most regular attenders were 'selected for trial' and a matron appointed to super-intend the arrangements.[60] Hardly surprisingly, the parents were not keen to cooperate with this scheme. Moorhouse rejoiced when, in December of 1843, 'four fresh children' were sent along voluntarily, and reported this as 'an improvement upon the past, for all the children that had previously been received had to be taken almost in direct opposition to the wish of the parents'.[61] In April 1844 Moorhouse was still positive about this scheme and reported that none of the girls had 'slept out of the matron's house since the 20th of February'.[62]

In the same report Moorhouse mentioned a second school for Aboriginal children which was shortly to be opened at Walkerville, a village a small distance to the north-east of the city. This was designed to cater for the children of the River Murray people who had been regularly visiting Adelaide, especially in the colder months, since the stationing of a Sub-Protector at Moorundie in 1841. Their relations with the less numerous Adelaide Kaurna people were not cordial, and although Moorhouse wished to extend the same bene-fits to all, he soon found the situation impossible. The school at the Location was deserted as the Kaurna fled from the Murray people and there were violent battles in the Adelaide parklands as the Ramindjeri from Encounter Bay, allies of the Kaurna, sided with them against the Murray people.[63] At first the official reaction was to encourage the Murray Aboriginals to stay in their own territory. Sub-Protector Eyre at Moorundie tried to re-inforce this intention by providing rations only to those who were 'well-behaved' and stayed away from Adelaide.[64] This proved ineffective, however, as Adelaide seemed to be an irresistible magnet for the River Murray people until the spread of population provided employment and other attractions in the rural areas.[65] Thus, the establishment of a school for the River Murray children may be seen as an attempt to achieve something pos-itive from what was otherwise a dilemma.

The Walkerville school conducted its classes in English, unlike the school at the

---

59 Report of Protector of Aborigines, 8 July 1843, GRG24/6/1843/812

60 ibid.

61 Report of Protector of Aborigines, *SAGG*, 11 January 1844, pp.14–15

62 Report of Protector of Aborigines, 10 April 1844, *Despatches of the Governors of the Australian Colonies, with reports of the Protectors of Aborigines, Parliamentary Papers*, House of Commons, 1844, pp.361–2

63 For details of these disturbances see Foster, 'The Aborigines' Location in Adelaide', pp.26–7.

64 Report of Sub-Protector of Aborigines, 20 January 1844, *Despatches of the Governors of the Australian Colonies, with reports of the Protectors of Aborigines, Parliamentary Papers*, House of Commons, 1844, pp.352–5

65 See Report of Protector of Aborigines, 4 October 1843, GRG 24/6/1843/1234. Subsequent reports indicate that the attrac-tions of Adelaide continued to exert a powerful influence throughout the 1840s and 1850s, especially in the winter months.

Aborigines' Location where teaching was undertaken in the vernacular. In 1845 it boasted a considerably larger average attendance than the Location school: 15 boys and 23 girls, compared with nine boys and 10 girls, with the largest number in attendance at any one time being 98. These children were making similar sorts of progress as those reported on earlier, being acquainted with 'sin and its consequences, the nature of future rewards and punishments, and the objects of our Saviour's mission, as well as with the alphabet and fundamental arithmetic processes'.[66]

A Sunday School for Aboriginal children was opened by members of the Methodist New Connexion Church at the Walkerville School in July of 1844. While the instruction it provided was described as catechetical, it was also a form of literacy training and it seems reasonable to assume from the reports of each that the day and Sunday schools complemented each other. Indeed the decision of the Governor to permit the church to conduct the Sunday School was on the assumption that it would aid the government in its efforts at secular and religious education.[67]

While reports of the Sunday School do not list advances syllable by syllable as Moorhouse's school reports do, they offer interesting assessments of the perceived nature of the intellectual and moral progress of the children who attended. For example, in December 1844, the directors of the Sunday School reported that the children had 'made an almost incredible advancement in intelligence in the space of a few months'. While acknowledging that it would have been premature to claim spiritual victories, they nevertheless took heart from the following:

> One of our most intelligent boys having left the school clandestinely, to accompany his parents into the bush, returned shortly afterwards, and said he could not be comfortable to remain away because the persons in the vicinity of whose house he had been stopping were in the habit of swearing and working on the Sabbath, whilst, since he had been to the Sunday School, something within told him that it was not right to do such things.[68]

In the same report, the Sunday School directors advanced some general opinions of the Aboriginal children in their care. They believed they possessed a capacity for learning 'not at all inferior to the best class of European children to be found anywhere in a mixed community', and were eager to learn and to persevere with education 'except when the influence of parental authority is brought to operate upon the predisposing inclinations'. They were confident that their vagrant habits would soon be replaced by more industrious ones, and that their own missionary efforts would be richly repaid.[69] A year and a half later, after 'uninterrupted work' and the involvement of teachers from other denominations, the report of the Sunday School was markedly more sober. Although the directors could claim that 80 children were 'theoretically acquainted with the way of salvation', they also confessed:

66 Report of Protector, *SAGG*, 17 July 1845, pp.173–4

67 Report on Sunday School for Aboriginal children, *SAGG*, 5 December 1844, pp.275–6

68 ibid., p.276

69 ibid., p.276

we have not yet been encouraged with an instance in which a decided change of heart appears to have taken place, but several we believe are seriously enquiring after better things ... We are yet only on the threshold of our work: a very small portion of the rubbish has yet been cleared away which blocks up the passage to the soul.[70]

They admitted that the girls were lost to the influence of the Sunday School by 14 and the boys by 16 years, and that they then relapsed into 'the degrading habits of savage life'. In contrast to their earlier optimism, they were resigned to the view that the Aboriginal 'predilection for vagrancy' was 'an almost insurmountable barrier to permanently beneficial education'. Yet their Christian commitment to evangelism and to hope remained: 'to overcome this [barrier] must be the great object of all who are engaged in endeavouring to ameliorate the condition of this portion of our race'.[71]

By mid-1845 the school building at Walkerville was in such a state of decrepitude that Moorhouse decided to combine the two schools and establish a new one, known as the Native School Establishment, at the Royal Sappers and Miners Barracks in Kintore Avenue in the centre of Adelaide.[72] After refurbishment, the buildings were ready for occupation in January 1846. The teacher from Walkerville took charge, providing education in English for children from Adelaide, the River Murray and from other settled districts.[73] For this to have succeeded, the antagonisms that earlier caused conflict among the groups must have become less marked. It seems reasonable to assume that they were eroded by time and receded before the perceived advantages of being in or near Adelaide.

Insofar as the schooling provided for the Aboriginal children was designed to equip them with useful skills and habits of industry, Moorhouse could from time to time claim some evidence of practical success. He wrote about attempts at 'domestication' in July 1843 and reported that one girl had been employed as a domestic at Government House since March 1841.[74] His report for the second quarter of 1849 revealed that the girls had made 36 pairs of trousers, 24 cotton shirts, 28 chemises, 18 red shirts, 36 pocket handkerchiefs and 24 shawls at school.[75] In the following year, he reported that two boys were employed as messengers at the Government Printing Office, nine were occupied at the Government Domain, and one was a messenger to the Governor. The girls, meanwhile, were still sewing.[76] Pleasing as all this was, he was ready to acknowledge the equivocal nature of the results to which he could lay claim:

One is open to admit that these have not been as encouraging as we desired they would have been. There is, however, reason to hope that the instructions have not been altogether in vain.

---

70 Report on Sunday School for Aboriginal children, *SAGG*, 27 May 1847, p.169

71 ibid., p.169

72 GRG 57/7/1, 29 May 1845

73 Foster, 'The Aborigines Location in Adelaide', p.27

74 Report of Protector of Aborigines, 8 July 1843. GRG/24/6/1843/812

75 Report of Protector of Aborigines, *SAGG*, 19 July 1849, p.313

76 Report of Protector of Aborigines, *SAGG*, 17 January 1850, pp.46–8

During the nine years' operation of the school, only one child who has been instructed in it, has been arraigned in a Court of Justice.[77]

In the face of such modest success, Moorhouse pursued other strategies. As early as 1846, he was recommending marriages among those children at the Native School Establishment who were, according to native custom, old enough to be married. He saw this as the only means available to him to prevent their return to the bush and the re-establishment of parental and customary influence.[78] Although his plan was declared unworkable since, according to British law, the children were under age and could not be married without parental consent,[79] Moorhouse continued to pursue the idea, and in January 1850 reported:

> in order to prevent the children returning absolutely to the bush, a trial has been made of marrying them, and inducing them to engage in the Port Lincoln district, where they would be removed from the influence of parents and friends.

Five couples had been married and had volunteered to make the move, although four of these had refused to embark on the ship when the moment of departure arrived.[80]

Moorhouse's hand was strengthened by a proposal from Anglican Archdeacon Matthew Hale in June 1850 to establish a training institution for Aboriginal young people near Port Lincoln. Hale had arrived in the colony in 1848 with the first Anglican Bishop of South Australia, Augustus Short, and the two men shared a vision of a 'Christian village', isolated from the undesirable influence of most Europeans, in which attempts to civilise and Christianise the natives might bear greater fruit than had so far occurred. This proposal drew a prompt and spirited response from Moorhouse. He believed that it would be acceptable to the young people and it coincided with his cherished goal of removing them from two sets of undesirable and corrupting influences: their families, and Adelaide. Indeed it was a welcome beacon of hope, after many disappointments:

> It is very disheartening and somewhat humiliating to see all our attempts at improving the Natives assume the aspect of failure. All legitimate means have been used, but this one of separation, and it is very desirable that it should be tried.[81]

Hale's project, which was backed by his own resources, attracted in addition the support of the colonial government, the Society for the Propagation of the Gospel, and a small group of Adelaide settlers who were disturbed by the impact of colonisation on the original inhabitants. The government allowed Aboriginal reserve land to be resumed for

---

77 Report of Protector of Aborigines, *SAGG*, 19 July 1849, p.313

78 Report of Protector of Aborigines, 30 April 1846, GRG 24/6/1846/520

79 Advocate-General, 7 May 1846, GRG 24/6/1846/567

80 Report of Protector of Aborigines, *SAGG*, 17 January 1850, pp.46–8

81 Report of Protector of Aborigines, 21 June 1850, GRG/24/6/1850/1346

the proposed settlement and provided a loan to cover establishment coasts and to pay the wages of key staff. Moorhouse dispatched 'graduates' of the Aboriginal school in Adelaide to Port Lincoln ahead of Hale, to work as servants while awaiting the establishment of the new venture. Hale sailed to Port Lincoln in September 1850, and after judging his first choice of location, Boston Island, unsuitable because of inadequate fresh water, established his Native Training Institution on the mainland at Poonindie, about 11 miles north of Port Lincoln.[82]

Hale understood the purpose of his Native Training Institution to be 'the moral and industrial training and Christian instruction of aboriginal natives'. He clearly believed the natives to be educable, but harboured no high hopes for what they might achieve. In his first formal report to the government he wrote:

> ... it forms no part of my plan to look to the natives for the performance of any great or impor-
> tant work as principals. As helpers or, as I may term them, second class labourers, we have occu-
> pied them in a variety of ways; and thus employed they have worked with considerable
> steadiness, and have cheerfully performed their duties.

He reasserted his view that the best hopes for civilising and Christianising the Aboriginals lay in gaining access to them when young and keeping them separated from their own people. His experience with one adult man proved

> that it is possible, under favourable circumstances, and by a proper adaptation of means, to
> induce a native who has grown to manhood in almost a wild state to settle down and conform
> to civilized habits of life

but he argued that 'it is not consistent with a wise economy of means to adopt this mode of action'.[83]

Hale's initial plan to accept only young people who had already been educated at the Native School Establishment in Adelaide was soon abandoned. The effect of several intakes to Poonindie, together with the continuing decline of numbers of Aboriginals in Adelaide as settlement spread and offered opportunities further afield in the colony, was the forced closure of the Native School Establishment, for want of numbers, in 1852. The government school for Aboriginal children established in Port Lincoln under the missionary Clamor Schurmann in 1850 also closed in 1852 and its functions were transferred to Poonindie at the beginning of 1853. Within a short time, Hale was required by the government to accept not only children, but also adults from the troubled Port Lincoln district, where violence between the indigenous population and the settlers was rife, and to operate Poonindie as a ration depot a well as a training institution.[84]

Moorhouse visited Poonindie in 1852, and in December of that year reported that it had 21 'inmates', and that it was

82 Peggy Brock, *Outback Ghettos: a history of Aboriginal institutionalisation and survival*, Cambridge University Press, Cambridge, 1993, pp.24–6

83 Matthew Hale, Report on the Native Training Institution, Poonindie, *SAGG*, 24 July 1851, pp.511–12

84 Brock, *Outback Ghettos*, pp.26–7

gradually and steadily improving [them] and raising them very perceptibly in the scale of rational beings. The evidence of their improvement which is most tangible, and which it is impossible to gainsay, is the constancy and steadiness with which they adhere to the habits of civilized life and the striking improvement in their manner of performing the various duties of the station.

By then there had been a death at the institution, and Moorhouse, perhaps mindful of earlier reports of 'deaths in great numbers' from a 'complaint of the lungs' among the indigenous population of Port Lincoln considered it

> very remarkable how any kind of complaint amongst them seems, sooner or later, to turn to a complaint of the chest, and how soon the constitution gives way when attacked in this quarter.[85]

Such reports were to become commonplace. In March of 1853, when the numbers of residents at Poonindie had risen to 45, Hale was regretting five deaths in four months, and asking for a medical man:

> to watch very narrowly [their] general health ... and he might then be able to discover, whether amongst the peculiarities of their habits, and manner of life in this place, there is anything that can be specially fixed upon as being detrimental to health.[86]

The deaths continued, and in 1854 Hale was reporting 'a remarkable and unlooked for result': the natives, as well as making 'very rapid moral, intellectual and physical advancement' were showing 'resolution and steadfastness in seeking the way of eternal life'. The reason for this, he suggested, was that:

> sickness and death have been constantly busy amongst us; and thence, by the Grace of God, these persons have learned to see the extreme folly of setting the mind upon anything on this side of the grave as the ultimate object of their aims.[87]

Hale continued to report deaths at Poonindie and to attribute them either to the native constitution or to the will of God. However, Octavius Hammond, a qualified medical practitioner who in 1856 took over as superintendent when Hale was appointed Bishop of Perth considered that the appalling sanitary conditions were the more likely cause.[88] By that time, 29 of the 110 persons who had been admitted to Poonindie since its establishment had died, with most of the deaths occurring among infants and young children.[89] It had not been an auspicious beginning for Hale's experiment.

---

85 Report of Protector of Aborigines, *SAGG*, 30 January 1851, p.79; 23 December 1852, p.774

86 Matthew Hale, quoted in Report of Protector of Aborigines, *SAGG*, 24 March 1853, p.193

87 Matthew Hale, quoted in Report of Protector of Aborigines, *SAGG*, 23 February 1854, p.151

88 Matthew Hale, quoted in Report of Protector of Aborigines, *SAGG*, 24 August 1854, p.620; Brock, *Outback Ghettos*, p.35

89 Brock, *Outback Ghettos*, pp.34–5. Brock, using data provided to the government by Hammond, shows that mortality rates were as high as 50 per cent for the period 1856–60.

Reports of illness and of high death rates among the Aboriginal population, such as those reported from Poonindie and from government stations throughout the colony, must have been discomforting to Moorhouse. As Protector, he was responsible for the health of the Aboriginals, and even if health is narrowly understood as meaning absence of disease, he did not succeed in offering them much protection. Vaccination against smallpox was available in Adelaide from 1839, but plans for a native hospital to treat diseases requiring the confinement of the patient seem not to have materialised.[90] From very early in his period of office he was aware of and concerned about the spread of venereal disease, which 'raged' among Aboriginals in centres of European population remote from Adelaide, but powerless to do anything about the circumstances which promoted it. His annual report of 1843 noted, perhaps disingenuously, that the Aboriginals were subject to 'those diseases common to the human race' such as phthisis, scrofula and venereal diseases.[91] These diseases had not been known among the indigenous population before the arrival of Europeans. That they had rapidly become prevalent since then, and were associated with high levels of serious illness and death was evidence of the social and economic dislocation and marginalisation which had become the lot of the original inhabitants. Rather than being 'common to the human race' these, and many other diseases, were much more likely to be found, and to be deadly in their effects, among the poor and dispossessed.[92]

When Sub-Protectors were appointed to the outlying districts, they reported regularly on sickness among the Aboriginals in their charge and on numbers of births and deaths, although there appears to have been no attempt to discern causation or trends, or even to calculate rates. There is a tone of resignation in much of this reporting and little evidence of any concerted effort on the part of government to respond to the problems, except through the provision of rations and blankets, and sometimes medicine. The use of rationing to care for the sick and destitute was clearly established by about 1850. Sub-Protector Scott reported from Moorundie at the beginning of 1851 that he was using rations to relieve 'the wants of the sick, aged and destitute'. A report from Yorke Peninsula a few months later noted that the women there were 'in a fearful state of disease'. The disease, coyly unnamed, but said to be communicated by Europeans, had affected three-quarters of the indigenous population who had been given medicine and a flour ration since they were 'so much affected as to be unable to leave their huts'.[93]

In September of 1852 Moorhouse replied defensively to a memorandum from the Lieutenant-Governor enquiring about the prevalence of disease among the natives. Moorhouse pointed out that the information which had prompted the Lieutenant-

90 JP Litchfield, Inspector of Hospitals, *SAGG*, 18 July 1839, p.1; Report of Protector of Aborigines, 9 October 1839, *Fifth Annual Report of the Colonization Commissioners*, p.351

91 Report of Protector of Aborigines, 4 October 1843, GRG24/6/1843/1234

92 As indicated in chapter two, above, the evidence for this is substantial. For an indication of class- and socio-economic status-based health differentials in the nineteenth century, see, for example, Wohl, *Endangered Lives*.

93 Report of Protector of Aborigines, *SAGG*, 30 January 1851, p.80; 17 April 1851, pp.264–5

Governor's enquiry was from Port Lincoln only, and that 'the opinion that there are not twenty male and female adults free from it [venereal disease] is, I am inclined to think, a very erroneous one'. He claimed that medicines and treatments were available from the local doctor or directly from the Protector, and that all those who made use of them were cured. He asserted further that the 'natives receive as much attention as circumstances will permit; they are never overlooked', and drew the attention of the Lieutenant-Governor to regular reports from the Sub-Protectors which, he claimed, demonstrated this. He specifically mentioned the extra rations of flour and medicines regularly given to the sick and indigent among their charges. And lest the Lieutenant-Governor be still unconvinced, he added:

> I have attended all the Natives who will submit to medical treatment during the thirteen years I have been in contact with them. In Adelaide alone I have cured 2000 cases of itch and as I have a supply of medicines allowed, I attend all cases. When I am absent, the Colonial-Surgeon always attends if required.[94]

Moorhouse probably did do as much 'as circumstances [would] permit'. But the circumstances were not conducive to the health of the indigenous population. The Sub-Protectors were not doctors, nor effective controllers of the working and living conditions of their charges or their relations with the European population. They shared the fatalism about the miseries of the lowest social ranks and the lack of understanding of the preventability of much suffering that was common in their time. No official action was taken in response to the alarming mortality at Poonindie and it seems to have been rare for the reports of illness from any of the government depots to have aroused much official concern.[95]

At that time of course, medical treatment for poor, non-indigenous South Australians, especially in rural and remote areas, was scarce and of variable quality and limited efficacy. It is difficult to know how much better off they were than the indigenous population in terms of access to medical treatment, or to get a clear picture of how different their profile of morbidity was. What we do know, however, is that, despite various assaults on its health, the European population grew steadily, and not just as a result of immigration. The Aboriginal population, on the other hand, declined. In short, colonisation was killing them. It was also having other effects, such as removing their independence and control, producing dependence, limiting economic choices and opportunities, and communicating negative judgements about their culture and abilities. We now recognise that these things have a profound, complex and long-term negative impact on people's health. At the time, among those with responsibility for the welfare of the Aboriginals

---

94 Report of Protector of Aborigines, 8 September 1852, GRG/24/6/1852/2609

95 The Lieutenant-Governor's 1852 memorandum to Moorhouse is an obvious exception. The only other example of a direct government response to illness that I have come across in this early period was in response to a request from Sub-Protector Mason at Wellington for medical advice about a woman with a diseased breast. The Commissioner for Crown Lands, who assumed responsibility for Aboriginal affairs from 1857, instructed him to seek advice in this case and for all cases 'when he may consider such advice to be absolutely necessary'. Report of Protector of Aborigines, *SAGG*, 14 April 1859, p.352.

there was some evidence of partial understanding of this impact, or at least a degree of dis-appointment and frustration that they had been unable to provide the original population with more protection from the ill-effects of colonisation.

Moorhouse had other worries apart from the high levels of sickness and death among his charges. He shared the frustration of his Sub-Protectors over their inability to control the movements and activities of the indigenous population as they would have liked and the consequent development of what he saw as a significant problem in Adelaide. His reports indicate continual movement, especially of the Murray people, to and from Adelaide. This was largely seasonal, with an influx during the winter when employment opportunities in the country were scarce. In Adelaide, there was no employment for them, and apart from the Aborigines' Location, where Moorhouse's attempts to establish order and pro-ductive activity had not met with much success, nowhere for them to live without raising the ire and offending the sensibilities of the colonists. Thus they became vagrants with ample opportunities to succumb to the 'evil' of intoxication. Access to alcohol was one of Adelaide's powerful attractions for the Aboriginals, and the behaviour associated with its public consumption helped cement negative attitudes towards them among the colonists. Moorhouse was frustrated in his attempts to suppress either the supply of or the demand for alcohol, or to induce the natives to return to the interior for work.[96]

Adelaide had other attractions beside alcohol. The annual distribution of rations on the Queen's Birthday, a practice established by Governor Gawler in 1838, continued to attract several hundreds each year, but eventually, with the establishment of rations depots and the growth of employment opportunities outside Adelaide, the closure of the Adelaide school, and indigenous fears of the forced removal of young people to Poonindie, these numbers diminished. In 1853 Moorhouse expressed his pleasure that there were fewer present for the distribution than he had seen in any previous year. He had 'wished it to be so', and took it as an indication that many more of them were usefully employed in the country districts.[97] By 1855, there was virtually no Aboriginal population remaining in Adelaide. Small numbers visited for short times, especially during winter, and camped in the Parklands. At such times, 'Frequent cases of intoxication occurred to the annoyance of many Europeans and, in several instances, attended with danger to the natives them-selves.' In September 1855, still finding it 'impossible' to convict those who supplied them with the liquor, Moorhouse was threatening to have the Aborigines whose interests he had tried so hard to protect banned from Adelaide.[98]

As it turned out, this was the last quarterly report filed by Matthew Moorhouse in his role as Protector of Aborigines. The fact that, within less than twenty years since the estab-lishment of European settlement, he was conceding that there was no longer a place for Aboriginal people in Adelaide is a poignant indication of the extent to which he had failed to realise the ambitious goals of his protectorship and of the extent to which the original

---

96 Report of Protector of Aborigines, *SAGG*, 15 July 1852, p.424; 23 December 1852, p.772

97 Report of Protector of Aborigines, *SAGG*, 28 July 1853, p.498

98 Report of Protector of Aborigines, *SAGG*, 20 September 1855, p.718

South Australians had been confirmed as not part of the public. Reports from his Sub-Protectors around the same time were further evidence of the gap that had opened up between the government's periodic proclamations of policy and intent and the realities of the lives of the indigenous population. It was clear that those who had come into contact with Europeans and European institutions had not experienced the happiness, enlightenment, justice and opportunity to share in the benefits of 'civilisation' so easily promised by Hindmarsh and Gawler. For most people within European society, these benefits accrue in part through the protection of the law and in part through remuneration for work. Underlying racist assumptions and hostilities, incompatible economic aspirations and failure to accommodate cultural difference ensured that neither of these mechanisms operated to benefit the Aboriginals. Gawler's glib assurance – 'If any white man injure you, tell the Protector and he will do you justice'[99] – had proved empty, despite Moorhouse's good intentions and consistent efforts. Instead, a culture of mutual distrust had been established: the settlers expected criminal activity from the Aboriginals, and the Aboriginals knew from bitter experience that they had little chance of asserting their rights against the authority of the police and the courts.

Nor had Moorhouse's desire to encourage industrious habits among his charges and to foster the notion that rations were remuneration for work and not merely 'handouts' met with much success. This was hardly surprising given the behaviour of some settlers towards the Aboriginals[100], and the inconsistency of the government's own actions in relation to rationing. The distribution of rations was a powerful tool of government and could be used to pursue various policy ends, not all of them compatible with one another. First conceived before the establishment of the colony as a form of compensation for loss of land, rations quickly became a means whereby the colonisers, from the Governor down, attempted to communicate with the indigenous population and gain their confidence. As settlement spread into the interior, rationing became a means of 'pacification' and extension of government control. Eventually, as a result of the social and economic disruption attendant upon this extension of colonial influence and authority, rationing became a response to ill health, dependence and destitution.[101] In short, by the 1850s it was being used to alleviate problems which had been produced by the process of colonisation and by earlier forms of rationing. In all of this, its potential as a coercive instrument of assimilation is quite clear. It is also clear, given these powerful alternative uses of rationing, why Moorhouse's hope that it would assimilate the Aboriginals into a culture which linked payment with work was not realised.

---

99 Governor Gawler's speech, 1 November 1838, *South Australian Gazette and Colonial Register*, 3 November 1838, p.4

100 Moorhouse believed that indolence had been encouraged by inappropriate handouts before he arrived, and was frustrated by the continuation of this trend. See above, pp.61

101 For an account of rationing practices and Aboriginal responses to these in the early years of the colony, see Robert Foster, 'Feasts of the Full-moon. The distribution of rations to Aborigines in South Australia: 1836–1861', *Aboriginal History*, vol.13, no.1, 1989, pp.63–78; Allan Pope, 'From Feast to Famine: the food factor in European-Aboriginal Relations, South Australia, 1836–1845', *Forum, Journal of the History Teachers Association of South Australia*, July 1988, pp.47–54.

Work for the indigenous population remained a problem, for reasons beyond Moorhouse's control and unconnected with the practice of rationing. By the mid-1850s settlers were pushing further into the interior. Mineral discoveries in South Australia and in the eastern colonies were encouraging immigration and providing a rapidly expanding market for labour and for agricultural produce. Despite this, as Timothy Coghlan indicates in his monumental historical survey of economic conditions in the colonies between 1788 and 1901, the 1850s in South Australia were marked by short-term imbalances which meant that employment opportunities for labour, by which he means European labour, were by no means stable, especially for those not able or willing to seek work outside the cities. In an unregulated and non-unionised environment this led to hardship and destitution for some.[102] Coghlan has almost nothing to say about the employment of the Aboriginal population, seeing them merely as a stopgap rural labour force who could be made use of during short-term shortages of European labour. He notes, for example, that in 1852, when European farmers and labourers left in droves for the Victorian goldfields, there was a marked reduction in the area of land under crop, and:

> the area would have been still less were it not for the employment of the aborigines, who were at that time fairly numerous. They proved useful servants, though as a rule they were incapable of remaining steadily at work.[103]

He records that, in 1853:

> there were few able-bodied European shepherds remaining in the country. The work of tending, shearing, and dressing sheep was done very largely by the aborigines, who were paid at the rate of 12 shillings a week with rations. In some districts no white shepherds were to be found.

If the Aboriginals were useful, they also represented a saving to the employers, since Coghlan tells us that wages for European sheep workers rose from £35 to £50 per annum during 1853, that is from about 13 shillings and sixpence to over 19 shillings a week.[104] Official reports from the period, while not providing a comprehensive picture, indicate that for Aboriginal people employment opportunities were typically precarious, highly variable, seasonal, insufficient to support dependents, and characterised by conditions and expectations different from those which applied to non-indigenous workers.

The regular reports of the Sub-Protectors of Aborigines provide glimpses of indigenous involvement in the colony's rural workforce. For example, Sub-Protector Minchin, reporting from the northern district in 1854 reported the Aboriginals as 'showing a willingness to work, and an advancing skill'. He thought that 'their ideas seem more steadily fixed on self-exertion', and ventured that this might be the result of the discontinuing of rations.[105]

---

102 Coghlan, *Labour and Industry*. For the 1850s, see vol.ii.

103 ibid., vol.ii, part iv, chapter vi, p.675

104 ibid., vol ii, part iv, chapter vii, p.747

105 Sub-Protector Minchin, *SAGG*, 25 May 1854, p.412

At the same time, Scott, at Moorundie, was seeing things differently. Aboriginals in his area were working for the squatters, 'in a slight degree', their labour, 'in the absence of European labour, [being] of some importance'. He regretted that 'as the country of the aborigines becomes more thickly populated by Europeans the number of the former decrease' and was asking for more rations and 'extras' as a reward for 'the exemplary manner in which the aborigines of this district have behaved for the last twelve years'.[106] Brewer, at Guichen Bay in the South-Eastern Districts, reported that, since there was a scarcity of European labour, many of his charges were 'constantly in the employ of the settlers, by which means they obtain plenty of food, good comfortable clothing, and many of them money wages'. On the strength of this he proposed discontinuing the monthly flour ration to men, but continuing to supply it to women and children. Apparently what the men earned was not sufficient to provide for their dependents as well.[107] Mason, reporting from Wellington, claimed that Aboriginal workers who worked for European farmers at harvesting were well paid, returning with an 'abundance of clothing, and blankets, netting twine, and fish-hooks and lines, and other useful articles, which will give them the means of procuring food during the winter season'.[108] However, other reports from Mason indicate the unreliability of work opportunities and the dependence of the Aboriginals on European needs and priorities that were sometimes highly specific, non-continuous and involved only small numbers. For example, in January 1851, he wrote:

> During the months of September and October [1850] six natives were employed in rowing the boats used by his Excellency the Governor, in his expedition to and from the Darling, the whole of the time they were so employed their conduct was exceedingly good, and was highly approved of by his Excellency. The severe labour of rowing the boats nearly one thousand miles, five hundred miles of which was against a stream running two miles an hour, and for the first twenty-three days without resting a day, all this was endured without murmuring, and equally as well as white men could have done.[109]

Mason's pleasure at being able to report this short-term, high-profile work for six Aboriginals is evident. In 1853 he again reported on work opportunities provided by proximity to the colony's main river system. The 'natives', this time their numbers not noted, were 'employed at cutting and stacking firewood for the river steamer which is shortly expected', keeping open a channel from Goolwa to the Murray mouth and replacing beacons on the shoals of Lake Victoria. For this they were being paid in rations, fish hooks and money. Whether this payment was sufficient to meet the needs of others in their community is not clear, but may be guessed at by Mason's mentioning, in the same report, 'much sickness', mainly rheumatism and complaints of the chest.[110]

While it is not possible to gauge accurately the impact of such employment

---

106 Sub-Protector Scott, *SAGG*, 25 May 1854, p.413

107 Sub-Protector Brewer, *SAGG*, 28 July 1853, p.499

108 Sub-Protector Mason, *SAGG*, 25 May 1854, p.413

109 Sub-Protector Mason, *SAGG*, 30 January 1851, p.80

110 Sub-Protector Mason, *SAGG*, 28 July 1853, p.499

opportunities, it is important to set the positive reports alongside others which tell a different story. Mason, for example, did not always report positively. In 1851, he complained of a lack of food for the Aboriginals at Wellington. He put this down in part to the effects of severe weather on fish supplies, but also to the destruction of food-bearing vegetation by the colonists' sheep and cattle. Furthermore, he noted:

> there are no settlers in their country who can give them employment, and being nearly in a starving state, they have taken every opportunity of stealing the food they could not obtain honestly.[111]

Some had been imprisoned as a result. This was an example of the intractable dilemma that had been disturbing the peace of the colony since the earliest days of European settlement: indigenous responses to loss of livelihood and to limited options led to behaviour that was deemed by the authorities to be criminal and deserving of punishment, thus establishing a vicious cycle of need, misunderstanding, mistrust and violence.

In all districts summer was the period of highest employment. The young and healthy moved away from the ration depots for a season of shearing or harvesting and learnt to rely on the government to care for their dependents. For example, Mason reported in 1855:

> As is usual in this season a number of sick and aged natives, unable to travel to the harvest-fields, have been left by their friends in my care; to such I have given a daily allowance of one pound of flour each, when they applied for it.[112]

This situation continued. The long-serving Mason, who was a regular and informative reporter, provided an informal summary in 1858. He wrote of 'constant employment' for some, as 'stock-keepers, shepherds, horse-breakers, bullock-drivers, and whalers', of 'occasional employment' for others, when the settlers were prepared to offer sufficient pay, and of dependence of the sick, aged and infirm on the care and rations provided by the government.[113] In the following year he recorded his opinion that many of the Aboriginals were 'exceedingly industrious' and 'useful', and commended a couple of local European employers for their fair treatment: 'in justice to these gentlemen I must say that they pay the natives, and use them equal in all respects, to the white people'. It was at best an ambivalent judgement. Nevertheless, Mason, who confessed to having little faith in what could be achieved 'as regards religious instructions', concluded that 'in fact from what I know of the natives, after living twenty years amongst them, I think industry will advance their civilization more than anything else'.[114] However, as he knew well, opportunities for industry were limited. On the other hand, dependence and indolence had been induced in many of the indigenous population by the practices of the colonial government and been entrenched as a new way of life, replacing the ancient one that colonisation had destroyed.

---

111 Sub-Protector Mason, *SAGG*, 23 October 1851, p.714
112 Sub-Protector Mason, *SAGG*, 8 March 1855, p.204
113 Sub-Protector Mason, *SAGG*, 19 August 1858, pp.616–617
114 Sub-Protector Mason, *SAGG*, 13 January 1859, p.28

The end of an era was signalled by the gazetting of Matthew Moorhouse's resignation and retirement on 3 April 1856.[115] Moorhouse returned to England[116] with, in all probability, ambivalent feelings about his achievements as Protector of Aborigines in South Australia. He was not replaced, and after the elections of 1857 which followed the establishment of responsible government in South Australia in 1856, the office of Protector was suspended. Official responsibility for the welfare of the indigenous population passed to the Commissioner of Crown Lands and Immigration. Under this new dispensation, some of the rations depots were closed, causing major disruption to the lives of many indigenous people and significantly diminishing the numbers being provided for by the government. In March 1859, Edward Hitchin, secretary of the Crown Lands and Immigration Office, reported on a tour of Aboriginal stations.[117] The report is a telling indication of minimalist government activity and crude assimilationist judgements of the behaviour and social worth of the indigenous population. There were by then three government depots and three officers – two of them police troopers and the other Sub-Protector Mason – 'supervising' all the River Murray natives, who were many fewer, especially at Moorundie, than had been the case a few years earlier.[118] The tone of the report suggests that every reasonable and kindly effort to further the interests of the indigenous population had been made by the government and settlers, but the Aboriginals, not knowing what was best for them, had, for the most part, declined to grasp the opportunities offered. For example, Hitchin did not see much evidence that 'the greatest kindness in protecting and instructing even young natives' had 'eradicate[d] their naturally-implanted taste for an unsettled and idle life'. As an instance of this regrettable situation he reported:

> On questioning some quite young lads, who were pointed out to me as having been inmates of the Poonindie mission, as to whether they would consent to return to the institution to finish their education, they most unhesitatingly declined.

More worthy of his approval were some 'remnants of the Adelaide tribe who had been persuaded to leave Port Adelaide to live permanently at Willunga', a village about 28 miles south of Adelaide:

---

115 *SAGG*, 3 April 1856, p.247

116 Moorhouse later returned to South Australia, where he lived for the rest of his life. See 'Moorhouse, Matthew (1813–1876)', in Douglas Pike (ed.), *Australian Dictionary of Biography*, vol.5, Melbourne University Press, Carlton, Victoria, 1984 [1974], pp.283–4.

117 Edward J Hitchin, Report on the Aborigines of the Murray and Lake Districts, *SAGG*, 17 March 1859, pp.258–9

118 Hitchin does not provide the comparative figures. However, as Raynes has noted, the 55 natives he mentions as being at Moorundie, where the depot had been closed for over two years (1856–58), represent merely 10 per cent of the number recorded five years earlier by Sub-Protector Scott. Even at Wellington, where there had been no closure of the depot, numbers were half what they were when Mason was first appointed, Hitchin, *SAGG*, 17 March 1859, p.258; Raynes, '*A Little Flour*', p.17.

Two young couples, members of this tribe, were brought up in the Adelaide School, and are certainly the most advanced specimens of aboriginal improvement I have seen, the males being good workmen, and all four having decided European ideas and tastes.[119]

Hitchin's report is striking in its lack of insight and compassion. It reveals no awareness of the historical processes that had been at work in South Australia since the establishment of the colony. It mistakes the results of complex social and economic change for 'naturally-implanted' disposition. It is oblivious to indigenous attachment to land and kin. It assumes without question the superior value of European culture. It implies, in unmistakable fashion, that the only acceptable Aboriginals – the only ones with a future as part of the public – are those who, against the odds, manage to assimilate themselves to European ways. This sits oddly with the picture painted by Sub-Protector Mason who, alone among Sub-Protectors and government agents, continued to report regularly throughout 1859 and 1860. He wrote of 'good conduct', but also much sickness, deaths that outnumbered births, inadequate shelter, the continuing need to provide daily rations, sometimes to people from outside his area, erratic and insufficient employment, further restrictions to livelihood as a result of European land acquisition, and periodic violence and unrest.[120] This was a picture of a people whose health and perhaps even survival had, within the space of 23 years, been put at grave risk by the establishment of a colony whose government had promised them protection, justice and advancement.

By the end of the 1850s, the South Australian Government, locally elected by a narrow franchise of the wealthiest colonists and in charge of its own affairs, had come close to washing its hands of responsibility for the original population. There were, however, South Australians with other views and a preparedness to act and to goad their government into action. The next chapter explores the impact of their thinking and activity on indigenous well-being.

---

119 Hitchin, *SAGG*, 17 March 1859, p.259. The last remaining group of Aboriginals in the vicinity of Adelaide were required to quit their Port Adelaide camp in September 1858 and were transferred to a reserve at Willunga, where they were expected to remain.

120 Sub-Protector Mason, *SAGG*, 13 January 1859, p.28; 14 April 1859, p.352; 12 May 1859, p.418; 14 July 1859, p.603; 22 September 1859, p.869; 20 October 1859, p.953; 9 February 1860, p.126; 17 May1860, p.452; 19 July 1860, p.6331; 1 November, 1860, p.1013

Chapter 4

1858–1911:
Missionaries and Protectors

As Christians it is our privilege – and as colonists it is our duty – to endeavour to Christianize and thereby to civilize the aborigines of the province; and though there may be differences of opinion as to whether or not our might is our sole right to the land there can be none as to the fact that we do owe these unfortunate beings a debt – a debt which I trust we shall be found anxious to pay by uniting cordially in endeavouring to raise and ameliorate their condition spiritually, morally and socially. **Fred Monk, Secretary, Aborigines' Friends' Association, 1861**[1]

At a public meeting held in Adelaide on 31 August 1858 the Aborigines' Friends' Association (AFA) was established. The object of this organisation was 'the moral, spiritual and physical well-being of the natives of this Province'. It enjoyed vice-regal patronage and was led by a large committee of clerics and prominent citizens.[2] The foundation of the association had been preceded by a series of preliminary meetings, beginning with one held on 28 July 1857, to which were invited 'persons interested in the welfare of the aborigines'.[3] The Bishop of Adelaide, Dr Augustus Short, presided over that initial meeting and set a positive tone for its deliberations by reporting on the work of the Native Training Institution at Poonindie:

the results of [this work] had clearly proved that the aborigines of this colony were not only perfectly capable of being moulded into very useful and trustworthy members of society, but of fully understanding and receiving into their hearts and minds the truths of Christianity.[4]

---

1 *Observer*, 22 February 1861

2 *Observer*, 4 October 1858. Patron: His Excellency the Governor, Sir Richard Graves MacDonnell; President: Hon George Fife Angas; Vice-Presidents: the Bishop of Adelaide, Dr Augustus Short, Mr Justice Boothby and Hon FS Dutton; Treasurer: Messrs N Oldham and GW Hawkes; Secretary: Mr CB Young; members: Messrs William Giles, FS Monk, William Milne, MP, Samuel Goode, James Smith, FH Faulding, Thomas Padman, Charles Smedley, William Peacock, George Prince and Daniel Kekwick; Captain Watts, Dr Mayo, Revs Archdeacon Woodcock, CW Evan, R Haining, J Gardner, W Ingram, J Lyall, G Stonehouse, AR Russell and R Needham.

3 *Register*, 24 July 1857, p.1; 28 July 1857, p.1

4 *Observer*, 1 August 1857

In the light of the low level of government activity in relation to the indigenous population – one speaker referred to the 'supineness which had generally prevailed' – and in particular the failure of the South Australian Government to retain the office of Protector, the
meeting agreed that 'some further efforts should be made with a view to ameliorate the
physical and spiritual welfare of the aboriginal inhabitants of the colony'. In seconding this
motion, George Fife Angas, prominent pioneer and politician, argued that the 'desultory
nature' of current efforts in relation to the Aboriginal population resulted from:

> the want of a permanent association of a few persons who would take a deep and permanent
> interest in the welfare of the natives, and keep alive an interest in the minds of the colonists
> generally.[5]

A committee was established forthwith, resolving to meet monthly and to gather information on which to base a decision about which area of the colony it should concentrate
its attention on. As a result of these enquiries, it decided to focus on the area around the
mouth of the River Murray, a gathering place of significant numbers of Aboriginal people
of the Ngarrindjeri clan, who were in a 'pitiable condition ... owing to their tribal territories having been invaded and appropriated by the white settlers'.[6] A deputation from the
committee waited on the Commissioner of Crown Lands and secured a promise that the
government would defray the cost of rations provided to needy Aboriginals among whom
the AFA proposed to work and to the children who attended the school it planned to open.

At the meeting of 31 August 1858 at which the AFA was constituted these plans were
formally launched. By January 1859 the government's and the public's response to the
association's appeal for funds had been sufficiently generous for it to resolve to establish
immediately 'an institution ... for the education of the young, and a home and training
centre for those who were older'. By the beginning of April 1859 George Taplin, a Port
Elliot school teacher and Congregational lay preacher, had begun work as the AFA's missionary agent, and by the end of that month had chosen a site for the institution on the
shores of Lake Alexandrina at Point McLeay. Taplin wasted no time in visiting and
gaining the confidence of Aboriginals in the surrounding districts and in embarking on a
program of building to provide living quarters for himself and his family, and a school
room, dormitories and kitchen to support his educational work among the children.[7]

This series of events underlines the extent to which the indigenous population were
seen as a people apart and not part of the public. The government's response to the impact
of colonial expansion on the Aboriginals was, as we have seen, minimal and lacking in
coherence. Although they were critical of this 'supine' response, the focus of the concerned
citizens who formed the AFA was less on the reform of government policy and practice

---

5 ibid.

6 CE Bartlett, *A Brief History of the Point McLeay Reserve and District*, Aborigines' Friends' Association, Adelaide, 1959, p.1

7 Gordon Rowe, *A Century of Service to the Aborigines at Point McLeay, SA*, Aborigines' Friends' Association, Adelaide, 1859,
   pp.5–6. George Taplin was a person of considerable ability and insight. For details of his early life and preparation for
   his missionary role see Graham Jenkin, *Conquest of the Ngarrindjeri*, Raukkan Publishers, Point McLeay, South Australia
   [1979] 1995, pp.74ff.

and more on what could be achieved through philanthropy, undergirded by modest government support. They construed the issue as a welfare matter, amenable to redress through the efforts of 'a few persons who would take a deep and permanent interest in the welfare of the natives' and committed themselves to raising public awareness of it in these terms. The government appeared willing to concur in this approach, letting the AFA make the running and merely responding to its requests for help rather than developing its own position and program. It was to adopt a similar position in relation to other Christian missions established in South Australia over the next half-century: the Moravian and Lutheran missions in the remote Cooper Basin at Kopperamanna and Killalpaninna (1867), the Yorke's Peninsula Aboriginal Mission, established at Point Pierce (1868), and the Lutheran mission at Koonibba on Eyre Peninsula (1901).[8]

The period from the establishment of responsible government in South Australia in 1856 until the passage of the *Aborigines Act* in 1911 was one in which organised activity relating to the indigenous population was shared between missions and government. Within this largely unplanned and somewhat haphazard partnership it was frequently the missions and their supporters who took the initiative, raised some public concern and goaded reluctant governments into limited action.

The resources which governments directed towards Aboriginal affairs during this period were small. The office of Protector, suspended after Moorhouse's departure in 1856, was filled by Dr John Walker from 1861 until his death in 1868. It then remained unfilled again until EL Hamilton was appointed Protector in 1880. In the interim, government activity in relation to Aboriginals was carried on by clerks in the Aborigines Office within the Department of Crown Lands and Immigration and by an expanded band of Sub-Protectors, police officers, station owners and other responsible citizens who were authorised to distribute rations to Aboriginals at various locations around the colony, designated as ration depots. The distribution of rations under stringent conditions was the nearest approach to government policy during this period. It had the effect of encouraging the concentration of the Aboriginal population in particular areas and of providing them with opportunities, albeit unequal and highly constrained, for assimilation into the colonial economy. As a system it was characterised by a huge power imbalance and was replete with opportunities for abuse and exploitation of the indigenous population. However, it did allow some of them to continue living on or near their country and to maintain aspects of their traditional culture, while providing the means of survival in the face of bad seasons and of agricultural and pastoral expansion into their traditional hunting and gathering grounds.

Another government initiative which, from 1851, worked in concert with the rationing system to provide some Aboriginals with opportunities to maintain links with country and culture was the inclusion within pastoral leases of a clause 'recognising the undoubted right of the natives to dwell upon the land, and to follow their usual customs

---

8 The name of the Yorke's Peninsula Aboriginal Mission was Point Pierce until the government took over the mission in 1915. From then, for reasons unknown, the spelling was changed to 'Pearce'. I follow this usage.

in search of food'.[9] This far-sighted provision stands in stark contrast to late twentieth-century fears about whether the interests and rights of pastoralists and indigenous people can 'coexist' on pastoral leases.

Robert Foster, in a careful analysis of the impact of government activity in this period, argues that, while Aboriginals were regarded as intruders in towns and as 'moral patients' on missions, the ration system and the provisions within the pastoral leases which recognised at least their economic links with their land allowed them 'a place' within rural society, while at the same time providing settlers, especially pastoralists, with a subsidised labour force.[10] The significance of this has frequently been overlooked, since it was the missions who were the activists in the cause of Aboriginal 'uplift' and 'advancement', and missionary activity that generated the most 'noise' about Aboriginal issues during the second half of the nineteenth century. Reports of missionary activity, relayed to supporters through mission societies, churches and philanthropic organisations and to the general public through the secular press loom large in the archival record. This can be misleading, since, as Foster notes:

> the majority of Aboriginal people in colonial South Australia had little or no experience of missionary life. But despite their slight direct influence on Aborigines ... the influence of missionaries on public perception, through their publications and the work of supporting agencies such as the Aborigines' Friends' Association, was considerable. Just as importantly, much of our contemporary understanding of aboriginal society and race relations comes to us through a dense filter of missionary perceptions.[11]

In fact, most Aboriginal South Australians who, in the second half of the nineteenth century experienced sustained contact with European society, did so through the expanding rural economy and the government's practice of rationing.

This chapter traces some of the major activities – often intertwined and symbiotic – of missions and governments in South Australia between the late 1850s and 1911 and their impact on the well-being of the indigenous population. It shows how these developments occurred within a context characterised by a balance between, on the one hand, apathy and neglect in which, especially for colonists in Adelaide and the areas of closest settlement, out of sight was out of mind, and, on the other, a sense of duty towards a hapless race who, although assumed to be dying out, nevertheless deserved to be offered the benefits of Christianity and 'civilisation'. It argues that this history effectively limited the involvement of most of the indigenous population in South Australia's civic life and 'progress' and undermined their capacity to maintain independent, productive and healthy lives. By 1911, legislation had formally confirmed them as not part of the public and had established a complex regulatory system which defined and controlled them as separate and other.

---

9 Robert Foster, 'An Imaginary Dominion: the representation and treatment of Aborigines in South Australia, 1834–1911', PhD thesis, University of Adelaide, 1993, p.195. *SAGG*, 30 January 1851, p.79

10 Foster, 'An Imaginary Dominion', p.215

11 ibid., p.215

Perhaps nudged into action by the AFA and by evidence of some humanitarian concerns in the community, or by the perception that the Aboriginals constituted a vexing political problem, the government, in 1860, appointed a select committee of the Legislative Council on 'The Aborigines'. The committee's brief was 'to take evidence and report on the present condition of the natives, and to suggest means by which that condition may be ameliorated'.[12] Chaired by the Hon. George Hall, it sat on 14 occasions in September and October 1860 and heard evidence from 20 witnesses: clerics, missionaries and supporters of mission societies, former and current Protectors of Aborigines, police officers, long-term residents of the colony, the Commissioner of Crown Lands and 'certain natives'.

The Anglican Bishop of Adelaide, Dr Augustus Short, was the first witness to be examined. Despite his association with Poonindie Native Institution and with the AFA, his view of the situation was uncomplicated and naïve. He claimed that, when he arrived in the colony in 1847, the natives were 'in a perfectly savage state', but by 1860, some progress was apparent. He put this down to 'the protection of kind and attentive settlers', and to the effect of schooling:

> I know that the natives at Port Lincoln, who were brought up in the school at Adelaide from childhood, and transferred to Mr Hale's care at Poonindie, were superior in moral character, intelligence and skill in labor.

In the place of 'the wild savage', Poonindie had produced 'the tame black, useful to society'. Short recommended that schools for Aboriginal children be established in other districts and that care be taken to reduce contact between children and 'the wild natives', since such contact resulted in 'moral and physical injury'. He noted that 'the Adelaide tribe is gone', but revealed little insight into the reasons for its disappearance: 'I cannot account for it except that they get more meat, and their blood must be in a hotter state'.[13]

The Hon. JT Bagot, the Commissioner of Crown Lands, was officially responsible for the well-being of the indigenous population. His evidence made it apparent that he had not made this a priority, or had even achieved a clear view of the situation beyond concluding that less was being done than was previously the case:

> ... the whole care, with respect to the aborigines appears to me to be rather less, and not much system in it ... I have not had time to give it any attention.

---

12 *SAPP* 1860, vol.3, no.165, Report of the Select Committee of the Legislative Council upon 'The Aborigines' together with Minutes of Evidence and Appendix, p.3. Harris argues that the Select Committee Inquiry initiated by the Hon. John Baker was 'a thinly disguised attempt to discredit the Point McLeay mission', John Harris, *One Blood. 200 Years of Aboriginal encounter with Christianity: a story of hope*, (2nd edn), Albatross Books, Sutherland, New South Wales, 1994, p.356. Certainly Baker's speech in parliament calling for the establishment of an enquiry was extreme in content, vitriolic in tone and highly critical of the AFA and of Taplin. *SAPD*, 4–5 September 1860, pp.743–5. The members of the committee were the Hons George Fife Angas, John Baker, Samuel Davenport, George Hall (chair), and George Waterhouse.

13 Augustus Short, Bishop of Adelaide, Select Committee Evidence, *SAPP* 1860, vol.3, no.165, pp.1–7

He assured the committee, however, that it was 'a matter' he was 'much interested in', and if he were 'in the same position long' he would 'give [his] attention to it'.[14]

George Mason, Sub-Protector at Wellington since 1839, had a much clearer idea of the situation and forceful views about appropriate strategies for improvement. He preached the gospel of work as he had always done in his regular reports to government, and rejected the accusation that he produced indolence by distributing rations. His policy was to provide food and care for the old and infirm, but to encourage the able-bodied to look after themselves: 'Let them go to work; there is plenty of work for them around the lakes'. While this may have been a glib judgement on the availability of appropriate and sufficient employment opportunities, in other matters he revealed detailed insight into when independence could be expected and when help was needed. For example, he rejected the suggestion that huts should be provided, insisting that the Aboriginals could provide these for themselves, using the abundant supply of pine and reeds. On the other hand, he believed that 'one of the greatest gifts the government could confer on them would be to give a canoe to each family', since the purchase of land by settlers had blocked their access to bark from suitable trees, thus reducing their opportunity to build canoes and to use them to procure their own food. He also believed the Aboriginals needed better access to medical care. He was authorised to engage 'a medical man' in extreme cases only, but that involved travelling 30 miles to Strathalbyn, where a Dr Blue was prepared to see Aboriginal patients 'for nothing', and to bill the government.[15] He believed more schools were needed, but was adamant that schooling should not involve child removal, because of the great love between family members and the likelihood that children sent away to school would pine for their country and friends, and abscond. In any case, parents did not value education for literacy, which they associated with removal to Poonindie, and told their children that 'learning to sheep-shear, reap corn, and bring the money home to them is better than Poonindie'. When asked whether 'someone should have the inspection of all establishments, for the benefit of the aborigines', Mason was unequivocal: 'Yes, it would do a deal of good. When Mr Moorhouse had it years ago, he did a deal of good, a great deal'.[16]

Matthew Moorhouse had by then returned to South Australia, where he spent the rest of his life, and so was able to present his own evidence to the Select Committee. He did so in a courteous and moderate fashion, but there is no mistaking that he thought the South Australian Government had lost its way in relation to Aboriginal affairs. 'It is impossible', he suggested, 'to do the natives justice, unless there be someone in the [Crown Lands] office whose duty shall be to attend to all such points.' He recommended the reinstatement of a Protector with the powers of an itinerant magistrate and duties in the districts beyond the jurisdiction of the local courts. When it was suggested that members of the clergy might be sufficient to this task, he indicated scepticism by referring pointedly

---

14 Hon. JT Bagot, Select Committee Evidence, *SAPP* 1860, vol.3, no.165, p.50

15 This was Dr Sinclair Blue, MD Glasgow1837, and registered as a medical practitioner in South Australia in 1854. Reece Jennings, 'The Medical Profession and the State in South Australia, 1836–1975, vol.2, p.6, MD thesis, University of Adelaide, 1997

16 Sub-Protector George Mason, Select Committee Evidence, *SAPP* 1860, vol. 3, no.165, pp.78–87

to the complex and multifaceted nature of his own work as Protector. Indeed, he was not sanguine about the prospects of whatever could be done. He believed that Aboriginal reserves should continue to be set aside and leased so that revenues from them could be used for 'maintenance' of the natives, but saw no hope that they would themselves settle on reserves, and, in fact, believed institutionalisation and keeping them in one place was 'incompatible with their lives and health'. He judged half-castes to be 'decidedly' more intelligent than 'the natural aborigine' but concluded:

> As far as educating the native in civilization, I believe, in most instances, it is utterly hopeless. The only thing that can be done for them is to soften down their life, and, by humanely treating them, to make it as easy as possible.[17]

This view, which clearly revealed his disappointment with his own attempts at 'civilising', was to become much more widely shared as time passed and was to profoundly influence government and public attitudes and action, and, indeed, inaction.

In 1860, however, it was a view not shared by George Taplin. Taplin, as we have seen, was the Superintendent of the recently established mission station at Point McLeay, on the shores of Lake Alexandrina. He was subjected to lengthy, detailed and at times hostile questioning by members of the Select Committee. The tone of the interrogation was doubtless connected to the fact that the land that Taplin had recommended as the site for the mission included 'three good sections' of a neighbouring pastoral run leased by one of the members of the committee, the Hon. John Baker. Baker insinuated that the natives had been 'less tractable' since Taplin's arrival, which perhaps reflected Taplin's concern that the Aboriginals not be cheated of pay and that no one be allowed to 'make an unfair profit' from them.[18]

Taplin reported positively on the work at Point McLeay. There had been an excess of births over deaths since he took up his position in April 1859 and he claimed that the people were better off physically, even though they suffered from seasonal health problems, including rheumatism and pulmonary complaints and also from 'excessive smoking' of tobacco bought with wages and income from fishing. There was no medical practitioner closer than a journey of ten miles by boat followed by 60 on land, and so Taplin provided what care he could himself, relying on a supply of castor oil, linaments, salve, senna, rhubarb and iodine of potassium. Questioned closely about his use of government rations, he insisted that 'a small portion only require to be supplied with rations – the larger number get their own living'. He refused to endorse the view that rations were compensation for loss of land and used them instead as payment for work on the mission in order to encourage habits of industry:

---

17 Matthew Moorhouse, Select Committee Evidence, *SAPP* 1860, vol.3, no.165, pp.94–9

18 George Taplin, Select Committee Evidence, *SAPP* 1860, vol.3, no.165, pp.61, 66–7. Taplin was careful not to accuse Baker of any specific wrongdoing, but did claim to be aware of instances of Aboriginals being cheated. He reported that he had dispensed with the services of his own cousin because he did not deliver the Aboriginals a fair price for the fish he sold at market for them.

> We give them labour as it is injurious to him to keep him in flour and let him live in idleness; and even as a kindness, I would give him work. It would be neglectful and wrong to encourage him in idleness.

For example, he had employed six Aboriginals for three months to build the school house at Point McLeay and paid them one shilling per day, plus flour, tea and sugar at each meal. He judged the indigenous population to be 'as capable of enduring continuous labour as the European' and recommended fencing, farming, shearing, harvesting and the supplying of wood and stone as suitable occupations. In an optimistic mood that was later to be undermined by the harsh realities of life at Point McLeay he resisted all suggestions that the mission site was poor and was never likely to provide all the food and work that was needed to sustain a settlement there.

When asked whether he thought the efforts of the government in relation to the Aboriginals were in general commensurate with its responsibilities, Taplin's answer was unequivocal: 'I hardly think so. I think more labour might be advantageously employed in civilizing and Christianising the aborigines'. 'Christianising' was his fundamental concern:

> I would first attack their superstitions and endeavour to influence them to give up their religion – to cast aside superstition and adopt Christianity ... nothing but their conversion to Christianity would ever satisfy me that we had met with what I should call success.

However, he was clear that attempts at conversion must be accompanied by concern for material needs, if only for the sake of consistency:

> ... I think it would be inconsistent to teach them Christianity, and neglect their physical wants ... If I taught them the precepts of the Christian community that we should relieve the distressed, and be merciful and kind – I should be bound to exhibit an example of benevolence.

Taplin thought that a protector should be appointed 'to itinerate throughout the colony', and was critical of rationing as 'destructive to industry' even though he admitted that in the absence of employment there seemed to be no alternative. He advocated the 'training' of half-castes, but was opposed to the forced removal of children from their homes.[19]

At its final sitting the committee sought evidence from 'certain natives'. These were two men and a woman of unknown age who identified themselves as being from Port Lincoln, which presumably meant Poonindie, but who were originally from Moorundie. The questioning was brief and inept and failed to elicit much information, or, in some instances, any response at all. The witnesses confirmed that rations and blankets were distributed only to the sick and old. They also said that they liked to be in Port Lincoln because this meant being away from 'the old black fellows' and because they did 'not like to be wicked'. When asked what they meant by 'being wicked' they listed fighting,

---

19 George Taplin, Select Committee Evidence, *SAPP*, 1860, vol.3, no.165, pp.50–62, 62–71

robbing, swearing and drinking.[20] There was evidence of some accommodation here, but whether it was to the values of the mission or to what the witnesses presumed to be the expectations of the Select Committee is not clear.

The Select Committee report acknowledged that the indigenous population, notwithstanding that they were 'nomadic and uncivilized tribes' who had not made 'the best use of the land', nevertheless had 'an equitable title' to it, and had been 'virtually dispossessed'. The committee's aim had been to compare the condition of the Aboriginal population at the time of European possession with their present condition, and their conclusion was forthright:

> All the evidence goes to prove that they have lost much, and gained little or nothing, by their contact with Europeans, and hence it becomes a question how far it is in our power, or what is the best possible means of compensating them for the injuries they have sustained, or of mitigating the evils to which, so far as they are concerned, our occupation of the country has led.

They considered 'the present state and condition of the aborigines' to be 'unsatisfactory'. 'The attempts made to ameliorate that condition' were 'not commensurate with the duties devolving upon the community'; indeed there was an 'almost entire absence of any system for the protection and support of the aborigines'.[21]

The evidence presented to the Select Committee, taken together, certainly reveals a lack of system. It demonstrates that the government was doing almost nothing in relation to the indigenous population, that most of what it did was reactive and dependent on the initiative of the few agents employed and that these agents were not always of a similar mind. The attitude of the Select Committee members to those working with the Aboriginals was nit-picking and somewhat mistrustful, especially in relation to Taplin. The questioning reveals a level of suspicion about how rations and other forms of government support were being used. It appears designed to highlight alleged tensions between Mason and Taplin and to portray Taplin as neglectful of some of the more isolated Aboriginals within his area of influence. Against this negative and blame-shifting background, and despite the forthrightness of its introductory remarks, the report's recommendations seem much like a re-run of strategies already found not to have worked under Matthew Moorhouse.

The report recommended the appointment of a Chief Protector 'to watch over the general interests of the aborigines', and to 'dispense justice, summarily, in all matters of dispute between the natives themselves, as also between natives and Europeans'. Sub-protectors should be appointed 'in different districts, where the natives are numerous', to care for physical needs, especially of the aged, sick and infirm, to 'train them to steady industrial habits of civilized life', and 'to endeavour to eradicate their vile superstitions and barbarous rites, leaving the mind open for the reception of the simple truths of Christianity'. To avoid the 'great evils arising from collecting different tribes from a great distance to a central depot', settlers in outlying areas who were known to be 'well intentioned towards the blacks', should be subsidised to distribute rations to local Aboriginals, subject to the regulations and inspection of the Chief Protector. Thus

---

20 'Certain natives', Select Committee Evidence, *SAPP* 1860, vol.3, no.165, pp.99–100

21 Select Committee Report, *SAPP* 1860, vol.3, no.165, p.3

the Government would always be in possession of the fullest information respecting the aborigines, and be enabled to carry out, or assist in carrying out, any scheme that might appear feasible, whose object would be the future and permanent benefit of the natives.[22]

The report also recommended a more faithful adherence to the policy of using income generated by the resumption of Aboriginal reserves for the benefit of the Aboriginal population. Using the 'very incomplete' public records at its disposal, the committee estimated that 'the greater proportion' of the 8000 acres set aside as Aboriginal reserves since the establishment of the colony had been resumed, that is, leased to European settlers, and that the annual income of £1000 from these leases had been 'merged in the General Revenue'. Once 'merged' in this way, funds had not been forthcoming to meet the needs of the Aboriginals who consequently experienced 'considerable suffering'. The report therefore recommended 'that the fund for the relief of the aborigines should be a special one', based on income from already resumed reserves and augmented by income from additional reserves, 'until the amount ... derivable from that source equals the necessary expenditure of the aborigines department'.[23]

The next section of the report noted that the colonial authorities were instructed to respect indigenous rights to and 'enjoyment of' land, and that on the 'cession' of their lands to the colonial powers, the Aboriginals were to be compensated 'not only with food and shelter, but with moral and religious instruction' and 'gratuitous medical assistance and relief'.[24] Finally, the report offered an assessment of the current efforts, including the government's, to provide for the welfare of the Aboriginals, and found them all wanting. The influence of Mason, the only Sub-Protector appointed by the government solely 'for the purpose of protecting the interests of the aborigines', was acknowledged, but he was judged to have failed to attend to 'the physical necessities' of many of those under his protection. This was because of distance, government parsimony and 'lately a laxity in the performance of his duties'. Poonindie's management and financial position were declared unsatisfactory and the committee members wondered whether it should give up its location and farming interests and move to a location where it could isolate itself from 'the local Port Lincoln tribe', which was alleged to be 'inferior in every respect to any other known in South Australia'. Point McLeay was described as having 'more of the character of a private establishment for Christianizing the natives than a public institution for the support and protection of the aborigines', and while Taplin's 'zeal' was not questioned, his 'system' needed to be 'greatly modified':

> The Committee are of [the] opinion that the attempt to instill Christian principles into the minds of a portion of a tribe by day, and allow them to retire and mix with others in wurleys at night, is not judicious.

In fact they concluded by stating 'their strong conviction' that:

---

22 ibid., pp.3–4
23 ibid., p.4
24 ibid., p.5

permanent benefit, to any appreciable extent, from attempts to Christianize the natives can only be expected by separation of children from their parents and evil influences of the tribe to which they belong. However harshly this recommendation may grate on the feelings of pseudo-philanthropists, it would in reality be a work of mercy to the rising generation of aborigines.[25]

The Report of the 1860 Select Committee is a highly instructive document. On the one hand it is unequivocal in acknowledging the harm and loss that the indigenous population had suffered since the establishment of the colony of South Australia. It focuses directly on the question of land and the extent to which existing arrangements fall short of the original intentions or hopes of the colonial authorities and short-change the Aboriginals. On the other hand, however, the only plan it can envisage for financing provision for Aboriginal needs rests on the acquisition and control of more land. Current and future instances of dispossession are seen as requiring compensation, but the compensation is in the form of food, clothing, housing and health care, things with which the rest of the population would expect to be provided not as compensation for loss but as a consequence of being part of society and participating in the economic opportunities that that entails. Furthermore, the culture of the Aboriginals is summarily dismissed as barbaric and worthy only of destruction. The Aboriginals are to be 'Christianised' and 'civilised', although precisely what is meant by these uninterrogated code words is never entirely clear. It is clear, however, that the process will involve conformity to European standards, especially as these apply to 'habits of industry', and the relinquishing of their own history, identity and autonomy. And, despite the testimony of some well-informed witnesses against child-removal, the report recommends this as a 'work of mercy' crucial to 'the advancement of the race'.[26]

It is difficult to read this report as being genuinely concerned with 'the advancement of the race'. If 'Christianising' and 'civilising' are taken to mean becoming like the rest of South Australian society, there is nothing in the Select Committee's recommendations or in the circumstances obtaining in the colony to indicate any real opportunity for this to happen. The proposals of the Select Committee about the provision that the government should make for the indigenous population are not about opportunities for 'advancement', for choice, or for sharing fully in the life of the colony; they are proposals merely for survival – and perhaps only short-term survival – and for producing a level of conformity consistent with the Aboriginals not being any kind of burden or unsettling influence. Thus the 1860 Select Committee Report and its recommendations established and legitimised an agenda of inequality, of non-inclusion, of lack of autonomy and of radically differential claims on civic goods. What we now know about the determinants of health in populations, and especially about the complex links between social inequalities and health, confirms this as a long-term agenda for poor health.

The 1860 Select Committee upon the Aborigines is instructive in another way. In both the evidence and the report we see the emergence, in an embryonic form, of various ideas that gathered momentum during subsequent decades and powerfully shaped public

25 ibid., p.6
26 ibid., p.6. As indicated above, Mason and Taplin argued strongly against taking children from their families.

opinion and government policy. These include the notion that the Aboriginal population was dying out, that the primitivity and barbarism of their culture made them irredeemable, that attempts, therefore, to 'Christianise' and 'civilise' were unlikely to meet
with much success, and that the situation was being complicated by the appearance of
mixed-race people, 'half-castes' whose intelligence and social worth, compared with 'the
natural aborigine' became a matter of energetic and unresolved debate. These ideas were
a crucial aspect of the context in which government, missions and the South Australian
community dealt with issues relating to the indigenous population.

Despite its shortcomings, the report of the 1860 Select Committee on the Aborigines did
encourage some government initiatives which developed simultaneously with the expansion of missionary activity. The office of Protector of Aborigines was reinstated and
Dr John Walker was appointed Protector in November 1861.[27] He set out immediately on
a tour of inspection of the south-eastern district of the colony 'for the purpose of acquiring
full information respecting the Aborigines' which could be the basis for the establishment
of 'a regular system for the relief of [their] physical and temporal wants'.[28]

Although clearly a man of energy who took his role as Protector seriously, throughout
his term of office Walker revealed limited insight into the underlying causes of the conditions he observed among the indigenous population. In the final report of his 1861–62
information-gathering tour he concluded that while many Aboriginals were 'tolerably well
clothed', had an 'abundance of food' and enjoyed 'wonderfully good' health, given 'the
anti-hygienic circumstances to which they are exposed', there was:

> still much in their condition to excite feelings of the deepest commiseration, and enough
> both of want and disease to demand increased and more widely diffused efforts for their
> relief.[29]

Their numbers were generally agreed to be decreasing and he put this down to various diseases, of which tuberculosis was the most fatal, and to female infecundity and infanticide.
He thought the direct causes of the diseases from which the indigenous population suffered were insufficient or unsuitable food, abuse of alcohol, 'immoderate smoking', loitering about towns, 'intense indolence' and 'the want of that muscular exertion and
mental exhilaration which the chase afforded in their savage state'. Since some of these
arose out of 'the wretched social conditions and vicious habits of the Natives' any 'system
for the amelioration of their present state' needed to focus on 'their moral and social ele-
vation'. He expressed his belief in Christianity as 'the best instrument for the suppression

27 *SAGG*, 21 November 1861, p.970. Walker (1812–68) was a medical practitioner, who qualified in Scotland in 1833, was
     registered in South Australia in 1855, and practised briefly at Mount Barker. On his death, the obituary in the *Advertiser*
     recorded that he had taken a 'leading part in public affairs in this settlement', but made no mention of the nature or quality
     of his work as Protector of Aborigines, *Advertiser*, 28 September 1868.
28 John Walker, General Report on the Aborigines, GRG 35/1/342, 18 February 1862; GRG 35/1/791, 13 April 1863
29 John Walker, General Report on the Aborigines, GRG 35/1/791, 13 April 1863

of crime and vice amongst the Natives', and also 'the only effective instrument of Civilization'.[30] His practical suggestions, however, were mostly about rationing.

Walker believed there was a need for more ration depots across the colony, but concurred with existing government policy that rations should be distributed only to those in demonstrable need, since 'it is an injury instead of a benefit to the healthy and strong, as it encourages them in that indolence to which they are naturally inclined'. The rations should consist of one pound of flour, two ounces of sugar and a quarter of an ounce of tea daily for eligible Aboriginals, rice only as a 'medical comfort', and meat or other extraordinary items only when 'certified to be absolutely necessary by any qualified Medical Practitioner'. In addition, more blankets should be provided, since 'no greater boon can be conferred on the Natives than a large warm blanket to each on the approach of winter'. While Walker was sanguine that these suggestions, if followed, would prevent much illness, he also recognised the need for medical treatment and recommended that in the most populated districts, medical practitioners be appointed on an annual salary to offer 'advice and medicines' to all sick Aboriginals from their district who applied for help.[31]

In subsequent quarterly reports Walker consistently reported on illness among the Aboriginals. However he had little to say about its cause, beyond simplistic, behavioural explanations, or its remedy, beyond the administration of government rations, simple medicines and 'contributions of cast-off clothes, boots etc which are generally given away by the white man' but which could be 'carefully distributed among those who are deserving objects'.[32] On occasion he was more expansive, but his analysis did not progress much beyond that of his earliest reports: he noted the seriously 'injurious' effects of alcohol, the undesirable influence of towns, the 'unsteadiness' and proneness to fatigue of Aboriginal workers, and the unfortunate impact on young people of elders who 'still cling ... to their former mode of life, and their gross superstitions'.[33]

During Walker's term of office, the system of rationing, designed to protect Aboriginals from privation without undermining incentive to work, was strengthened, as he had recommended. The Queen's Birthday distribution of rations in Adelaide, established by Governor Gawler in 1838, was abolished in 1861, but ration depots outside the capital proliferated. There were 58 by 1866, many of them on remote pastoral stations far beyond the Murray and lakes districts that had been the focus of earlier government initiatives. It was convenient for the government to make pastoralists dispensers of rations and it was an arrangement welcomed by many of them. By providing rations the government was not only effectively subsidising the pastoralists' employment of Aboriginal workers but also providing them with a means of control and surveillance of Aboriginals on their land. Missions too were designated ration depots, and missionaries dispensers of

---

30 ibid.

31 ibid. This long and detailed report is preserved as a handwritten docket. While various of Walker's suggestions attracted brief marginal comments from government officials who perused it, the only substantial notation refers to the exact specification and possible source of supply of blankets to be provided to the Aboriginal population.

32 Report of Protector of Aborigines, *SAGG*, 5 January 1865, pp.7–9. In this instance, Walker is quoting Dr Clindening, Medical Officer responsible for Aboriginals at Mt Gambier.

33 Report of Protector of Aborigines, *SAGG*, 20 October 1864, pp.886–8; 23 March 1865, pp.266–268; 29 June 1865, pp.580–3

rations. By 1879, when there were 50 ration depots operating, five were on missions, and these were responsible for more than one-third of all the stores distributed.[34] Thus the system linked government, pastoral and missionary activity by making station managers and missionaries 'surrogate protectors and policemen'.[35]

While missions and ration depots were places where Aboriginal people gathered and in some cases made their homes, they were also places from which people came and went as they balanced other needs and priorities in their lives. Government agents inspecting depots sometimes reported that most of the Aboriginals were absent: the able-bodied had gone elsewhere in search of seasonal work or to attend traditional ceremonies, leaving only the frail and sick in the care of the government. On missions, this kind of movement occurred as well, even though the missions worked hard to build a sense of community and commitment to place by offering services, especially education, and providing what work they could. While some indigenous people accepted the opportunities and constraints offered by the mission communities, made permanent homes there and lived and worked according to the missions' structures and expectations, others exhibited a more equivocal and partial response; still others steadfastly remained on the margins within the ambit of the missions' care and concern, but preferring to retain their freedom, even though it meant a wurley rather than a stone cottage. It was not a neat system, and the 'success' that the missionaries sought was by no means guaranteed. The diversity of indigenous responses was evidence of agency and capacity for choice that is sometimes overlooked.

Walker died in 1868, and the government, despite the extension of its activity during his protectorship, did not appoint a Protector to succeed him. The system of maintaining and controlling the indigenous population through the mechanism of rationing continued. It was administered centrally through the tiny Aborigines Office that continued within the Department of Crown Lands and Immigration and in the field through the established team of quasi Sub-Protectors. However, it seems that beyond that, the government 'had once again lost interest in the Aborigines'.[36] By this time, however, interest was growing in other quarters, and missionary activity was on the increase.[37]

———————

Although the period after 1860 is one in which government activity in relation to the Aboriginal population seems confined to rationing, and in which missions come into prominence and appear to be the effective policy-makers and providers of services, this is an over-simplified view. It misses or downplays both the essential interdependence of government and missions at this time and the impact of the government's program of rationing. Missions were not independent of governments: they were frequently badgering them for money, land and other kinds of support and seeking endorsement for the direction of their work. As well as being clients of government, they were also its agents. By

34 Foster, 'An Imaginary Dominion', p.191

35 ibid., p.189

36 ibid., p.192

37 For a site-by-site summary of mission activity in South Australia, see Mattingley and Hampton, *Survival in Our Own Land*, pp.175–262.

providing basic education and training of children, and enough employment, as well as rations in the form of food and shelter, to avoid destitution among adults, they were carrying out the government agenda identified in the 1860 Select Committee report. In line with their own as well as government views, this activity was undertaken in segregated settings, even though its educational aspects were, in theory, designed to promote assimilation into the wider community.

Such missions have received a bad press in recent times. It is easy, and in some quarters fashionable, to deride them as purveyors of racism, destroyers of culture, and agents of the disintegration of Aboriginal communities. While elements of this reputation are deserved, blanket denigration of missions, which often rests more firmly on ideology than on research, is unsatisfactory on two important counts. In the first place, it ignores the argument, based on careful research into particular missions over lengthy periods, that far from destroying Aboriginal people, missions did, in some cases, act as havens or 'ghettos', as places and institutions that provided protection, produced loyalty, and developed identity and a sense of community among their residents. In the second place, it exhibits some of the racist and assimilationist characteristics that it derides by ignoring the variety of Aboriginals' responses to mission activity and their capacity to exercise influence and leadership as well as judgement and choice, albeit to a limited extent, within the mission context. Graham Jenkin's research on the relationship between the Point McLeay mission and the Ngarrindjeri, and Peggy Brock's on the links between missionary activity, institutionalisation and survival at three other South Australian sites – Poonindie, Koonibba and Nepabunna – provide a compelling and nuanced counter to the crudeness of the mission-bashing approach, without denying any of its legitimate criticism.[38] Similarly, in his influential study of the Ramahyuck Mission established by Moravian missionaries in Gippsland, Victoria, in the 1860s, Bain Attwood argues that, although missions could create 'prisons of inequality' in which Aboriginals were 'disenfranchised from the wider society', they did not have the capacity to destroy all independence or command required responses. On the contrary, they were instrumental in the emergence of new indigenous understandings of community and identity.[39] John Harris, in his comprehensive, frankly sympathetic but not uncritical history of Aboriginal missions throughout Australia, also recognises Aboriginal agency in a way that many critics of missions do not.[40]

Such readings of the histories of missions and the Aboriginal people whom they influenced are valuable in helping to create a basis for assessing the impact of the missions on health, where health is understood as being not merely about disease or its absence, but about all those things – nutrition, housing, education, employment opportunities, autonomy, sense of worth and self-esteem, control over one's life and capacity to command the respect and positive regard of others – that determine the well-being of individuals and of populations. Missions often had a comprehensive influence over these factors and therefore over the health of those in their care. In addition, as research from North America suggests, careful analysis of a range of post-contact experiences, which for many, but not all

38 Jenkin, *Conquest of the Ngarrindjeri*; Brock, *Outback Ghettos*

39 Bain Attwood, *The Making of the Aborigines*, Allen and Unwin, Sydney, 1989, pp.43–4, 118–19

40 Harris, *One Blood*

indigenous people, involve some experience of missions and institutionalisation, also guards against a simplistic misreading of this history as 'an uninterrupted, inevitable progression from autonomy to cultural disintegration and dependence'.[41] By recognising that, in their interactions with missions and other agents of colonisation, Aboriginal groups have sometimes been able to maintain significant levels of autonomy and self-sufficiency, but at other times been forced into major cultural accommodation, we may gain further insight into what contributes to or conversely undermines their resilience and well-being.[42]

Moravian (United Brethren) missionaries were active in the Australian colonies from 1850, having received invitations from government authorities to establish missions in New South Wales and the Port Phillip and Swan River districts.[43] A reformed church with fifteenth-century origins in what is now the Czech Republic, the Moravians were 'essentially a missionary fellowship' with a particular interest in 'the most remote, unfavourable and neglected parts of the surface of the earth'.[44] South Australia qualified as such a site. Between May 1865 and August 1866, four Moravian missionaries from Germany arrived in the colony, via Victoria, where they had been gaining experience on already established Moravian missions. The first two to arrive, Revs Gottlieb Meissel and Heinrich Walder spent time with Taplin at Point McLeay, and then Walder, with the third of the Moravians, Rev. Julius Wilhelm Kuhn, visited Yorke Peninsula, home of the Narungga people and site of a burgeoning copper-mining industry, centred on the towns of Wallaroo, Moonta and Kadina.[45] Kuhn remained there at the invitation of a group of settlers, who in 1866 formed a committee to establish an institution 'for the civilization and evangelization of the Aborigines on Yorke's Peninsula'. In February 1868 the Yorke's Peninsula Aboriginal Mission was established on 600 acres of pastoral lease at Point Pierce, 35 miles south of Wallaroo, with Kuhn as missionary.[46] Kuhn remained long after the Moravians had severed their connection in 1870; the mission subsequently continued to attract support from various Christian churches and the government.

Meanwhile, a fourth Moravian missionary, Rev. Carl W Kramer, had arrived in South Australia from Victoria and, with Walder and Meissel, travelled to remote Lake Kopperamanna, home of the Diyari people in the far north-east of the colony.[47] Arriving in December 1876, they discovered not only that Lutheran missionaries sent out from Germany by the Hermannsburg Mission Society and supported by the Australian Lutheran synods were

41 Edward H Spicer (ed.), *Perspectives in American Indian Cultural Change*, University of Chicago Press, Chicago, 1961, cited in Brock, *Outback Ghettos*, p.122

42 With reference to a later period, this point is also made strongly in relation to Aboriginals and the pastoral industry, in Anne McGrath, *'Born in the Cattle': Aborigines in cattle country*, Allen and Unwin, Sydney, 1987.

43 For a detailed summary of Moravian missions in Australia in this period, see Bill Edwards, *Moravian Aboriginal Missions in Australia, 1850–1919*, Uniting Church Historical Society (SA), Adelaide, 1999.

44 Stephen Neill, *A History of Christian Missions*, Penguin Books, Harmondsworth, 1964, p.237, cited in Edwards, *Moravian Aboriginal Missions*, p.9

45 Edwards, *Moravian Aboriginal Missions*, p.20. Edwards records his name as Kuehn, but in government records, and other secondary sources, his name is consistently spelt Kuhn. To avoid confusion I have adopted this usage.

46 Mattingley and Hampton, *Survival in Our Own Land*, pp.195–7.

47 The name of this people is alternatively spelt 'Dieri'.

establishing themselves in the same area, but also that relations between Aboriginals and European settlers in the area were dangerously tense. The Moravians and the Lutherans were each leased 100 square miles of 'waste land', that is, the country of the Diyari, as Aboriginal Reserve land, and despite considerable dangers and difficulties, they established two missions, the Moravians at Kopperamanna and the Lutherans at Killalpaninna. However, by May 1869 the Moravians had abandoned the cause, leaving Kopperamanna to become an outstation of Killalpaninna.[48] In 1868 the Hermannsburg missionaries at Killalpaninna, JF Goessling and E Homann were joined by a schoolteacher, W Koch, and subsequently by other clergy and lay staff. They learnt the Diyari language, used it as the medium of instruction in their school, and translated sections of the Bible and other Christian material. In addition to dealing with the financial pressures which were the lot of all missions, they battled an extremely harsh physical environment, in which long periods of drought were interspersed with devastating floods. But they stayed.[49]

The story of intertwined government and mission activity in relation to Aboriginals during the period 1859–1911 can be told through government and mission records, although it is a story with gaps and imbalances. Missions in receipt of government support were required to report regularly to the government, and officers of the government deemed it important to visit and inspect at least those that were closest to Adelaide. Thus government records provide an ongoing account of the work of some missions and of government opinions about their work, and about the condition of the indigenous population in general.

Within this historical record, then, some missions loom larger than others, for a range of reasons. Proximity to Adelaide tended to mean greater surveillance by the Protector or the Aborigines Office. Some missionaries were more assiduous and expansive than others in their reporting habits. Some mission support bodies had their base in Adelaide, and therefore ready access to politicians and the press, and others did not. Some missions, by virtue of being supported by independent coalitions of Christians and philanthropists, rather than being answerable to the mission boards of a particular denomination, had greater freedom to appeal directly to the government and to the public. For all these reasons we can learn most from government records about the AFA mission at Point McLeay in this period, somewhat less about the missions at Poonindie and Point Pierce, and less still about the Lutheran missions at Killalpaninna and, by the end of the period, Koonibba. The AFA's own records of their work at Point McLeay were more public than the records of the other missions. The annual general meetings of the AFA were held in prominent venues in Adelaide and were reported in detail in the secular press. Moreover, the government seemed more aware of it than of other mission bodies. The mission itself was

---

48 Edwards, *Moravian Aboriginal Missions*, pp.20–2. Edwards suggests various reasons, apart from the immediate environmental challenges, for the failure of the Moravian mission at Kopperamanna.

49 The Killalpaninna mission suffered many setbacks but survived until 1915. For a detailed account of its difficulties and achievements, and its relationships with the Lutheran church, the South Australian government and the Diyari, see Christine Stevens, *White Man's Dreaming: Killalpaninna Mission, 1866–1915*, Oxford University Press, Melbourne, 1994. See also Harris, *One Blood*, pp.376–83, Mattingley and Hampton, *Survival in Our Own Land*, pp.189–94, and for a first-hand missionary reflection, see below, Appendix 3.

considerably less remote than any of the others, and since it could be reached in less than a day's journey from Adelaide, supporters often visited and sometimes had their reactions published in the press. In addition, groups of Aboriginals from Point McLeay were brought to Adelaide from time to time to perform concerts and demonstrate craft activities.

The tendency for some voices to be heard above others does not apply just in the case of missions and missionaries. Government officials and other citizens with responsibility for Aboriginal people also made a differential impact within the government records. Some medical officers, for example, reported more regularly and more expansively about health among Aboriginals in their area than did others. Similarly, some police officers who acted as *de facto* Sub-Protectors had more to say in their reports to the government than others, while the voices of many station managers, who were also *de facto* Sub-Protectors, were seldom heard.

The greatest silence of all was from the Aboriginal people themselves. Government and mission records and much secondary scholarship reported on and discussed them, but failed to accord them agency or give them a voice. Their identity was hidden and homogenised behind such labels as 'the natives' and 'the blacks'. Periodically, named individual Aboriginals appeared in the records, usually when they had a specific request of government, but for the most part individuals did not emerge from the group or appear to be exercising independence or leadership within their communities.[50] Nor were the groups usually distinguished from each other, except geographically. There was little use of clan names or evidence of interest in cultural differences between, say, the Ngarrindjeri, the Narungga and the Diyari. Increasingly, the only differences of interest to the non-Aboriginal community were those between 'full-bloods' and 'half-castes', or 'wild blacks' and 'mission Aborigines'. Recent scholarship has suggested that Aboriginal independence in this period was ignored or under-reported. For some indigenous people, engagement with the settlers, especially through employment, provided a measure of independence, assertiveness, literacy and the know-how to negotiate the European world. This was not something that missionaries or protectors usually recorded in their reports.[51] However, while acknowledgement of such independence as existed is important, it should not be overstated or allowed to cloud the more general picture of dependence and radical disadvantage.

Careful use of government and non-government records, as well as recent secondary research on hitherto hidden aspects of colonial race relations can fill in some gaps. However, the story will still never be fully told. Distance, isolation, and the primitive means of communication and surveillance that prevailed in the past, as well as apathy and neglect, have left us with an incomplete picture. In addition, at the time those phenomena had the

---

50 When individual Aboriginal people were identified it was much more likely to be in non-public, unpublished departmental correspondence than in published reports appearing in, say, the *South Australian Government Gazette* or *South Australian Parliamentary Papers*.

51 For evidence of greater indigenous independence and leadership in South Australia than is usually acknowledged, see Jenkin, *Conquest of the Ngarrindjeri*, Brock, *Outback Ghettos* and Jude Elton, 'Comrades or Competition? Factors affecting union relations with Aboriginal workers in the South Australian and Northern Territory pastoral industries, 1878–1958', PhD thesis (2006), University of South Australia, and personal communication, 8 March 2004. Similar evidence for other parts of Australia is found in Attwood, *The Making of the Aborigines*, and McGrath, *'Born in the Cattle'*.

capacity to produce some independence from central policy and some capacity to remain uninfluenced by it. Thus the comparative silence in the historical record about many places of Aboriginal settlement outside the missions and the areas closest to Adelaide alerts us to the possibility that what was happening in these places might have been different from what was happening in those which received more attention. While few Aboriginals could escape the macro effects of colonisation, some must have been unaware of or in a position to ignore the micro elements of Aborigines Office policy.

These caveats notwithstanding, there is much that we can learn about the impact of non-indigenous policies and practices on the health of indigenous people in the period between the 1860 Select Committee and the 1911 *Aborigines Act*. The historical record provides evidence of specific issues relating to health and illness, but much more about complex underlying, long-term determinants of health. These were not identified as health issues at the time, and have usually not been seen as such in secondary literature either. My purpose is to focus on these in the light of the understanding now available to us through the public health research summarised in chapter two.

Throughout the period various commentators regularly identified specific health issues – or more properly illness issues – similar to those identified earlier by Moorhouse and his Sub-Protectors, by Hale at Poonindie, and by Walker when he took office as Protector of Aborigines. Dysentery, diarrhoea, catarrh and various chest ailments, colds, influenza, rheumatism, pneumonia and skin diseases were frequently mentioned. However, 'the native scourge', consumption, caused the greatest concern and was responsible for the greatest mortality.[52] The Report of the Aborigines Department for the half-year ended June 1874, for example, mentioned sickness and death from consumption in many districts throughout the colony.[53] It was frequently assumed to be something to which the Aboriginals were constitutionally predisposed – 'when a cold settles on their lungs they are gone in a few weeks' – or which resulted from their behaviour – 'it takes them off rapidly, especially at this time of the year when they do not take good care of themselves' – rather than the result of their living conditions. It should be noted, however, that consumption, that is, tuberculosis, was the leading cause of adult deaths in Australia during the colonial period and remained so well into the twentieth century. Its prevalence was greatest among the poorest sections of the community and it was associated, not, as was once supposed, with the immorality or constitutional weakness of the poor, but with the circumstances of poverty, especially poor nutrition and over-crowded and poorly ventilated housing. Thus it is hardly surprising that it became such a problem among dispossessed Aboriginals, or that arguments about their 'consumptive predisposition' were common.[54]

---

52 Taplin referred to consumption as 'the native scourge'. Report of Protector of Aborigines, *SAGG*, 20 August 1868, p.1144.

53 Government reporting was minimal for several years after the death of Walker in 1868, but became more regular and expansive after the appointment of EL Hamilton as Sub-Protector in September 1873.

54 Report of Sub-Protector of Aborigines, *SAGG*, 20 August 1874, pp.1667–74. See Judith Raftery, 'Health', in Wilfrid Prest (ed.), *The Wakefield Companion to South Australian History*, Wakefield Press, Adelaide, 2001, pp.244–7; Judith Raftery, 'Keeping Healthy in Nineteenth-Century Australia', *Health and History*, vol.1, no.4, 1999, pp.274–97.

Alcohol was another frequently reported health issue, and concern about it was often linked with recommendations about keeping the indigenous population away from the undesirable influence of towns. In 1864 Walker argued that:

> the effects of spirituous liquors are so injurious to the natives, that I think their visits to our
> towns, and their residence in the neighborhood of public-houses should as far as possible be
> discouraged.[55]

He recognised that the problem was one of supply as well as demand, and called the supply of intoxicating liquor to Aboriginals 'a great source of disease and misery among them', which 'destroy[ed] almost every chance of doing any good for them either physically or morally'.[56] It was a recurring refrain. Dr Clindening reported from Mt Gambier in 1865 on the 'great and growing evil' of drunkenness, and its 'heart-sickening' results.[57] In 1868, Walker noted that there was 'a great deal of spirit drinking' in the Blanchetown area, and in 1874, the rations issuer from Tarpeena reported some arrests for drunkenness, noting that when they had money the Aboriginals went into the townships in order to get drink.[58] In 1866 Taplin was rejoicing in the 'increased disposition' of Aboriginal people to settle at a 'a place so far from public houses' as Point McLeay was, but in subsequent years was linking increased drunkenness among his charges with the influence of the nearby town of Meningie.[59] In 1874 he claimed that, while the health of the Aboriginals had, on the whole, improved, 'those who suffer most are those who now frequent the townships and public-houses' and that 'those who hang about Adelaide always return . . . in a low state of health'.[60] Even the acquisition, in 1876, of some much-needed extra land at the Needles Reserve on the Coorong was a mixed blessing, since there, removed from the surveillance in place at Point McLeay, they were able to procure 'a great deal of intoxicating liquor', and then came to the ration depot, 'shaking and trembling with the collapse of the system'.[61]

Recognising these problems was one thing; doing something about them was another, and those who cared about them often lacked the resources to make a difference. Sub-Protector JP Buttfield, who was stationed in the Northern District from 1866 and who also inspected conditions in the Western District, reported that 'much sickness prevails among the blacks' and asked plaintively whether, at least in the case of well-understood diseases,

---

55 Report of Protector of Aborigines, *SAGG*, 20 October 1864, p.887

56 Report of Protector of Aborigines, *SAGG*, 11 November 1864, p.7

57 Report of Protector of Aborigines, *SAGG*, 23 March 1865, p.267

58 Report of Protector of Aborigines, *SAGG*, 20 August 1868, p.1145; 20 August 1874, p.1669

59 Report of Protector of Aborigines, *SAGG*, 26 July 1866, pp.718–19; 11 July 1867, p.664. AFA, Minutes of General
    Committee, 3 January 1969, SRG 139/2, vol.1

60 Report of Sub-Protector of Aborigines, *SAGG*, 20 August 1874, p.1667

61 Mattingley and Hampton, *Survival in Our Own Land*, p.183; Report of Sub-Protector of Aborigines, *SAGG*, 20 March
    1879, p.794

something might be done to mitigate their sufferings ... Might not medicines be prepared and supplied to the different depots throughout the Colony? Thus the poor sufferers would at least have their passage to the grave made less rugged.[62]

Taplin reported on the positive effects that improved housing had on the health of the Aboriginals, especially infants. But the records of the AFA show how difficult it was to find the money for even the most basic of cottages at Point McLeay, even though the provision of cottages could be linked not only to health improvement but to the Christianising and civilising goals so widely espoused.[63]

It seems that there was never enough money from any source, whether government or non-government, to provide for the indigenous population in anything other than the most basic and niggardly way. This was often not sufficient to guarantee good health. Nor was there much will in the community to do what might have been needed or helpful, or much imagination about how to deal with some of the problems which impinged directly on the health of the indigenous population, for example, the illegal supplying of alcohol and the 'corruption' of Aboriginal girls and women by non-Aboriginal men. Walker, in the most reflective report he wrote during this term as Protector of Aborigines, suggested that there needed to be stronger sanctions against those who supplied alcohol to Aboriginals, such as loss of their licenses, and that flogging would be an 'adequate punishment' of Aboriginals who consumed liquor.[64] The police-and-punish theme was echoed by Taplin. He believed that:

> many of the drunken natives are quite as blameable as the whites, and deserve to be punished. Nothing would so much stop drunkenness among the natives as to punish them sharply for getting drunk.[65]

Later he concluded that:

> the placing of a police trooper at Meningie had the very best results – it restrained unscrupulous whites from tempting natives addicted to drink, and strengthened the hands of those opposed to intemperance.[66]

However, in relation to the other, sometimes linked problem, he was at a loss:

> I cannot think what is to be done with the bad white men who corrupt the native girls. I know of one now who is flagrantly addicted to it, but it appears there is no law which will reach him.[67]

---

62 Report of Protector of Aborigines, *SAGG*, 26 July 1866, p.721

63 See for example, AFA, Minutes, 1 June 1866; 4 June 1867; 21 January 1868; 15 May 1873, SRG 139/2, vols 1 and 2. See also Report of Protector of Aborigines, *SAGG*, 20 August 1868, p.1144; 18 March 1875, p.507

64 John Walker, General Report on the Aborigines, 13 April 1863, GRG 35/1/791. The margin of the report has been annotated with an emphatic 'No!!!' at this point.

65 Report of Protector of Aborigines, *SAGG*, 11 July 1867, p.664

66 Report of Sub-Protector of Aborigines, *SAGG*, 18 March 1875, p.507

67 Report of Protector of Aborigines, *SAGG*, 11 July 1867, p.664

An increase in government interest in the welfare of the Aboriginal population was signalled by the appointment of a Sub-Protector in the Aborigines Office in January 1873,
and the reinstatement of the office of Protector in 1880. EL Hamilton, formerly teacher
of the Mount Lofty District School and clerk of the courts of Gumeracha and Mount
Pleasant in the Adelaide Hills, was appointed Sub-Protector in September 1873, promoted
to Protector in 1880, and remained in that office until his retirement in 1908.[68] He was
energetic and opinionated and the reports he wrote and gathered from others provide a
vivid picture of what was happening to indigenous people, at least in those areas of the
colony where there were mission stations or ration depots. They also provide insight into
the changing context of ideas, theories and debates in which policy was made and services
provided. In addition, while they continue the established pattern of providing comments
and data about specific, immediate health and illness problems, they also frequently
address broader, underlying issues, such as education, employment and land, which had
long-term and complex impacts on health.

Perhaps encouraged by Hamilton's appointment and by information about 'a probability of the government introducing some special legislation for the aborigines', Taplin
took the opportunity in August 1874 to present not merely a routine report but a list of
recommendations for policy.[69] He recommended that groups of Aboriginals be given
'a clear right to some portions of the land', since as settlement advanced they were
being 'pushed off their country' and such reserves as existed were often in unsuitable
locations. In addition, individual Aboriginals should be able to claim legal tenure of
certain sections of land, and 'occupy their land of right and not merely by sufferance'. He
believed they should be compelled to send their children to school, and that 'a law to facilitate the adoption of half-caste and quadroon children by benevolent white people would
do much good', if it prevented the children from returning to the tribe. There should be
harsher penalties for supplying the indigenous population with alcohol and punishment
for those who were guilty of drunkenness. There needed to be a law forbidding the
selling of poison to Aboriginals and another to control the number of dogs they could
own. There should be a means of summary trial and conviction of Aboriginals 'in the far
interior' who commit crimes, and when Aboriginals were brought to court, there should
be an interpreter provided. He recommended the prohibition of 'native customs which are
injurious and a nuisance to either natives or whites', and thought that the Aboriginal
population should be forbidden to 'frequent' Adelaide, which was 'a fruitful source of evil
to them'. It seems odd that Taplin made no recommendation about employment, since
this was a constant concern of his. In the same report he expanded on the difficulties of
finding other than seasonal work for more than a few of the available Point McLeay men
and implied that employment was central to their inclusion in the community and even
to their survival:

---

68 Raynes, 'A Little Flour', p.21; *SAGG*, 6 April 1865, p.299; 4 September 1873, p.1458; *Quiz*, 19 February 1904, p.13
69 See below, Appendix 4.

... if the natives are fraternally cared for and provided with employment I do not think they need become an extinct race. I forsee that if employment is provided for them, and homes, they may yet become a useful class of the community.[70]

It is not known what Hamilton thought of Taplin's eclectic policy agenda, although the record shows that he admired the missionary and his achievements at Point McLeay, and ideas he put forward in 1875 echoed some of Taplin's. Hamilton claimed that the condition of natives was 'not so satisfactory as could be desired'. As a result of their contact with Europeans they were less active and more helpless than they had been 'in their wild state', and census data showed that they experienced high rates of mortality, 'from causes that might, to a great extent, be preventable'. Their hunting grounds had been greatly diminished, they had periodic difficulty in finding employment, and the practice of supplying them with food and clothing, without labour in exchange, was demeaning and pauperising. He saw a great need for education and training for children and regular employment 'in profitable industrial pursuits' for adults. He judged the current system 'for the protection and support of the natives' to have 'accomplished a good deal' in 'ministering to their physical necessities and alleviating the hardships of their position', but considered that it had 'failed in checking the high rate of mortality by arresting the causes that are operating in producing the premature decay of the race'. He did not specify what these causes were but his report clearly implied that they were related to 'the injurious effects of our occupancy of their country'.[71] Nor did he specify which Aboriginals he was talking about, but continued the usual pattern of referring to them all as though they were one homogeneous population, and as though their experience of colonisation was the same in all parts of the colony.

However, the report went on to suggest that 'a much better state of affairs' existed at the mission stations at Poonindie, Point McLeay and Point Pierce, where mortality rates were lower and birth rates higher than elsewhere, and where the residents were 'instructed and usefully employed'. He claimed that at these missions

> the difficulties attending first attempts to bring savages under new conditions of life, and accustom them to civilized usages, seem in a fair way to be overcome, and the systematic efforts made at these institutions are gradually producing substantial results.[72]

This positive assessment was not wholly accurate. Hamilton's views probably involved some wishful thinking and a selective response to some of the details reported from Point McLeay, Point Pierce and Poonindie at that time. Taplin wrote of 'exceedingly good' conduct, increased numbers of children and the improved quality of life of children whose parents lived in cottages. The Rev. WJ Kuhn at Point Pierce rejoiced in a 'much more friendly response from the natives', and claimed that all of those on the station were employed at shearing, fencing or building. He was also employing 'wandering natives' as kangaroo shooters, in order 'to bring them under station influence'. He, too, judged the

---

70 Report of Sub-Protector of Aborigines, *SAGG*, 20 August 1874, pp.1667–8

71 Report of Sub-Protector of Aborigines, *SAGG*, 18 March 1875, p.506

72 ibid., p.506

conduct of the natives as good, but deplored the 'evil influence' of the nearby towns. At
Poonindie not many 'wurley natives' remained, as they were employed by settlers and,
according to the superintendent, the Rev. RW Holden, there were no complaints about
their conduct.[73] However, it was not the case that on those missions the residents were all
'instructed and usefully employed', and nor could they be, given either the inadequate size
of their land-holdings, or attitudes in the surrounding community, or both. Ironically,
Poonindie, where the ideal of self-sufficiency was the closest to being realised and where
Aboriginals were, to a larger degree than elsewhere, part of the regular economy, was soon
to be destroyed because of its very success.[74]

Nevertheless, Hamilton's recommendation was that similar stations capable of sustaining pastoralism and agriculture be established in other parts of the colony – in the
Northern district, on the Murray, in the Western District near Streaky Bay, and in the South-
East. Claiming to base his plans on encouraging evidence from Victoria, where 'the wise
liberality of the Parliament of Victoria' had ensured that the Aboriginals were 'prosperous'
and had 'pretty good' health, he painted a beguiling picture of what could be achieved:

> The object of primary importance should be to make these stations self-supporting in a few
> years. To accomplish this, reserves would be required of several thousand acres, carefully
> selected with regard to situation and soil, so that not only pastoral and agricultural pursuits
> could be followed, but also to enable hops, arrowroot, and *tous-les-mois* to be grown, which,
> under favourable conditions would be the most suitable and profitable industries; silk culture,
> if possible, should also be attempted. Occupation of a light and varied nature would thus be
> provided for both old and young, adapted to the peculiar disposition of the aboriginal.
>
> To aid in making these efforts a success it would be desirable to introduce special legislation
> of a paternal character, which would provide for native schools, making education compulsory,
> to prevent the children being kept away by their parents.
>
> A system of certificates might be adopted with great advantage, under which the natives
> could leave the stations and enter the service of an employer for wages, and obtain redress in
> the event of attempts being made to deprive them of their earnings. Evil disposed persons
> would also be prevented from withdrawing willing and industrious aboriginal laborers from the
> stations under false pretences.[75]

No such stations were established, but legislation of the 'paternal character' envisaged by
Hamilton was eventually passed, along with a raft of regulations which controlled the lives
of the indigenous population in circumstances which kept them apart from the rest of the
population and failed to deliver prosperity, good health or self-sufficiency.

A year later Hamilton was silent about the proposed new stations, and focused
instead on two threats to the well-being of the natives. The first was continued exposure
to 'the evils of wurley life', but of greater danger, to judge by the greater attention he paid
to it, was the impact of 'western civilization'. This led to increased vulnerability to disease

---

73 ibid., pp.507–9

74 For details of Poonindie in this period, see Brock, *Outback Ghettos*, pp.44–9, and also Harris, *One Blood*, pp.334–50.

75 Report of Sub-Protector of Aborigines, *SAGG*, 18 March 1875, p.506

and high mortality rates. He noted 140 deaths for the year ended 31 December 1875, 38 of them from consumption and 55 from measles. He also noted that European medical treatment was difficult to apply effectively. Aboriginal drunkenness, and the supply of alcohol by whites were still problems. He predicted that the extension of pastoral activity in the remote Musgrave, Mann and McDonnell ranges would spread the adverse effects of European culture, and characterised the motivation for the establishment of a Lutheran mission on the Finke River as being to protect indigenous interests from such effects.[76] This report also indicated something of the reach of the ambivalent blessings of white welfare: there were 54 depots for distribution of blankets, rations and medicines, 21 of them on pastoral leases, 22 at police stations, six at mission stations, and five in private hands.[77]

Sub-Protectors around the colony echoed some of Hamilton's concerns. Drunkenness was reported from several centres, there had been much illness and death from measles, and although there were many reports of employment of the Aboriginals over the summer months, opportunities for work were by no means universal. For example, from Streaky Bay, in the Western District, it was reported that 'some of them are employed on sheep stations, but the greater number do no work'. In Wallianippie, also in the Western District, 'there has been very little work done by them, from the simple reason that there was not much to do – in value, possibly not exceeding £70'. From the Lutheran Mission Station at Kopperamanna CA Meyer reported a little more fully on some of the issues involved:

> A great deal more could be done for the natives, were there not some financial difficulties.
>
> There is a great need for the natives to be supported, because game and food in general are very scarce up here, besides there are a great number of old, infirm, blind and cripple, who are unable to go for food. The young blacks cannot find much work now, as most runs are fenced; we make them go wild-dog hunting and pay them for the scalps they bring in; but in a hot season like this, they are not able to go far from want of water.
>
> We have succeeded in sinking wells, and have now a good supply of water in our station. We employ as many natives as possible in dam-making, building, shepherding, etc., but are not able to supply work for all.

These reports stand in contrast to the reports from Point Pierce and Poonindie where more favourable physical circumstances, the persuasiveness of the mission culture and the artificial economy of the mission produced different results. At Point Pierce, Kuhn had kept a 'hunting party of about forty of the wandering natives' throughout the winter months when employment opportunities were characteristically at their lowest, and paid them 'market price for their [rabbit] skins'. He said that 'every inducement is held out to every native to settle at the station', where they received rations, and 'regular wages, according to merit'. Similarly at Poonindie – 'a home open to all well-conducted natives, wurley or otherwise,

---

76 Missionaries supported by the Evangelical Lutheran Synod of Australia and the Hermannsburg Mission Society, Germany, left Adelaide on 22 October 1875 and arrived at their chosen site on the Finke River, in the Northern Territory, on 8 June 1877. Harris, *One Blood*, pp.383–407.

77 Report of Sub-Protector of Aborigines, *SAGG*, 6 April 1876, pp.636–7

providing constant employment, with payment for work done, in cash' – every able-bodied Aboriginal was expected to earn his living, 'idleness being strictly forbidden in the institution'.[78]

This is an important report. It implies that the place for Aboriginals is somewhere between the wurley and western civilisation. But where is this place? It seems that both Hamilton's and the missionaries' answers were that it was the missions or similar segregated and regulated settlements such as Hamilton had proposed in 1875. Opinions varied about the nature and purpose of such settlements. Were they a permanent solution to indigenous displacement? Or were they merely a staging post, until the wurley was left behind and safe entry to the west assured – through the assimilation of culture, attitudes, and aptitude? Evidence that this transition was being made was patchy and unconvincing, and its supposed drivers – education, employment and the embrace of Christianity – persistently difficult to achieve. In fact, during the last decades of the nineteenth century, hope about the transition from wurley to western civilisation co-existed with an increasingly articulated pessimism about the irredeemability of the indigenous race and its likely extinction.

It would be naïve to accept all the reports furnished to the government at this time at face value. The internal contradictions and superficiality seen in many of them raise questions about the extent to which officials applied a different set of standards and expectations to the indigenous population, and lend weight to the argument that they were presumed to have lesser and simpler needs than Europeans. The regular reports of Dr RB Penny, Medical Officer for Aborigines in the Tatiara District in the colony's south-east, for example, are difficult to reconcile with other sources of information about the health and well-being of the indigenous population. They have a tone of unperturbed complacency about them. In 1875 he had no complaints: the natives were contented, industrious, working for wages, using the proceeds sensibly, enjoying good health, were not fighting, and in most cases were not dependent on government rations. Three years later, nothing had altered his optimism or his glib reporting style. All were content and very industrious, and there had been no epidemics and no police complaints. This happy state continued throughout the next year, during which the males were all 'more or less employed' and all his charges were content and wanted for nothing.[79]

Periodic reports of the 'excellent medical attention' available to Aboriginal people are further examples of different standards being applied to their needs. Serious cases of illness were from time to time treated at the Adelaide Hospital, where according to an early report of Hamilton, Aboriginal patients received good care.[80] But this was not the norm. Some Aboriginal people could receive attention from medical practitioners, who were paid by the government to provide a minimal level of care. But as already noted, this attention was often difficult to access and was to be used in extreme cases only. Much of the time the only medical attention that Aboriginals could access was via the modest medicine chests of medically unqualified missionaries and Sub-Protectors, and in some areas even this was not available.

Complacency, capacity for self-deception and double standards were apparent not just

---

78 ibid., pp.639–40

79 Report of Sub-Protector of Aborigines, *SAGG*, 6 April 1876, p.638; 20 March 1879, p.795; 12 February 1880, p.544

80 Report of Sub-Protector of Aborigines, *SAGG*, 18 March 1875, p.507

in the field but at the level of the Aborigines Office as well. Sub-Protector Hamilton concluded in 1879 that the system was working well. Although other stations did not enjoy the advantages and natural resources of the colony's oldest, Poonindie, most were working towards the amelioration of the natives' lives. Missions still appeared to be the most effective mechanism for dealing with the natives, but he believed that the status of the native schools might be raised by making them state schools, as had already happened in Victoria. However, his judgement that the system was working well was belied by the 1876 colonial census figures which had shown the number of Aboriginals in the settled district to be 3953, of whom only 217 males were recorded as in the employ of settlers. Indeed, in the same report, Taplin once again named unemployment as the main problem at Point McLeay, and noted that it was exacerbated by the Aboriginals' unwillingness to leave their own country as well as by their inability to cope with white competition for jobs. Many found themselves in necessitous circumstances because of this and, deprived of much of their old hunting grounds, almost starved when fish and game were scarce.[81]

Nevertheless, in his next report Hamilton continued to insist that needs were being met: the able-bodied had no difficulty in finding employment, rations were distributed judiciously to the old, the sick and the infirm, 'every attempt' was being made to care for the sick by the Medical Officers who were responsible for the care of the natives as well as of the destitute, and at least in the regions of the Lower Murray and the Lakes, the natives were making quite a lot of money. However, unlike Dr Penny's exemplary charges, they were wasting most of their money on alcohol, and Hamilton wondered if establishing a savings bank for their use would be a good idea. A similarly contradictory picture was painted in the same report by Mr Joseph Shaw of Poonindie. The natives there, he claimed, were 'remarkably well cared for', and had 'all the necessaries of life supplied', including 'excellent free medical attention'. On the other hand, they could readily obtain alcohol, and the wurley natives, ageing and producing few children, would soon die out.[82]

Work or lack of it was a constant item in government and mission reports. The role of employment in advancing the well-being of the Aboriginals seems to have been taken for granted, and the encouragement of conditions that allowed it to be sustained was asserted to be one of the important functions and responsibilities of mission and government action. However, as indicated above, it was, from the beginning, a goal that was largely unrealisable.[83] Mission stations, as part of their plan of protection and acculturation and in order to survive as economic entities, attempted to find work for 'their' Aboriginals on the stations themselves. In most cases, this was bound not to succeed; nor was it easy to find sustained outside work. The experience of Point McLeay serves as an example.

---

81 Report of Sub-Protector of Aborigines, *SAGG*, 20 March 1879, pp.791–2, 794

82 Report of Sub-Protector of Aborigines, *SAGG*, 12 February 1880, pp.542–5

83 See above, pp.74–6. For an account of the very earliest examples of the inclusion of Aboriginals in the South Australian labour market, and the decline of some opportunities from as early as the 1840s, as a result of mechanisation and the extension of fences, see Allan Pope, 'Aboriginal Adaptation to Early Colonial Labour Markets: the South Australian Experience', *Labour History*, no. 54, May 1988, pp.1–15.

The financial difficulties of the mission were apparent from the late 1860s.[84] In 1867 Taplin reported his hopes that farming at Point McLeay would eventually make the station self-supporting, while at the same time provide employment for the natives and cultivate 'habits of industry, forethought and economy among them'.[85] But employment and economic self-sufficiency depended on land and Point McLeay never had enough, and what it had was not very productive.[86] The minutes of the AFA and Taplin's reports to the Aborigines Department frequently mentioned poor seasons and failed crops, and, as Jenkin makes clear, the small size of the property in relation to the numbers living there meant that serious underemployment was always the norm no matter what was tried.[87] From the earliest days, work on the mission station had to be supplemented with outside work. While seasonal jobs – usually shearing, wool-washing and harvesting – were relatively easy to obtain, they often involved considerable travel and did not provide an income sufficient to maintain the mission population at other times of the year. On the mission itself, as well as farm work, there were opportunities for fishing, carpentry, stone masonry, saddlery, blacksmithing, baking, domestic work, and even some teaching and missionary activity. For low wages and rations, the Ngarrindjeri built the plant of the mission – church, school, dormitories, workshops, store – as well as, in some cases, their own cottages. Thus they supported the 'civilising' and 'Christianising' program of the AFA, established a home and an opportunity for western education for themselves at Point McLeay, and at the same time locked themselves into the closed and artificial economy of the mission.

The AFA and its employees tried from time to time to engage some of the Ngarrindjeri in the external economy, but only within narrow parameters and without much success. They were repeatedly defeated by lack of funds and unsympathetic community attitudes.[88] The one thing that would have made a real difference – the granting of a substantial portion of productive land – did not occur. Writing about this in the 1970s, Jenkin foreshadowed more recent public health understandings and unwittingly reinforced the theme of this book:

> Had the tiny sum been spent in the 1870s that would have enabled the Ngarrindjeri to become
> independent and self-sufficient farmers, it would have saved countless thousands of dollars which,

---

84 AFA, Minutes, 14 April 1868, 12 May 1868, SRG 139/2, vol.1. These spoke of 'pecuniary embarrassment . . . such as to cause the gravest alarm for the continuance of the work'.

85 Report of Protector of Aborigines, *SAGG*, 11 July 1867, p.664

86 It was much less well endowed with land than other mission stations. The comparative data recorded by Hamilton in his 1879 report show that Point McLeay, with twice as many Aboriginals reliant on it than was the case at Poonindie and three times as many as at Point Pierce, had less than one-third as much land as Poonindie, and somewhat more than one-third as much as Point Pierce, Report of Sub-Protector of Aborigines, *SAGG*, 20 March 1879, p.791.

87 Jenkin, *Conquest of the Ngarrindjeri*, p.109. The property at Point Mcleay, at its largest, was an average-sized holding for the district, but it attempted to support up to 300 residents, not, as was the usual case, one farming family.

88 Jenkin discusses, for example, largely unsuccessful attempts at procuring apprenticeships and places as domestic servants for boys and girls from Point McLeay; a commercial fishing venture that never lived up to Taplin's hopes; an initially promising bootmaking business that did not survive in the open market, *Conquest of the Ngarrindjeri*, pp.110–11, 127, 207–8.

in the 1970s, the present government has to spend each year on some of their socially, mentally and physically sick descendants.[89]

Even the most successful of the many ventures attempted at Point McLeay were short-lived, and at best made only a meagre contribution to the well-being of the mission and its people. Wool-washing – of their own clip and that of surrounding properties – was begun at Point McLeay in 1881. Of course this work, like much other available to Aboriginal workers, was seasonal and it was limited in scope. In 1892, when there were about 150 residents at the station and between 150 and 200 'wurley natives' relying on it for monthly rations[90], wool-washing employed 16 men for six weeks, and in 1894, 20 for three months. This meant £200 per annum for the AFA and was 'the most remunerative and reliable source of employment' to that date. However, because of the increased saltiness of Lake Alexandrina caused by the construction of barrages at the Murray mouth, the venture was destroyed by 1902.[91]

One other source of occupation for the Ngarrindjeri and income for AFA at this time stands in telling and poignant contrast to the failed attempts to establish 'mainstream' businesses. The women used their traditional skills to make reed mats, baskets and other items to sell at mission bazaars in Adelaide. By this means £209 was raised for the AFA in 1900, the money being spent on repairs and additions at the mission station.[92] In similar vein, from time to time groups of Point McLeay and other Aboriginal people visited Adelaide as members of concert parties to publicise the work of the mission or to raise money. A group of 35 Aboriginals, unidentified except for 'about a dozen of the Yorke's Peninsula blacks' staged two performances of a 'Grand Corroboree' at Adelaide Oval in 1885 for a total audience of perhaps 20,000, including the governor and his party. In 1895 a small group from the Point McLeay Glee Club sang at the Adelaide Town Hall and at Government House.[93] Such activity, which aroused curiosity and drew positive responses from church and philanthropic groups in Adelaide, confirmed the indigenous population in the eyes of the broader community as a people apart: quaint, separate, members of a disappearing culture, people for whom special arrangements had to be made but whose needs were simple – in short, not part of the public.

While the mission at Point McLeay struggled financially from the start, the Native Training Institution at Poonindie achieved self-sufficiency by the 1870s. Through a flourishing farming operation it was able to pay wages to its Aboriginal and non-Aboriginal employees, to support those unable to work and to provide basic education and medical services. It

---

89 ibid., p.209

90 Sources providing some quantification of activities and provisions at Point McLeay at this time include a report in the *Christian Colonist*, 1 July 1892, of a visit to the station, and the Annual Report of the AFA delivered at its annual general meeting on 1 December 1892, and reported in the *Register*, 3 December 1892.

91 Jenkin, *Conquest of the Ngarrindjeri*, pp.177, 206

92 ibid., pp.177, 211

93 *Advertiser*, 30 May 1885, pp.1, 6; 1 June, p.5; *Register*, 12 December 1895. The tone of the reporting of the corroboree was condescending. The singing was 'a nasal drone', the music 'not the highest development of musical art' and the whole performance, 'although it might have been highly dramatic to the native minds, to the educated Caucasian it seemed to be what the Yankees call a 'very one-horse show'.

became increasingly less isolated geographically as land around it was taken up for farms and pastoral runs, and less isolated economically as Poonindie people succeeded in finding and maintaining outside work.[94] Brock argues that Poonindie's uniqueness rested on more than its economic strength. Its history of being peopled originally by young Aboriginals sent from Adelaide before they were thoroughly immersed in the culture of their own clan group and its subsequent inclusion of mixed-race children from the Port Lincoln district and local Pangkala people who went there by choice, meant that

> the Aboriginal community that grew up at Poonindie had no roots in any particular pre-European society ... the community which evolved ... was, in many senses, a new Aboriginal community. It started with nothing and over the years built up a thriving farm. It became self-supporting and offered friendship to its inhabitants out of which a new set of family and extended family relationships developed.[95]

This probably made what happened to the Poonindie people in the 1890s harder to deal with. From the 1880s, pressure mounted among local non-Aboriginal people and in parliament for the Poonindie land to be resumed and the Poonindie population to be moved further into the interior. They had been too successful. Their land was clearly fertile, and therefore, in the eyes of many, more appropriate for European use. The Poonindie people could move to the desert, which, despite evidence to the contrary, was conveniently deemed to be the natural habitat of all Aboriginals. The depression of the early 1890s increased pressure on the government to make the land available to non-Aboriginals and, in a pattern that has become familiar on every occasion where there is conflict between Aboriginal and non-Aboriginal economic priorities, non-Aboriginal interests took precedence. The Anglican trustees of Poonindie caved in to the pressure, the institution was disbanded in 1894, and by 1896 all the land had been sub-divided and sold – but not to Aboriginal claimants. Aboriginals who attempted to buy land were told that others had stronger claims, although as Brock argues:

> it is hard to imagine non-Aboriginal people could have a stronger claim on the land than those people who had lived on it for the past 44 years and 'improved' it from scrubland to agricultural and pastoral land. One can only conclude that it was considered that white people had a prior claim over non-white.[96]

The Poonindie people were dispersed: dispossessed and, with no return on their past stake in the land and no future stake in it, most opted to move to either Point Pierce or Point McLeay.[97] But they did not go without protest or miss the opportunity to admonish

---

94 Brock, *Outback Ghettos*, pp.44–9

95 ibid., p.39. This distinguished it from Point McLeay, established for the Ngarrindjeri, and Killalpaninna, established for the Diyari.

96 ibid., p.56.

97 A small number made other choices, but had to contend with considerable opposition and uncertainty. See Brock, *Outback Ghettos*, pp.57–9

the non-Aboriginal community. The following letter, signed by John Milera and Fred Wowinda, was published in the *Advertiser* late in 1894:

> Sir, we would like the people of South Australia to know of the refusal of the land board to grant our application for a few acres of native land for the purpose of making homes, as we are compelled to leave the place where we have lived and laboured for over a quarter of a century.
>
> We are ignorant of the principles by which the board is guided, but cannot help looking on our position as hard in the extreme. Away from here a few miles we will be wandering strangers, homeless and helpless, and yet we must go to join the crowd looking for work.
>
> We appeal to all fair and right-thinking men just to give our case a little thought and say if it is not a barren and hopeless outlook, and whether, keeping in view the dispossession of our race, it does not savour strongly of inhumanity.[98]

Soon after the mission at Poonindie was closed, and at a time when the capacity for the missions at Point McLeay and Point Pierce to resist government take-over was increasingly in doubt, the Lutherans began a new mission at Koonibba, near Denial Bay on Eyre Peninsula. A celebratory in-house account of the early years of this mission, published in 1926, describes an enterprise characterised by evangelistic zeal, naivety and a lack of engagement with the political and intellectual currents of the times. A late-comer on the missionary scene, in an area where there had already been about 40 years of European influence[99], the mission provides an interesting example of the capacity for a range of contradictory ideas to coexist and for new ventures to be oblivious of the lessons to be learnt from older ones.

In 1897 the Evangelical Lutheran Synod of Australia leased 16,000 acres from the government at Koonibba, where large numbers of Kokatha, Wirangu and Mining people were concentrated. This concentration was the result of pastoral intrusion on their traditional lands since the 1860s and more disruptive agricultural intrusion in the 1890s. By the end of 1898, the mission, as yet without a missionary, was in charge of ration distribution and employed a farm overseer who had set some Aboriginals to work clearing the land. Brock notes that numbers in the vicinity of the mission fluctuated, as the Aboriginals gathered for ceremonies or for work and then dispersed, using Koonibba 'as they would any other camp'. They visited out of curiosity, to get water during droughts, and because it was a traditional ceremonial ground – now with the added attraction of rations. It was a mutually satisfactory arrangement, especially in relation to the work needed to establish the mission. The farm overseer reported to the Lutheran mission board in 1899 that the Aboriginals had done for the cost of £30 work that would have cost £91 if non-Aboriginals had done it.[100] In this way:

---

98 *Advertiser*, 20 November 1894, p.6. Milera identified himself as 'Born and lived at Poonindie 29 years', and Wowinda as 'aged 38 years; 26 years at Poonindie. Sent there by the late Bishop Short'.

99 The first pastoral station in the vicinity was established at Yalata in 1858–60 and a ration depot was established at Fowlers Bay in 1862. Brock, *Outback Ghettos*, p.64

100 ibid., p.67

by the end of 1900, 600 acres of land had been cleared and 300 of them fired, a four-roomed stone house had been built, as well as a smithy, an iron hut, a stable, a hayloft and a wagon shed roofed with pepper bush and three tanks capable of holding 32,000 gallons.[101]

A missionary was harder to come by than a farm overseer and indigenous workers. CA Wiebusch, the first to take up the post, was by no means the Lutherans' first choice. He arrived, not yet ordained, from the United States of America in 1901 to take up what he called 'our Foreign Mission at Koonibba'. He was given no articulated policy to follow and he appears to have proceeded straight to Koonibba without orientation or communication with others working with Aboriginal people. His goals were frankly evangelistic. The focus of the education he established – teaching children by day and adults by night – was Christian conversion, rather than preparation for participation in the wider community. He taught in English, 'a tedious task' made difficult by the ignorance, superstition and 'very active and often antagonistic heathenism' of his charges, and regretted their continuing interest in 'their miserable corroboree dances and songs', which he described as 'lewd' and consisting of 'the vilest obscenity'.[102]

Many of the Aboriginals were reluctant to be converted. As Brock argues, their own religious and ceremonial life was still intact and vibrant, and conversion would have involved loss of adult status within their own culture. For them, Koonibba was a convenience and its attractions economic rather than religious. Wiebusch tried to deal with their reluctance by linking conversion to material rewards in a way that appears astonishingly crude, even by the standards of the time:

> Both Aboriginals and missionaries were united in a desire to maintain Koonibba as a refuge, but they divided the land into the two poles of mission and camp. Camp people received rations for work but were not constrained by the mission, coming and going as they pleased. Those in the mission settlement were hedged about by obligations and were punished if these were not fulfilled. If a person decided to be baptised – and for many it was a joyful and important event – there were benefits of better food and clothes, better presents at Christmas, increased wages and eligibility for a cottage. On the mission, they advanced from second-class to first-class citizens.[103]

Despite these inducements and the use of punishment and withdrawal of privileges for 'wrong doing', the elders and the traditional culture continued to exert some authority over the behavior and choices of the Koonibba Aboriginals, including those most under the influence of the mission.[104]

In time Wiebusch was joined by a school teacher, an assistant missionary, and a matron

---

101 ibid., p.68

102 CA Wiebusch, 'The Early Days of the Mission, 1901–1916', in *Koonibba Jubilee Booklet 1901–1926*, Lutheran Publishing Co., Adelaide 1926, pp.11–17.

103 Brock, *Outback Ghettos*, p.71

104 ibid., p.76. Brock notes, p.71, that this was less the case among those who were of mixed descent, who were uninitiated minors, who had had more contact with non-Aboriginals, or who were immigrants to the area. Not surprisingly, most of the earliest converts were from these groups

for the Children's Home which was built in 1913. He left Koonibba in 1916. In 1926, when assessing the achievements of his term of office, he mentioned the buildings, the size of the 'native congregation', and 113 baptisms, but had nothing to say about farm production, employment of the adults, the fate of the children educated in the school, relationships with the rest of the West Coast community or the long-term socioeconomic goals and plans of the mission. This stands in contrast to reporting from Point Pierce, Point McLeay and Killalpaninna where such issues had been articulated as matters of concern for many years. Although the situation changed somewhat in later years, there is a strong sense in Lutheran writings about Koonibba during its pioneering period, that salvation of souls really was all that mattered. The problematic context in which this occurred was not scrutinised. The mission, and the closed social and economic system it established were ends in themselves. 'The purpose of our mission is to bring the Bread of Life to lost and condemned sinners', wrote one of the early missionaries. While the government worried about what to do with the native children, at Koonibba it was all sorted out:

> we have struck the solution … Our Home serves as a feeder to our station school, to our church, to all the various departments of Mission activities: it is the hope of our Mission. It is the life, the education and the training of the Home that so appreciably assists in moulding the characters of our natives, that aids in making them reliable Christians.[105]

This reflected fundamental Lutheran teaching about the 'two kingdoms'. This teaching distinguished between the role of the church which was to preach the salvation of individuals through faith in Christ, and the role of the state which was to maintain civic order and advance material welfare. The 'two kingdoms' were separate spheres and one was not to trespass upon the other. As it happened, this Lutheran orthodoxy meshed neatly with the assimilationist thinking that prevailed in the secular community. It admitted no hint of indigenous agency. The 'inmates' of the mission were clearly seen as a people apart, passive recipients of what non-indigenous Christians had to offer, without the same choice about their lives and futures as the rest of the population, which included the mission staff and their families.

While imposed routines of life continued for Aboriginal people on mission and pastoral stations, and traditional culture was maintained in the most remote regions which had as yet been little influenced by Europeans, ideas in the wider community about the indigenous population and their future did not remain static. There was an increasing awareness that Aboriginals had undergone significant changes as a result of colonisation, and that various differences and imbalances had emerged within their numbers that demanded a response. However, there was by no means agreement about what was happening, or why, or about what the non-indigenous population ought to be doing about it.

Evidence of the changing situation was before their eyes, and could be confirmed from official records. Although it appeared that the indigenous population was declining

---

105 C. Hoff, 'Koonibba since 1920', in *Koonibba Jubilee Booklet*, pp.38, 45

in numbers, there were increasing numbers of 'mixed race' people, especially at the centres of Aboriginal population most visible to the people of Adelaide, that is, Point McLeay and Point Pierce. How were these people to be regarded? They clearly were not 'whites', but were they 'blacks'? What was their likely future, and, in particular, what was society's responsibility to those in whom the quotient of 'white blood' exceeded the 'black'?

Estimating the size of the indigenous population has always been a difficult and contentious task.[106] In South Australia, the earliest estimates varied considerably. In the 1840s, the Protector of Aborigines, Matthew Moorhouse, thought there were about 4000 who were in contact with Europeans, but his Sub-Protector at Moorundie, Eyre, believed that the figure was more like 6000. JD Woods, writing in 1879 but using data from the earliest years of settlement, including Moorhouse's and Eyre's, claimed there were as many as 12,000 in 1836.[107] There was a regular census in South Australia from 1844, but Aboriginals were not included in the count until 1871. However, estimates of the numbers of Aboriginals in 'settled districts' sometimes appeared in the annual statistical registers. For example, in the early 1850s, when the non-Aboriginal population rose from approximately 63,000 to 92,000, Aboriginal numbers were recorded as being around 3700. At the 1891 census, when the non-Aboriginal population had grown to 320,431, the indigenous population was recorded as 3134. There were, however, many gaps in the county-by-county summary, and no enumeration was attempted in the Musgrave Ranges or in other remote areas in the east and north-east of the colony.[108]

Despite many deficiencies in the record and a lack of clarity about who was being counted, it is impossible to read the available data for the colonial period as other than evidence of numerical decline in the indigenous population. The first *Commonwealth Yearbook* (1908) contained statistics for the period 1901–07, including those generated by the first commonwealth census of 1901, which enumerated 3702 Aboriginals, identified as 'full-bloods and half-castes living with full-bloods' in South Australia. The *Yearbook* maintained that Aboriginal numbers were 'never at any time large' and that in the face of European settlement they had 'shrunk to such an extent that in the more densely populated States aboriginals are, in point of numbers, practically negligible'. It noted that in South Australia, as in Queensland and Western Australia, there were 'considerable numbers of natives still in the 'savage' state' and warned that numerical information about them was

---

106   This is not only because of inaccurate or inconsistent records, but because of the complex political and ideological issues involved. These are particularly apparent when historians and others have attempted not merely to estimate indigenous population numbers but to account for their decline during the colonial period. A valuable contribution to scholarship and debate in this area is Bain Attwood and SG Foster (eds), *Frontier Conflict: the Australian experience*, National Museum of Australia, Canberra, 2003. While this focuses on the more specific issue of the effects of frontier conflict on population numbers, it also illuminates some of the broader issues in estimating and understanding numerical shifts in population. For the most comprehensive historical-demographic analysis of the population question see LR Smith, *The Aboriginal Population of Australia*, Australian National University Press, Canberra, 1980, especially pp.69, 143–56.

107   *Official Yearbook of the Commonwealth of Australia 1924*, Commonwealth Bureau of Census and Statistics, Melbourne, 1924, p.690; JD Woods (ed.), *The Native Tribes of South Australia*, ES Wigg and Son, Adelaide, 1879, pp.x–xi

108   Census of South Australia, 1891, *SAPP*, 1891, vol.3, no.74, tables II, XV

the result of 'mere guessing'.[109] An historical summary in the *Commonwealth Yearbook* of 1924 was prepared to be more specific. It suggested that in 1900 there where only 24 Aboriginals remaining in an area where Moorhouse had estimated there had been 1000, 'half a dozen' in Port Lincoln, and that it was 'doubtful' whether any Ngarrindjeri, who numbered about 3000 in 1840 and 600 in 1877, remained.[110]

That radical, and on the surface of it, unsupportable claim reflected a view – and an uncertainty – about who were Aboriginals and how they should be defined and regarded. By the end of the nineteenth century, at least in the settled districts, the notions of 'Aboriginality' and of clearly defined groups, such as signified by the names 'Ngarrindjeri' or 'Narungga', had been complicated by the emergence of a mixed-race population and by the considerable mixing of clan groups, mostly as a result of forced movements of population. These historical developments were a challenge not only for the statisticians at the Bureau of Census and Statistics[111], but more immediately for the people of South Australia.

There was an increasing awareness in several quarters that the indigenous population was not a homogeneous whole as had once been imagined. Apart from pre-existing differences among people of different areas and cultural groups, the population was now distinguished by differences generated by the experience of colonisation. From the 1880s the notion that the remaining Aboriginal people represented a 'remnant' of a dying culture became more common. In 1887, for example, the AFA described its mission at Point McLeay as 'a home and refuge for the remnants of the Lower Murray and south-eastern tribes.[112] In July 1892, the *Christian Colonist*, in a report on a visit to Point McLeay, suggested that what had been achieved there 'should point to the duty of making similar efforts on behalf of those remnants of the native tribes which still exist in various parts of this colony'.[113] The AFA annual report of 1 December 1892 quoted the Minister of Education, who was at that time responsible for Aboriginal affairs, as claiming it was 'the duty of the white population to look after and instruct the remnants of tribes who once roamed at their own sweet will over the adjacent country'.[114] People who have become mere 'remnants' do not, by definition, have an assured future, and from this period the idea that the Aboriginals were doomed to die out was frequently articulated or assumed. Their fate was linked to the acceptance of some

---

109 *Commonwealth Yearbook*, 1908, p.144

110 *Commonwealth Yearbook*, 1924, p.690

111 For example, discussion on the enumeration of 'Aboriginal natives' at the 1911 census defined them variously as 'full-blood aboriginals employed by whites or living in the proximity of white settlements', and as 'those in a civilised or semi-civilised condition'. Such definitions excluded many, and were ambiguous concerning half-castes. The 1921 census generated no data on half-castes, and commentary in the 1921 *Yearbook* explained that as 'half-castes living in the nomadic state, are practically indistinguishable from aboriginals, it has not always been found practicable to make the distinction, and further, ... no authoritative definition of 'half-caste' has yet been given', *Commonwealth Yearbook*, 1912, p.116–21; 1922, pp.1054–5.

112 AFA Annual Report, 21 November 1887, AFA Minute Books, SRG 139/2, vol.2

113 *Christian Colonist*, 1 July 1892, quoted in AFA Minute Books, SRG, 139/2, vol.3

114 AFA Annual Report, 1 December 1892, AFA Minute Books, SRG 139/2, vol.3

responsibilities, albeit vaguely conceived, by the non-Aboriginal population. Thus in July 1894, following a parliamentary visit to Point McLeay, the *Register* exhorted its readers:

> If, as some people suppose, our dusky-skinned brethren must inevitably die out, that circum-stance should but increase the natural obligation to treat them well. Let us make them happy while we may.[115]

And, increasingly, it was argued that the doom that awaited the Aboriginal remnant was linked to its primitivity, and was therefore unavoidable. The *Register*, reporting on the AFA annual general meeting in 1892, acknowledged the 'invaluable work' of the association, but suggested that:

> when the type of humanity is so low down in the mental and moral scale as that of the Australian aboriginal it is questionable whether it can ever be materially raised. Contact with the highest influences of civilization may give the native a veneer of the better qualities dis-tinguishing the white man; but it is easy to see how very thin in the great majority of instances is that veneer. Though the black is worse than slow in acquiring the white man's virtues, he is preternaturally keen in picking up his vices ... the best we are able to do for them seems to be to act in a rough and ready sort of way on the principle that the weak have special claims upon the generosity of the strong, and that we are bound alike by the dictates of justice and humanity to make the lot of the blacks as tolerable as we can – without unduly inconve-niencing ourselves – during that inevitable process of more or less rapid extinction to which they are being subjected.[116]

Although many commentators attempted the fine balancing act of acknowledging the value of missionary efforts while predicting the demise of the Aboriginal race, not everyone was so concerned. Frank Gillen in his evidence before the 1899 Select Committee Inquiry into the Aborigines Bill had no illusions about missions: they tried their best, but did no good beyond helping the old, the infirm and the sick. Speaking 'as one who takes the deepest interest in them', he declared: 'There is only one thing to be done with our Australian blacks ... You cannot do any more than make their path to extinction as pleasant as possible'. Since this was 'our obvious duty' it should be done in 'no niggardly spirit'.[117]

Embedded in such judgements were views that placed Aboriginals at the bottom

---

115 *Register*, 30 July 1894

116 ibid., 3 December 1892

117 *SAPP* 1899, no.77, Select Committee of the Legislative Council on the Aborigines Bill, Minutes of Evidence and Appendices, FJ Gillen, Select Committee Evidence, pp.94–101. Francis Gillen (1855–1912) was Post and Telegraph Station Master, and Sub-Protector of Aborigines and Special Magistrate in Alice Springs between 1892 and 1899. As a gifted amateur ethnologist, he assisted scientific expeditions in central Australia, and in partnership with the pioneering anthropologist Baldwin Spencer, made a significant contribution to knowledge about Aboriginal peoples and to the devel-opment of anthropological theory. See DJ Mulvaney, 'Francis James Gillen', in Bede Nairn and Geoffrey Serle (eds), *Australian Dictionary of Biography*, vol. 9, 1891–1939, pp.6–7.

of the evolutionary ladder, and deemed their situation to be irredeemable. They could neither escape nor withstand the impact of the higher civilisation that had taken over their land and compromised their culture and independence. However, many people, it seems, were able simultaneously to hold the view that individual Aboriginals were in a position to avoid the evolutionary fate of their 'race'. Missions were usually given the credit for this – or claimed it for themselves. Sub-Protector Hamilton, in a measured statement in 1880 commented on both the fate of indigenous culture and the saving power of the missions:

> Civilisation has proved very destructive to savage life ... 'The sun of civilisation extinguishes the feebler light of savagedom.' ... At the various mission stations a fair amount of progress appears to have been made, and the future prospects of these institutions are referred to in hopeful and encouraging terms. It would seem as if the new generation of aborigines were raising themselves above a mere animal existence, and becoming more susceptible to civilising influences, and showing an increased disposition to enter into useful and profitable employments.[118]

In 1888, the AFA suggested that a simple dichotomy had been created. There were 'two classes of aborigines: ... those trained in the habits of usefulness ... at the Mission Stations or elsewhere, and the wurley natives who must be more or less dependent'.[119] Of course, it was not as uncomplicated as that, even within the atypical and artificial world of the missions. The farm overseer at Point McLeay argued that mission-trained Aboriginals were 'far different from the natives of ten years ago', and that their education had produced some problems by fitting them 'for a higher and more intellectual kind of employment than that in which many of them are at present engaged'.[120] Indeed the question of what to do with mission-educated young people was to exercise the mind of missions and governments for many years to come.

Increasingly, such young people, but also others who lived not on missions but on remote stations or 'blacks camps', were of 'mixed race'. Questions about their future were especially challenging. 'Mixed race' or 'half-caste' children began appearing early in the colony's history. Their existence was recognised by an 1844 ordinance of parliament that made the Protector of Aborigines the legal guardian of all 'half-caste' children, and provided for their indenture as apprentices until the age of 21.[121] In 1865 George Taplin had indicated his distress about the proliferation of such children:

> I am sorry to say that the appearance of half-caste children is as frequent as ever. I wish much of it could be stopped. Do you think that any measures can be adopted with this object? I should recommend that a reward be given to the mother to tell who is the father, and that the man be punished on that information.[122]

---

118 Report of Sub-Protector of Aborigines, *SAGG*, 12 February 1880, p.542

119 AFA Annual Report, 17 September 1888, AFA Minute Books, SRG 139/2, vol.2

120 AFA Annual Report, 27 November 1890, AFA Minute Books, SRG 139/2, vol.3

121 'An Ordinance to provide for the Protection, Maintenance and Up-bringing of Orphans and other Destitute Children of the Aborigines', no.12 of 1844

122 Report of Protector of Aborigines, *SAGG*, 23 March 1865, p.266

While this kind of moral outrage was perhaps not widespread or long-lived, the historical record reveals some coyness or ambivalence about the existence of 'half-castes', and a reluctance to confront the circumstances that produced them, especially in the more remote areas.[123] Nevertheless, in the closing decades of the century there was no escaping the phenomenon, and in mission and government circles practical concerns about the future of mixed-race people and their place in society replaced moral discomfort about their existence. They were not dying out like the full-blood 'remnant', and many agreed with the assessment of the AFA that 'the extraordinary vitality of the mixed race is worthy of note'.[124] Their existence and assumed potential for assimilation prompted agitation for the passing of 'protective' legislation. On missions, in other areas where indigenous people were concentrated, in the Aborigines office, and in some sections of the broader community, two concerns emerged.

The first related to finding a place for educated young people of Aboriginal descent within the economy, since 'an idle native is very difficult to control'.[125] Hamilton, reflecting on the situation at Point McLeay and Point Pierce, acknowledged that:

> a number of young people, largely composed of half-castes and quadroons, are now showing intelligent progress generally, and deserve encouragement to become useful members of the community, or the greater number will lapse into a state of idleness and loafing about the stations.[126]

The Minister of Education agreed: his visit to the stations indicated that the 'half-castes' lived in 'comparatively forced idleness' after the age of 14 to 16, because of a lack of government action. The mission station at Point Pierce was seeking government funds to address this problem, describing it as 'an anomaly that the government should provide a teacher to educate the native children up to a fifth class standard and then do nothing further with them'. The mission's suggestion was for:

> a board of control, which might take the children – or at any rate the boys – when they leave school and place them in a position to learn some trade or occupation whereby they might improve and maintain themselves and become useful members of the community.

Hamilton wondered if the mission stations themselves could be given the legal status of 'reformatory and industrial institutions' with the power to 'manage a new race of educated half-castes and quadroons'.[127] These were complex questions, frequently asked, but no answers were forthcoming at this time.

The second concern related to 'rescuing' from a future among 'the blacks' mixed-

---

123 See for example evidence presented to the 1860 Select Committee on the Aborigines, and the 1899 Select Committee on the Aborigines Bill, *SAPP*, 1899, no.77.

124 AFA Annual Meeting, 17 September 1888, AFA Minute Books, SRG 139/2, vol. 2

125 WE Dalton, Secretary of AFA, Select Committee Evidence, *SAPP*, 1899, no 77, p.42

126 Report of Protector of Aborigines, 30 June 1904, *SA Aborigines Department, Report, 1902–03 – 1936–7*

127 Report of Protector of Aborigines, 30 June 1905, *SA Aborigines Department, Report, 1903–3 – 1936–7*

race infants and children whose 'whiteness' was assumed to make such rescue a moral imperative, and a future among Aboriginals unthinkable. Some of these children, especially those in remote areas, whose existence resulted from the unregulated conditions and marked power and gender imbalances of the pastoral frontier, were judged by non-Aboriginals to be neglected. However, there was no legislation to define them as such, and as Hamilton concluded, rather lamely, 'it is difficult to deal with them', since they 'wander around' with their mothers and 'their fathers are mostly unknown'. In the settled areas the issue was somewhat different, but the basic concern was still that 'half-caste' children be saved from the damaging effects of living with Aboriginals and kept within the influence of 'civilisation'. For example, Superintendents FW Taplin and D Blackwell at the Point McLeay mission were frustrated by the continuing influence of the local 'wurley natives' which resulted in Aboriginal and 'half-caste' children not attending school. While this had long been a cause for regret and regarded as a tragic waste, during this period it was increasingly being seen as a problem requiring government action. Taplin and Blackwell corresponded with the Protector, and the Protector with the minister, about the use of legal sanctions, including the withholding of rations and the invoking of the *Destitute Persons' Relief Act 1881*, in order to keep children out of the wurleys and in school, but to little effect.[128] Thus, ideas about 'protection' and control were clearly part of the policy context by this time, especially in relation to 'half-castes', but effective mechanisms for enforcing them were yet to be developed.

It was not just legal enabling mechanisms that were wanting. The capacity of the government to act on issues relating to Aboriginal people was constrained by lack of will as well as lack of legislation. While governments in other Australian colonies were passing legislation to 'protect' and control Aboriginals[129], the South Australian Government was slow to act and reluctant to make policy relating to its indigenous population a high priority. The delay in passing 'protective' legislation with extensive powers of surveillance and control could be regarded as a blessing – a kind of stay of execution – but the failure to act on other fronts exacerbated Aboriginal suffering and dependence. For example, insistent reports from the northern areas of the colony in the 1880s and 1890s about indiscriminate killing of Aboriginals, abuse of women and instances of neglect and near-starvation provoked some public interest and parliamentary debate but no constructive action. In addition, despite clear evidence that Aboriginal ventures often failed because of lack of land, nowhere more obviously than at land-starved Point

---

128 Raynes, 'A Little Flour', pp.26–7

129 Victoria: *Aborigines Protection Act 1869*; Western Australia: *Aborigines Protection Act 1886*; Queensland: *Aborigines Protection and Restriction of the Sale of Opium Act 1897*; New South Wales: *Aborigines Protection Act 1909*. For a summary of these acts and other legislation giving governments powers to control the lives of Aboriginals see Human Rights and Equal Opportunity Commission, *Bringing Them Home: report of the National Inquiry into the Separation of Aboriginal and Torres Strait Islander Children from their Families*, Commonwealth of Australia, Canberra, 1997, Appendices 1–7, pp.600–48.

McLeay, land was withdrawn from rather than extended to Aboriginal people during this period.[130]

In the face of government inaction, Protector Hamilton eventually took matters into his own hands, and in October 1890 submitted to the Commissioner of Crown Lands his 'Draft of a Bill for an Act for the Protection and Management of the Aborigines of South Australia'. The draft bill established no context for the powers it was proposing or indicated who needed to be protected from what. Defining 'aboriginal' to mean all aboriginals, 'half-castes' and children of 'half-castes' habitually associating with aboriginals, it proposed that the government should have the power to prescribe aboriginals' place of residence, the care, custody and education of their children, the conditions under which aboriginal children could be apprenticed, the distribution and expenditure of money voted by parliament, and the duties of local guardians of aboriginals, who would be appointed under the act. A Protector of Aboriginals would be appointed with full power to implement the act and its regulations, and there would be penalties for anyone acting against the act or obstructing the Protector in the execution of his duties.[131] This bill, and an amended version that Hamilton presented to the Minister of Agriculture and Education and the Northern Territory, who took over responsibility for the Aborigines Department in 1892, failed to excite the interest of government and no action was taken.

Eventually however, in 1899, an Aborigines Bill prepared by Charles Dashwood, Government Resident and Supreme Court Judge of the Northern Territory was introduced into the South Australian Parliament. It was widely regarded as inappropriate, reflecting conditions that applied in the Northern Territory, then administered by the South Australian Government, rather than in 'South Australia proper'. It was judged also to be impractical and unwieldy in its recommendations for a system of annual employment permits and for the control of the movement of Aboriginals from one district to another. However, it had the potential to provide the indigenous population with some protection against various kinds of abuse and many commentators agreed with the Hon. H Adams who reminded his parliamentary colleagues that:

> it must be remembered that they were not dealing with educated people, and just such protection as was reasonable in the case of children was only fair in the case of the aborigines.[132]

Debate on the bill in the Legislative Council was complicated by conflict of interests, as several members of the council were pastoralists who employed Aboriginal labour. The bill was referred to a Select Committee of the Legislative Council in August 1899 and the evidence of that enquiry is highly instructive in several ways.[133]

On many fundamental issues witnesses, who included pastoralists, farmers, mission-

---

130 Raynes, 'A Little Flour', pp.24–5

131 Hamilton to Commissioner of Crown Lands, GRG 52/1/286, 6 October1890

132 H Adams, SAPD, Legislative Council, 1 August 1899, p.43

133 Select Committee of the Legislative Council on the Aborigines Bill, Minutes of Evidence and Appendices, and Report, together with Minutes of Proceedings, SAPP, 1899, vol. 2, nos.77 and 77A. The members of the Select Committee were the Hons. F Basedow (chair), J Lewis, G McGregor, J O'Loghlin, W Russell, A Tennant and E Ward.

aries, clergymen, government officers and an ethnologist, held radically opposed views which did not provide the government with any clear direction on policy development. For example, some claimed that missions achieved a great deal, while others considered that they achieved very little; some believed that Aboriginal people were capable of being 'civilised', but others were adamant that they were not; some thought that protective legislation was urgently required to regulate conditions of employment, while others saw no need of it; some thought that 'blacks' and 'half-castes' should be kept apart, or that 'blacks' should be kept apart from 'whites', but others saw any such separation as an impossibility.

In other ways, however, the witnesses were in substantial agreement. Most considered that the indigenous people were of lesser intellect than Europeans, and like children who did not know what was best for themselves, needed a guardian to make decisions for them. They also implicitly agreed that the future of Aboriginal people within the broader community was a limited and circumscribed one. It seems that none of the witnesses envisaged lives for Aboriginal people other than on missions, pastoral stations or special reserves. None considered that the Aboriginals needed employment options or harboured material aspirations beyond those currently associated with casual and mostly unskilled labour, although several, including WE Dalton, the Secretary of the AFA and Pastor GJ Rechner of Kopperamanna and Hermannsburg Missions pointed out that even that limited involvement in the economy was in some instances hampered by lack of land.[134] The Rev. R Mitchell, formerly of Beltana in the colony's north, believed that the European takeover of Aboriginal land was 'more responsible than any thing else for their decimation', but his concerns were dismissed by his questioners, who attributed indigenous land loss to 'natural causes, incidental to the settlement of the country'. The issue of land and its relationship to Aboriginal employment or well-being was not seriously canvassed during the inquiry.[135]

No Aboriginal people were requested to give their views on the bill designed for their protection, underlining the perception that their needs were simple, and that non-Aboriginal people knew what they were. One Eyre Peninsula station manager suggested that as long as they were paid five shillings or seven-and-sixpence a week, 'they go to their camp and are happy', and a farmer from the north-west of the colony protested, 'Oh, leave them alone. The creatures are happy. Do not upset them. They will be alright'.[136] However, the bill allowed for the possibility that some Aboriginals might be exempted from its conditions and be treated as *de facto* 'whites'. This implied notions of acceptability, of making the grade: Aboriginals, unlike non-Aboriginals, had to be individually approved in order to become part of the public. Dalton was of the opinion that decisions about exemption should be 'more as to morals than anything else'; education would not be an appropriate guide since 'wickedness sometimes increases with education'. Although a policy of exemption did not eventuate at this time, the racist and assimilationist underpinnings of the notion were to remain influential for decades to come.

The Select Committee report recommended that the bill in its current form would be inoperable and possibly injurious to the indigenous population. In its place it proposed an

---

134 WE Dalton and Rev. GJ Rechner, Select Committee Evidence, *SAPP*, 1899, vol.2, no.77, pp.42, 44; p.10

135 R. Mitchell, Select Committee Evidence, *SAPP*, 1899, vol.2, no.77, pp.58–60

136 Clement Sabine and Christopher Wade, Select Committee Evidence, *SAPP*, 1899, vol.2, no.77, p.65, p.17

alternative bill which confirmed some existing provisions, such as services provided by missions and government support of needy and helpless Aboriginals. In addition, it provided for extended power for protectors to allow them greater control over the employment of Aboriginals and their movement around the country, as well as protection from various kinds of abuse that the inquiry had identified as occurring on the pastoral frontier. Once again, the government was not impressed. The bill was rejected and the matter was again allowed to slide.

During the first decade of the new century ministerial responsibility for the Aborigines Department continued to change frequently, as it had done in the 1890s, reflecting the low priority accorded matters relating to the indigenous population.[137] The reports of the Protector of Aborigines during that time, however, convey ongoing concerns about employment, education and a useful future, especially for the mission Aboriginals and 'half-castes'. Solutions were consistently seen in terms of greater government control and some of the missions saw their transformation into industrial training institutions as a logical and needed evolution. The issue of land and its relationship to the economic future of Aboriginal people featured frequently in Protector Hamilton's and the AFA's observations, but was never dealt with constructively. In 1903 FW Garnett, the superintendent at Point McLeay, reported on varied activity and cultural accommodation at the mission: 'socials, temperance meetings, entertainments, and young men's mutual improvement classes are held, and entered into with much spirit'. Furthermore:

> the men have been employed on the station [at] fencing, forestry, hedging, road-making, building, carpentering, blacksmithing, bootmaking, painting, rabbiting, and general farm work. A vermin-proof fence, four miles long, has been erected on the boundary of our Needles property. They have also been more or less employed by our neighbouring squatters and in the south-east, breaching, dugging, and shearing sheep.

This may have sounded very positive, but in fact the situation was grim. In the same report Garnett noted that, 'notwithstanding every economy', the increasing population, and the tendency of the mission to attract Aboriginal residents from elsewhere in the state, had 'completely overstrained the financial resources of this institution'.[138] Hamilton was aware of the problem. Land at the mission station was 'so limited ... as to seriously hinder the effort to provide remunerative employment for its large number of natives'. But he was distinctly unimaginative in finding a solution:

> Efforts are being made to overcome the difficulty experienced at Point McLeay in trying to provide its large number of inmates with remunerative employment by removing some of them to Point Pierce.

---

137 See Raynes, 'A Little Flour', pp.157–61 for a helpful tabular summary of government appointments and administrative arrangements in relation to the indigenous population from 1837–2000.

138 Report of Protector of Aborigines, 30 June 1904, *SA Aborigines Department Report, 1902–03 – 1936–7*

His relocation plans involved five families. The mission itself was of a similar mind, with Garnett reporting in 1905 that ten young half-caste men had been asked to leave Point McLeay and seek a living elsewhere.[139]

Such responses were pathetically inappropriate and ineffectual given the magnitude of the problem. The granting of a substantial area of productive land was clearly what was needed, but it did not occur. Some land which could have made a significant difference to Point McLeay did in fact become available around this time. The neighbouring Narrung Estate was sold in 1907, but the mission was in no position to buy any of it and the government failed to come to the party. The Point McLeay Superintendent was not impressed:

> It is a pity the Government could not have seen their way clear to have given us more land at the cutting up of the Narrung Estate for closer settlement, as with an increased area we would considerably help to make the mission self-supporting.

Hamilton's response was not to agitate for the purchase of some of the land but to worry about the impact of closer settlement on the mission, especially in relation to access to its customary supply of firewood and the possibility of a hotel being established nearby.[140] While this was significant as an episode in a history of government failure to take seriously the specific needs of the Ngarrindjeri at Point McLeay, or to plan for their long-term independence and well-being, it had broader significance as well. It was symptomatic of a more general government and community failure to confront the underlying causes of the issues – such as allowing the Aboriginals to become 'useful' members of society, controlling undesirable behaviour, and discouraging dependence and pauperism – which they claimed to be concerned about.

Perhaps this failure of serious intent was nowhere more clearly demonstrated than in the paucity of South Australia's annual expenditure on the indigenous population. The total government expenditure in 1905, based on an estimated indigenous population of 3745, which left many Aboriginals in the most remote areas of the state unaccounted for, was £1/2/10 per head, compared with £2/11/2 in New South Wales and £12/1/1 in Victoria.[141] However, this was an issue that was never faced. The assumptions of different and lesser basic needs that underpinned the niggardly annual budget for the Aboriginal population and the long-term effects of these assumptions on their well-being and their place in the Australian, and, indeed, human community were not what the policy debates were

---

139 Report of Protector of Aborigines, 30 June 1905, *SA Aborigines Department Report, 1902–03 – 1936–7*

140 Report of Protector of Aborigines, 30 June 1907, *SA Aborigines Department Report, 1902–03 – 1936–7*

141 Report of Protector of Aborigines, 30 June 1905, 30 June 1906. *SA Aborigines Department Report, 1902–3 – 1936–7*. Almost a quarter of the annual budget was needed regularly to subsidise the economically unviable activities at Point McLeay. Some sense of the paucity of the *per capita* provision may be gained by comparing it with the Australian basic wage, which in 1907 was seven shillings a day. This was deemed to be the amount required to keep a man, his wife and family in frugal comfort, and applied to all (non-indigenous) males working under Commonwealth awards. See Keith Hancock, *The Wage of the Unskilled Worker and Family Needs, 1907 and 1920*, National Institute of Labour Studies, Working Papers Series, no.152, June 2004, Flinders University of South Australia.

about. They operated on quite a different level and were chiefly concerned with the best means to control or minimise the problems – administrative, economic and, in a narrow and individual sense, moral – that had arisen from the colonial experience to that point.

The long-serving Protector of Aborigines, Hamilton, continued his efforts to secure controlling legislation right up until his retirement in 1908. Together with his successor, William Garnett South, and the AFA, he prepared yet another bill for a protection act, and this was introduced into the House of Assembly by John Verran's newly elected Labor government in 1910.[142] South, appointed to the position of Protector of Aborigines on 1 March 1908, made his position and priorities immediately clear:

> It will be seen that the aboriginal problem is rapidly assuming a different aspect than it bore some years ago. In comparatively few years the old type of native will probably have died out and be replaced by a race of educated half-castes with a sprinkling of blacks.

Many of South's ideas and proposals dealt simultaneously with the twin concerns of training and rescue that have already been discussed. He believed that the mission schools and the state schools which had taken over from them had 'worked wonders', since 'it is now seldom in the settled districts that one meets a native who cannot read and write'. However, they still lacked 'thrift and enterprise', and he was of the opinion that there was little hope of converting Aboriginal children into 'self-reliant, self-supporting people' unless they could be separated from 'the natives who still retain some of the old habits and customs of the race'. The solution was obvious:

> I am of the opinion that the young children – especially the half-castes – should be placed in an industrial institution, educated up to a certain standard and trained to useful trades and occupations and then apprenticed till they attain the age of 18 to 20 years. During this period they should not be allowed to mix with the other aborigines.

He warned that the current system 'practically teaches them to look to the missions and the government for help', and that unless radical action of the kind he recommended was taken, the state would 'long be troubled with an aboriginal problem in the shape of a lot of nomadic half-caste mendicants'.[143] In other words, South wanted Aboriginal children to become 'State children', and if this occurred, he looked forward with naive confidence to the disappearance of the race:

> In dealing with these children it should not be forgotten that each succeeding generation will undoubtedly become whiter, as the children of half-castes are as a rule much whiter than their parents; and no doubt the process will continue until the black will altogether disappear. There are now but comparatively few full-blooded natives left in the settled districts, most of whom

---

142 For discussion on this bill and the ensuing *Aborigines Act* of 1911, see below, pp.125–30. William Garnett South had been a clerk in the South Australian Police Department prior to his appointment as Protector of Aborigines, and before that had been in charge of police and Aboriginal trackers at Alice Springs. Raynes, *'A Little Flour'*, p.33.

143 Report of Protector of Aborigines, 30 June 1908, *SA Aborigines Department Report, 1902–03 – 1936–7*; *SAPP*, no.30, 1910

are old people; and in the far North a similar state of affairs is increasingly evident. The white blood, being the stronger, must in the end prevail, especially as some of the women are legitimately and illegitimately mating with white men. From this it is evident that the ultimate end of the Australian aboriginal is to be merged in the main population, consequently the sooner they are physically and morally improved the better for the elite race. I think that all half-caste children at least should be gathered in, instead of being left in the camps, where they are often subjected to the brutalising customs and ceremonial operations still prevalent in outlying districts.

South's attention extended beyond the children. He also had a solution for those old natives who hung around the city, begging and drinking, and thus were 'a source of trouble': 'they should all be placed and kept on a reserve by themselves, separate from the well-behaved natives'.[144]

Although there was still no legislation in South Australia for the protection and control of the Aboriginal population, some elements of 'protection' were nevertheless being achieved. In 1910 South reported that during the year several 'half-caste' children had been taken into care by the State Children's Department, 'with most encouraging results':

> The children are thriving and happy and will, I feel confident, grow up self-supporting members of the community, as they will know nothing of the habits of the aborigines and will be given an occupation.

He acknowledged that there had been some public opposition to this, but declared that it sprang from a failure 'to grasp the seriousness of the situation now facing South Australia'.[145]

His next annual report spelled out his thinking even more clearly. It was accompanied by photos of children, varying in age from infancy to perhaps 12 or 14 years, 'rescued' by the police from 'the Blacks' camps' in 'the interior', at the request of the Protector and the State Children's Council. The captions drew attention particularly to one nine-year-old-girl identified as a quadroon, with a half-caste mother and a white father. She was described as a prime example of a 'nearly white' child whom it would be scandalous to leave unrescued. The dress, hairstyles and stance of all the children had been carefully arranged to emphasise their assimilability. The report said that they were all 'doing well, and give every promise of growing up useful members of the community'. A year later, they were still doing well, and had 'apparently forgotten their former wretched surroundings'. To underline this assertion, a comment from the State Children's Council on the progress of these children was included in the 1912 report:

> It was with some degree of anxiety that the council undertook the work of training neglected half-caste aboriginals, but the result has so far justified the course adopted, and has made the council the more anxious to proceed. Those taken are doing well. One little fellow is the pet and joy of the whole family and of his school-fellows. One girl who came to the department a rough,

144 Report of Protector of Aborigines, 30 June 1909, *SAPP*, no.29, 1911–12
145 Report of Protector of Aborigines, 30 June 1910, *SAPP*, no. 29, 1913

uncouth, heavy child, is now a bright, intelligent-looking girl, who is rapidly assimilating the rudiments of an education. If she goes on as at present she will become a clever woman.[146]

However, Protector South warned, 'if they are left in the camps it will not be long before we shall have a race of nearly white people living like the aborigines'.[147] This was clearly unthinkable. It was also, of course, at odds with reality. The mathematically neat pattern of progressive whitening, imagined by South and many others, was a fantasy, since 'part-Aboriginal' persons did not always mate with non-Aboriginal persons who could contribute to the process of 'breeding out' the 'black blood'. There were many probable relationship combinations that maintained the quotient of Aboriginality, especially given the unlikelihood of white women marrying men of Aboriginal descent. However, these realities were not confronted by those who assumed that whiteness was a virtue universally to be desired, and who clung to a dream of racial assimilation via dilution of 'black blood', despite the contradictions in the policies by which they sought to pursue it and the clear evidence of alternative indigenous choices.[148]

There is no trace in the reports of the Protector of Aborigines from this period of any apprehension that separating children from their parents might be a source of grief or loss to them. South asserted that it would have been 'to say the least of it, cruel' to have left in the blacks' camp the nine-year-old quadroon girl, who was 'almost white' and 'had scarcely a trace of aboriginal features'. Once she and others had been 'rescued', scarcely any traces of their origins or parentage remained. The salvaging process stripped them of their history, their names, their familial and communal links, their language and culture, and fundamental choices about their future.

There is little doubt that at the beginning of the twentieth century most non-indigenous South Australians agreed with Protector South that such rescues were acts of kindness and mercy. With the eventual passage of the *Aborigines Act* in 1911 the government gave itself legislative power to establish extensive surveillance and control over the lives, not just of 'almost white' mixed-race children, but of all South Australians whom it defined as 'aboriginal'.[149] The next chapter traces how the implementation of this act continued to exclude Aboriginals from society and confirmed them as a people who, on the grounds of their race, were not part of the public.

---

146 Report of Protector of Aborigines, 30 June 1911, 30 June 1912, *SA Aborigines Department Report 1902–03 – 1936–7*

147 Report of Protector of Aborigines, 30 June 1911, *SAPP*, no.29A, 1913

148 The issue of social status, at a time when it was regarded as acceptable for women to 'marry up', but much less so for men to do the same, combined with racist views about the inherent inferiority of persons of Aboriginal descent, meant that there was no place in this scheme of 'whitening' for Aboriginal men. This was continually glossed over by proponents of assimilation by 'breeding out'. This is dealt with in more detail in chapters five and six.

149 *An Act to make provision for the Better Protection and Control of the Aboriginal and Half-caste Inhabitants of the State of South Australia*, no.1048 of 1911, assented to 7 December 1911

Chapter 5

1911–1939:
A Dying Race
and a Rising People

The pure-blooded Australian aborigine is fast dying out. Already over very large areas in the settled parts he has entirely disappeared. With the march of civilization only a few years will see, in all probability, the complete disappearance of pure-blooded natives.

John Burton Cleland, 1928[1]

The people I am concerned with are not really natives; they are a rising people ... The time is not far distant when they will all be white.

William Garnett South, 1913[2]

These half-castes and quadroons who have been taken over by the State Children's Department are, in most cases, doing remarkably well, and promise to develop into good citizens, as they do not come into contact with the aboriginals. Being nearly white they will have a good chance in life.

William Garnett South, 1917[3]

On 1 November 1911 the South Australian Parliament passed *An Act to make provision for the Better Protection and Control of the Aboriginal and Half-caste Inhabitants of the State of South Australia*, referred to thereafter as the *Aborigines Act, 1911*. The Chief Secretary, the Hon. FS Wallis, in his final remarks in support of the bill, noted the 'sad fact that when the aborigines come into contact with white people they began to die out'. He believed that they 'did not deserve to be classed as the lowest in creation', as some commentators had suggested, as 'there was a great deal of latent intelligence in the Australian aborigines'. Therefore 'anything that could be done to better conditions would be done', and the bill that he was commending was part of that effort.[4] This chapter explores how this new legislation operated – within a complex context of burgeoning

---

1 J Burton Cleland, 'Disease Amongst the Australian Aborigines', part 1, *Journal of Tropical Medicine and Hygiene*, 1 March 1928, vol.xxxi, no.5, p.53

2 WG South, Royal Commission evidence, *SAPP*, no. 26, 1913, pp.11–12

3 Report of Chief Protector of Aboriginals, 1917, *SA Aborigines Department Report 1902/03–1936/7*, p. 8

4 No. 1048 of 1911. FS Wallis, *SAPD*, House of Assembly, 1 November 1911, pp.420–1

missionary activity, major developments in scientific and anthropological thinking, and emerging humanitarian concern and indigenous activism – to maintain both the 'dying race' of 'full-blood' Aboriginals and the 'rising' 'mixed-race' population as people who were not part of the public.

The *Aborigines Act, 1911* gave the government the power to control the lives of indigenous South Australians. As discussed in the previous chapter, the Protector of Aborigines had been seeking such power for several decades. The act cast its net wide by defining an 'aboriginal' as an aboriginal native, a half-caste living with an aboriginal as wife or husband, a half-caste other than a spouse who habitually lived and associated with aboriginal natives, or a half-caste child under the age of 16.[5] The act established an Aboriginals Department, responsible to a minister, and charged with the responsibility for controlling and promoting the welfare of all aboriginals. What this meant was clearly spelt out in the act, which constructed the indigenous population as child-like, dependent, destined for limited futures not of their own choice, and liable to high levels of intrusion and control by government officers. It made them, quite literally, a people apart, separately governed, separately provided for, and not part of the public.

Under the act, parliament would continue to provide funds annually. The Aboriginals Department was to use these to purchase stock and implements to lend to aboriginals to whom land had been allocated; to distribute rations and other forms of relief or assistance; to provide as far as practicable for the supply of food, medical attendance, medicines and shelter for the sick, aged and infirm; to provide when possible for the custody, maintenance and education of the children of aboriginals; to manage and regulate the use of all reserves for aboriginals; and to exercise a general supervision and care over all maters affecting the welfare of the aboriginals, and to protect them against injustice, imposition and fraud.

A Chief Protector of Aboriginals was to be appointed and would be responsible for the administration and execution of the act. He would be the legal guardian of all aboriginal and half-caste children until they reached the age of 21, regardless of whether their parents were alive or not, except where such children were state children within the meaning of the *State Children Act* of 1895.[6] His guardianship responsibility included being empowered to seek financial support from fathers of half-caste children under the age of 18. Any funds secured by this means were to be spent as the treasurer of the state directed. Protectors answerable to the Chief Protector could be appointed in prescribed districts of the state and would be the local guardians of every child in their district. The act gave these local Protectors and the Chief Protector considerable power over the freedom of movement of the aboriginal population and many aspects of their daily lives.

---

5 In line with contemporary usage, the act did not capitalise 'aboriginal'. However, for reasons unknown, it replaced the more common form 'aborigine' with 'aboriginal', used as a noun as well as an adjective, including in the name of the department and the title of the Protector. In my direct summary of the content of the act I have replicated its use of 'aboriginal', but elsewhere revert to my normal usage, 'Aboriginal'.

6 No. 641 of 1895. Prior to the passing of the *Aborigines Act, 1911*, attempts to 'rescue' and 'protect' Aboriginal children under the powers of the *State Children Act* had been complicated by a lack of clarity about definitions relating to identity and to the notion of neglect.

The authority of the act was underlined by the fact that no warrant need be issued for arrests in relation to supposed offences against it.

The Chief Protector was responsible for the general care and management of any property of aboriginals, including the right to sell it, although not without consent of the aboriginals concerned. He could remove aboriginals to and from reserves, and aboriginals who refused to be thus removed were guilty of an offence. Protectors, justices of the peace and police officers could order aboriginals out of towns if they judged them to be loitering or not decently clothed, and Protectors could move aboriginals' camps any distance they saw fit away from towns. The act made it an offence for anyone else to remove any aboriginal or any female half-caste or any half-caste child under 16 years from one district to another without written authority of a Protector. However, there was provision for exemption from these removal clauses. Aboriginals who were legally employed, who held a permit to be absent from their reserve, or were females married to or living with non-aboriginals or were deemed by the Chief Protector to be satisfactorily provided for could all be exempted.

The act gave the Governor of South Australia the power to proclaim some areas prohibited to aboriginals and to declare, alter the boundaries of, or abolish reserves. It also empowered the governor to grant renewable 21-year leases of up to 1000 square miles to missions or similar institutions, at any rent he saw fit, and the minister, on the recommendation of the Chief Protector and the Surveyor-General, to allot blocks to aboriginals not exceeding 160 acres of Crown Land, or to buy land for them to occupy. In addition, the governor could make regulations consistent with the act, including *inter alia*: the care, custody and education of children; enabling any aboriginal child to be sent to and detained in an aboriginal institution or industrial school; the control and supervision of aboriginal children in institutions; prescribing terms and conditions for aboriginal apprentices and prisoners; exercising control over the distribution of payment for work to aboriginals living on reserves, to ensure that it was for their benefit; summarily punishing misdemeanours with up to 14 days imprisonment.

The act made specific provision in relation to health. Hospitals could be established for aboriginals and the governor could appropriate any part of any public hospital for treatment of aboriginals. In order to treat and contain contagious diseases among the aboriginal population, parts of hospitals could be declared 'lock hospitals' and patients could be removed to them under the care of any legally qualified medical practitioner. Furthermore, on the authority of the Chief Protector medical practitioners could enter any premises, medically examine any aboriginal and order him or her to be removed and detained in any lock hospital. Any aboriginal not cooperating with such direction would be guilty of an offence.

Perhaps surprisingly, given that it was a persistent and much remarked-upon problem, the act had nothing to say about employment, beyond specifying that employers of aboriginals were to be subject to inspection and enquiry by any Protector or police officer at any time, and that in the case of the death of an aboriginal employee, any wages due to him or her were to be sent to the Chief Protector. This omission almost certainly reflected the government's and the community's ongoing lack of imagination about or serious commitment to the assimilation of the indigenous population within the mainstream economy, despite repeated talk of apprenticeships and industrial training. It had an unintended consequence: since the act specified no separate conditions of employment for aboriginals it could not be used to exclude them from the conditions of industrial awards.[7]

The *Aborigines Act, 1911* marked the beginning of a new period of non-Aboriginal practice and policy towards the indigenous population. It provided the legal and administrative context for non-Aboriginal control of Aboriginal lives until the next significant piece of legislation was passed in 1939. It created in South Australia an official period of protection, although here, as in the other states which had enacted such legislation earlier, protection, while employing segregationist mechanisms, was, in deeply contradictory ways, always assimilationist in intent. The act purported to apply to the whole population it defined as 'aboriginal', yet it paid little attention to significant divisions which had emerged within the indigenous population, except those relating to the quotients of 'black' and 'white' blood, and was slanted much more to the assumed needs and problems of some sections of the population than others.

By the time the *Aborigines Act, 1911* was passed, the indigenous population consisted of four distinct groups in terms of their relationship with the rest of the state's population. None of these was 'part of the public', but the nature and extent of their separation from it and relationship to it differed. The first group were those who lived on or were connected to missions, where there was a high level of imposed order and control and where comparatively successful efforts at education and health care had been made. In some cases, two or even three generations of Aboriginal families had lived in such situations. The perceived problems of this group were how to encourage independence and employment outside the mission without the accompanying moral decay associated with drink, gambling and the evils of town life, and, most urgently, how to ensure that mixed-race children became less 'Aboriginal' and more 'white' in their habits, values and aspirations. More government money and concern was expended on this group than on any other,

---

7 How significant this was is open to speculation. New research is questioning common assumptions about indigenous exclusion from the workforce. It is claimed, for example, that significant numbers of Aboriginals were employed in the pastoral industry in this period. Jude Elton notes that pastoralism in the settled areas of South Australia meant sheep, not cattle. The wool industry was unionised early and Aboriginal shearers were frequently active and informed unionists, well-travelled, literate, and knowledgeable about what could be expected as a 'fair thing' in relation to pay and conditions. Especially if they worked in mixed, Aboriginal and non-Aboriginal teams they were likely to receive award wages and to benefit from improved 'white' conditions that resulted from collective organisation, for example in relation to food, water, lavatories and sleeping quarters. Jude Elton, personal communication, 8 March 2004; see also Elton, 'Comrades or Competition?'. By contrast, John Merritt, in his *The Making of the AWU*, which includes a history of the Amalgamated Shearers' Union of Australasia, makes no mention of indigenous involvement in the shearing workforce. Indeed, his only reference to Aboriginals as workers is to note that they were used as a source of cheap, casual labour in the early days of the colony, John Merritt, *The Making of the AWU*, Oxford University Press, Melbourne, 1986. For indigenous accounts of inclusion in the workforce, which indicate the limited, uncertain and exploitative nature of much indigenous employment, see Mattingley and Hampton, *Survival in Our Own Land*, pp.117–33.

and increasingly the focus of this attention was on what was seen as the 'half-caste problem'. The nature of this problem was complex, and was connected to deeply ingrained fears about the unity and 'whiteness' of the nation. A central concern was whether half-castes, who were growing in numbers, were 'civilisable' and could eventually be absorbed into the general community, or whether their 'black blood', however, diluted, would prove an intractable barrier to this.[8] The focus of the *Aborigines Act, 1911* on this group is apparent.

The second group were those who lived in or close to the settled districts but outside the mission stations. Many had learnt – through the removal of other survival options, most particularly their land – habits of dependence. Some were employed, but their work was usually insecure and poorly paid and not capable of guaranteeing their well-being or independence. All were susceptible to exploitation and abuse by unsupervised contact with non-Aboriginal people. During the period covered in this chapter, these people sometimes became the focus of attention of small, poorly resourced, evangelical religious groups who established minimal services for them, often with little in the way of cultural sensitivity or political insight. Their activity eventually focused more government attention on this group of Aboriginals.

In the more isolated areas were two more groups. The first were those whose lives were to some degree 'protected' by their place in the micro economy of the pastoral industry. This offered them a very limited assimilation into European society, while at the same time allowing them to retain some connection with their land and culture. This connection tended to diminish over time, with the extension of the pastoral frontier and as a result of the difficulties of trying to live within two worlds. These people were deemed to be less of a problem for the government and the rest of the community than the first two groups: they had employment, and their situation provided them with the semblance of an identity and some attachment to place.[9] There were some half-castes in this group, some of whom needed 'rescuing', but their numbers were not as great as on the mission communities and in the more settled areas, and they were not seen as such an issue.

The fourth group were those from the most remote areas of the state who were still largely uninfluenced by European culture. These people – and there were perhaps one thousand of them on the North-West reserve – were largely unknown at this time and took up little of the government's attention. The *Aborigines Act, 1911* was not about them and nor were the deliberations of the Aboriginals Department which it established. However, during this period they became the object of significant attention among scientists and anthropologists interested in understanding similarities and differences between races and in recording the culture of a group whom they regarded as both especially primitive in evolutionary terms, and likely to disappear. There was some understanding that while the isolation of this group constituted a benefit to them,

---

8 For a useful summary of perceptions of the 'half-caste problem', see McGregor, *Imagined Destinies*, pp.134–41

9 In his 1924 report, the Chief Protector of Aboriginals mentioned this non-troublesome group: if able-bodied they were 'useful and appreciated' on the cattle stations; if old, infirm or still children, they were provided for by the ration depots, *SAPP*, no.29, 1924, p.137.

they would eventually need to be buffered against the incursions that would inevitably come.[10] Their adherence to their own ways was not deemed a problem: they would soon die out, and in the meantime their behaviour did not impinge on or constrain any non-Aboriginal goals.

The *Aborigines Act, 1911*, despite the fact that it had been long awaited and had a clear focus, did not lead to significant immediate action. It appeared to have upgraded the status of Aboriginal issues by establishing a government department rather than an office within another department to deal with them, and by renaming the Protector the Chief Protector. But the new language was somewhat grander than the actual provision: the department had a staff of only two – the Chief Protector and a junior clerk – and the budget remained unchanged. However, by mid-1912, Chief Protector South was reporting some action taken under the provisions of the act, and mooting more. The Aboriginal camps which had existed around Adelaide had been 'broken up' and the 'old, disreputable natives' transferred to Point McLeay, 'where they are well provided for by the department, and are much better off and happier than while begging and drinking about the city'.[11] In the same report South wrote of serious discontent at Point McLeay and Point Pierce and outlined plans for their takeover by the government and the establishment of more efficient systems of employment, education and training. His plans, which ignored the chronic and intractable problems of trying to support too many people on too little land in situations that afforded only limited work opportunities, would, if implemented, 'soon solve the aboriginal problem'.[12]

There were others, however, who thought that the 'aboriginal problem' needed further investigation, and there were calls for a Royal Commission within less than a year of the passage of the *Aborigines Act, 1911*. The parliamentary debate that preceded the establishment of the inquiry made no mention of the act and indicated that politicians were at a loss about how to proceed. It revealed a multiplicity of views about the nature and needs of the indigenous population and an apparent lack of awareness that the questions which it was hoped the Royal Commission would address had been repeatedly considered by missionaries, Protectors of Aborigines and concerned members of the public during the previous decades, and, most recently, by the debate on the *Aborigines Act*.

In moving the establishment of the inquiry, William Angus, member for Victoria and Albert, noted that, although his original intention had been to limit its scope to the insti-

---

10 In his 1924 report, the Chief Protector of Aboriginals also made mention of the people of the North-West Reserve, who are 'away from the influence of the white man' and about whom, 'little is known'. He mentioned them again in 1933, after he had travelled with the Anthropological Research Expedition to the Musgrave Ranges in August of that year. Rations had never been supplied in this area, and he was of the opinion that 'the longer they can be kept outside the influence of white civilization the better for their moral and physical welfare'. *SAPP*, no.29, 1924, p.137; *SAPP*, no.29, 1933, p.41

11 Report of Protector of Aborigines, 30 June 1912, *SA Aborigines Department Report 1902–03 – 1936–7*, p.1. In the following year South again reported this action, claiming that the removed Aboriginals 'used to infest the city and suburbs', but at Point McLeay were 'quite happy' and 'behave[d] themselves well'. Report of Protector of Aborigines, 30 June 1913, *SA Aborigines Department Report 1902–03 – 1936–77*, p.1

12 Report of Protector of Aborigines, 30 June 1912, *SA Aborigines Department Report 1902–03 – 1936–7*, p.6–8. This is also to be found in *SAPP*, no.29B, 1912, pp.133–4.

tutions currently existing for the care of Aboriginal people, 'on going more fully into the question', he was convinced that it should be broadened to include 'questions affecting the welfare of the natives generally'. While the scope of the Royal Commission conformed to Angus's suggestion, the preliminary parliamentary discussion, the inquiry itself and the report focused on conditions and likely futures at the four existing missions – Point McLeay, Point Pierce, Killalpaninna and Koonibba – and the issues generally associated with 'mission Aboriginals'. Angus made much of the financial problems at Point McLeay and the fact that the AFA was carrying a responsibility that had become too heavy for it, and that in any case, properly belonged to the state. He decried the idleness and lazy habits that were induced in mission Aboriginals by a lack of employment opportunities and argued that government takeover of Point McLeay and Point Pierce would solve these problems and allow the missions to be run as 'industrial institutions'. He claimed that Aboriginals from the two stations were 'very discontented' and 'constantly asking' for such a solution. He also declared himself to be concerned about 'the deplorable condition' of half-caste and quadroon children: it would be 'a shame if they allowed such children to be reared as savages'. Accordingly, he wanted the Royal Commission to clarify the relationship between the Aboriginals Department and the State Children's Department and to strengthen their hands in regard to 'rescue' efforts. While 'full-blooded blacks' should be well-cared for, half-castes and quadroons 'should be trained to look after themselves by the labour of their own hands'. Finally, he noted that there was much sickness among the Aboriginals, in 'outside regions' as well as in the vicinity of the missions, and he advocated the establishment of special hospitals for them, since it was 'objectionable that the patients should be treated in ordinary hospitals'.[13]

John Verran, the former Labor Premier, was strongly in favour of a Royal Commission, in part because of a 'restless feeling' among the Aboriginals, especially those at Point Pierce who were asking for land of their own. He believed that mission Aboriginals had 'been trained to a bigger vision and a better understanding of citizenship' and 'if they did not deal with [them] by legislation, [they] would demand their rights in another fashion'. He also noted that 'about half of those whom Parliament had to deal with were half-castes' and implied that they had accrued some of the privileges and enhanced needs that were a corollary of whiteness:

> They must remember that a large proportion of the people were half-castes who must be edu-
> cated. Some young folk on the missions were as white practically as other people and they
> ought not to be allowed to grow up there.[14]

Other members of the house agreed with Verran about the need to provide training opportunities for mixed-race young people, thereby saving them from the 'comparative

---

13 W Angus, member for Victoria and Albert, *SAPD*, House of Assembly, 6 November 1912, pp.859–62

14 J Verran, *SAPD*, House of Assembly, 27 November 1912, p.1098. As Member for Wallaroo, Verran would have had an
awareness of the situation at Point Pierce. In an interjection during the previous session of debate on the Royal
Commission, Verran had indicated his understanding that the missions had 'outgrown themselves' by making their
residents 'citizens and not natives', *SAPD*, House of Assembly, 6 November 1912, p.861.

idleness' of the missions and the 'more or less vicious surroundings' of their families.[15] The motion was passed on 11 December and the Royal Commission established on 19 December 1912.[16] It turned into a long and drawn-out affair, meeting on 19 occasions between January and October 1913, eight more between January 1914 and April 1915, travelling to all the South Australian mission stations, requiring the Chief Protector to inspect, on its behalf, remote areas of the state, and examining 77 witnesses before submitting its final report in October 1916.

The first witness to appear before the commissioners was Chief Protector South. He was examined at length and his forthright views and comprehensive knowledge of the current situation established the parameters of the inquiry and subsequently strongly influenced the report. In terms of policy and government provision, he focused attention sharply on the mission populations and on mixed-race people. Other sections of the indigenous population demanded less attention. He declared that outback Aboriginals were well provided for, although 'one or two more depots might be opened'. Compared with the troublesome and spoiled 'half-castes':

> the natives in the interior, who work for their living on cattle stations, are a different and better class of people altogether. They are no trouble at all. They develop into good workers. I have seen stations worked entirely by natives.

He was in no doubt that the 'old full-blooded blacks' were dying out, and believed that the chief cause of this was 'driving them into settlements like Point McLeay where they have been herded in old wurlies'. They needed to be fed, sheltered and cared for, but beyond that presented no dilemma for the government.[17]

The mixed-race population, who then numbered about 800 compared with 4000 'full-bloods', were a different proposition.[18] South's concern about them was not just that they lived idle and unproductive lives on missions unable to employ or train them, and therefore constituted a drain on the taxpayer. He was also concerned that because they were partly 'white' they should have access to a different future. His concern about 'whiteness', as has already been noted, was apparent from his earliest days as Protector. In his Royal Commission evidence it emerged as his fundamental argument for government intervention. In his view, people who were 'practically white' and who were 'gradually developing into a white race' needed, indeed were owed, opportunities for training and for developing the habits and capacities of thrift and industry. They were 'a rising people' and it would be a waste and 'a pity' for them to be 'brought up amongst the natives'. In response to persistent, hostile questioning from the Hon. J Lewis, he put his cards openly on the table. Declaring 'the half-caste ... a better

---

15 Oscar Duhst, Member for Wooroora, *SAPD*, House of Assembly, 11 December 1912, p.1302

16 The commissioners were William Angus (chairman), James Jelley, John Lewis, George Ritchie and John Verran.

17 WG South, Royal Commission evidence, *SAPP*, no.26, 1913, pp.2, 8

18 These numbers are the ones consistently claimed by South and others working in the field at that time, and are the ones on which budgets and calculations of *per capita* expenditure were made. They do not include indigenous people living in the most remote regions who had no significant contact with the settler population.

man than the blackfellow' and 'the quadroon almost as white as we are ourselves', he claimed:

> The time is not far distant when they will all be white. If they were going to remain a race of aboriginals I would not trouble any more about them than merely feeding them. But you have another race to deal with and it is increasing in numbers.[19]

He was under no illusion however that this 'rising people' were as yet sufficiently 'white' to be treated as part of the general public, that is, as real 'whites', and outlined a program of government training and control that would aid them in their journey towards that end. In the first place, the government should assume control of the mission stations at Point McLeay and Point Pierce. These stations were 'too much of charity concerns' where the natives were 'reared in idleness' and not trained to be useful members of society. Indeed the mission upbringing had 'unsuited them to earn a living in competition with white men'. He was particularly critical of the 'ridiculous' industrial management at Point McLeay, where the people could 'come and go as they like[d]' and said he would 'put the natives on wages and expect a fair day's work for a fair day's wage'. He was also critical of the situation at Point Pierce, showing how its much-praised self-sufficiency resulted from the subletting of much of the mission's land to non-Aboriginal share farmers. While this arrangement was financially profitable, it deprived the Aboriginal residents of any stake in the land, and restricted their employment and earning opportunities to the extent that most were still partly reliant on rations. South's opposition to this system was substantial and complex. He had a philosophical objection to 'bring[ing] up natives on the earnings of white people', and to white farmers profiting from land which had been set aside for the benefit of Aboriginals. He believed the Aboriginals should have the opportunity of working the land themselves and acquiring a permanent stake in it. However, although 'they are not exactly natives, they are practically white people – intelligent white people, as good workmen as anyone else', the land should not be handed over immediately or to all comers. A deputation of Point Pierce men had waited on Premier Verran in April 1912, asking to be provided with 300-acre blocks, but South argued against this, since 'they have been brought up practically on charity, and I doubt if any of them would make a success on their own account'.[20]

South's suggested solution was for the government to take over the control of Point McLeay and Point Pierce missions, and to run them as industrial institutions. By this he meant that training in farming skills, trades and habits of industry and thrift be provided, and that the stations be places where:

> the old and infirm could and would be better cared for, and the able-bodied ones made to work for their own support. Charity could be entirely discontinued by paying regular wages, out of which they would have to support themselves and their families.[21]

---

19 WG South, Royal Commission evidence, *SAPP*, no.26, 1913, pp.6–7, 11–12

20 ibid., pp.3–5, 9–10

21 ibid., p.4

He insisted that the government could run the stations more efficiently than the missions, and provide better care and training opportunities for the Aboriginals, at only a little extra cost. When questioned about how government control could effect improvements, he said, 'I would put the natives on wages and expect a fair day's work for a fair day's wage'. What stood in the way of this at the present, he maintained, especially at Point McLeay, was the mission staff's lack of 'control of the natives'. This assertion followed immediately on a discussion of the chronic imbalance between numbers and land at Point McLeay. South was well aware of this imbalance and its effects on the capacity of the mission to achieve self-sufficiency or to provide work for its residents. He was also aware of the historic problems of finding work for them outside the mission, yet he still asserted that the government, if in charge, would be able to get the Aboriginals working. Questioning by the Royal Commissioners about this focused less on where the jobs were to be found and the barriers that existed in the community to the employment of Aboriginals, than on the presumed character and capacities of the indigenous population. South was convinced that the Aboriginals themselves would welcome government control:

> the people are discontented with their being kept at mission stations and fed on rations. I think
> if you are going among them you will find that they are not at all satisfied with being brought
> up on charity.

They needed 'a little nursing still', but this would take the form of 'lucrative employment', and later, as 'a reward to good natives when they have shown themselves worthy to receive it', some could be granted land.[22]

Indigenous testimony before the Royal Commission contributed significantly to the discussion about employment and land and provided a counter to some of South's views.[23] Men from Point McLeay confirmed claims that residents were often unemployed, but were clear that this was because of a lack of opportunity to work, or in some cases to inappropriate training, and not because of a native disposition to idleness. David Unaipon, later to be recognised for his leadership of his people and his creative talents and achievements, told the commissioners that he had done 'nothing in particular ... just odds and ends about the mission station, nothing very important', for ten or twelve years. He confirmed that there was dissatisfaction at the mission about inability to find work, lack of training for the children and a program that had 'unfitted many men for outside work' and had trained them to 'become parasites'. He favoured government takeover of the mission, believing it would lead to better training, more work and perhaps even more land.[24] Others from Point McLeay told a similar story. Daniel Wilson said there was no work and

---

22 ibid., pp.9–11. South's inconsistency about the economic basis of the problems at Point McLeay is all the more interesting in relation to his assessment of the short-lived private mission venture at Manunka, on the River Murray near Mannum. He was adamant that this had been a useless initiative, and had no patience with the 'herding' of Aboriginals on small pieces of land, to live 'in idleness' on government rations in a situation that offered no employment opportunities. pp.7–8. See also Mrs Janet Matthews (founder of Manunka mission), Royal Commission evidence, *SAPP*, no. 26, 1913, pp.57–8

23 The Royal Commission examined nine indigenous witnesses from Point McLeay, five from Point Pierce, four from Koonibba and two from Mount Serle station.

that 'we are simply knocking about the place'. John Wilson, senior, thought that there was work on the station for only half a dozen men, and Philip Rigney claimed that there were opportunities in the district, outside the mission, for only one-third of the mission's employable residents. Opinions differed about this outside work. John Wilson, senior, had been shearing for 37 years and claimed that there had been 'no objection whatever on the part of the whites to work with the natives at shearing or farm work'. Rigney noted that Aboriginal workers earned wages equal to those paid to non-Aboriginal workers in situations where a union rate applied, as it did in shearing. However, Pompey Jackson, who had worked at the neighbouring Narrung station for 33 years, had never had the opportunity to do shearing:

> I have found in my experience that there is an objection on the part of the white workers to working with the natives at shearing and farm work, because they do not want the natives to take the bread out of their mouths.

Closely questioned by the commissioners, Jackson remained adamant that there was not enough work to go around, and although at 64 years of age he considered himself ready to stop working, he was in favour of Aboriginals being given land they could work on their own account. The Point McLeay witnesses were of one mind that there were twenty men who could immediately make effective use of such an opportunity.[25]

The testimony of two men in particular constitutes a moving contrast to the assumptions of laziness and lack of initiative that were both implicit and explicit in the questioning of the Royal Commissioners and in the wider community attitudes that they reflected. Alfred Cameron had a 220-acre farm on the Coorong and a family of twelve to support. He told of his many abortive appeals to the AFA, the mission superintendent, the Protector of Aborigines and the Land Board in his effort to get more land, so that he could provide adequate pasture for his cows. Henry Lampard told a similar tale of thwarted hopes:

> I have been away from the mission station for 18 or 19 years. I tried my best because I wanted to get away from here with my boys. I have always thought that honestly earned bread is the best. I have a little piece of land – 120 acres – on the Coorong. It is fenced and I have a house on it. We have ploughed all of it that we can. We are growing hay and a little oats and barley. My boys are going on with dairying. Last year we had to come back to the mission station. I had to bring my stock from my farm on the Coorong to the mission station. And the

---

24 David Unaipon, Royal Commission evidence, *SAPP*, no.26, 1913, pp.32–4. For a summary assessment of Unaipon's life and achievements, see Philip Jones, 'Unaipon, David (1872–1967)', in John Ritchie (ed.), *Australian Dictionary of Biography*, vol.12, 1891–1939, Melbourne University Press, Carlton, Victoria, 1990, pp.303–5. A photo of Unaipon appeared in the Aborigines Department Report for 1907, under the caption 'An Ingenious Native'. The accompanying text referred to his 'neatly drawn design of a piece of mechanism which he claims can be attached to machinery and facilitate the attainment of perpetual motion', and said it was 'interesting to note that there are two other natives of a mechanical turn of mind at the Mission station *viz* Albert Karloan and Edward Kropinyeri'. See below, pp.165, 168, 171

25 David Unaipon, Pompey Jackson, Philip Rigney, John Wilson, senior, Daniel Wilson, Matthew Kropinyeri, Alfred Cameron, Henry Lampard, senior, Royal Commission evidence, *SAPP*, no.26, 1913, pp.32–8

mission is now helping me. I would like to get a piece of land. In the early days when I went to work the settlers treated me as a man. All the work the settlers give us now is a little bit in the harvesting time. The farmer must keep the work for his own sons and daughters. My cattle are at present here [that is, at Point McLeay] with Mr Cameron's.[26]

The Aboriginal witnesses from Point Pierce also stressed their desire for land and the independence they presumed it would bring them and their children. Some of them argued for this as a matter of justice. 'We looked upon it as ours', said Alfred Hughes. 'We are not quite satisfied. The other farmers came in and we considered we should have been here instead of them'. Joe Edwards agreed:

> We always understood this was our land, and looked upon it as our home … We are anxious to support ourselves. We have grown beyond the mission life, and if we remained here another 50 years we would not be any further advanced.

Tom Adams, senior, claiming that they were 'all very anxious that some of the most suitable ones should be put on the land', made a modest suggestion: 'give say half a dozen a start as a trial and we could judge by their efforts whether the scheme would be likely to prove successful'.[27] This fitted with the suggestions of the Point Pierce superintendent, Francis Garnett. Garnett was in favour of all the employable men being moved from the closed mission system and being placed on the land where they would benefit from the 'uplifting influence of a white environment', but suggested starting experimentally with just two men. He acknowledged that, as things were, with the Aboriginals dependent on the surrounding European population for work, 'the bulk of [his] boys' were under-employed. He put some of that down to racism:

> White men object to work at trades along with aborigines. The objection to colour comes in, and the aborigines often feel it. Even at shearing sheds for instance all around the lakes, possibly you know the station owner would allot one side of the board to the natives and the other side to the white men. It is necessary to separate them for the peace of the workmen. That becomes a practical difficulty in the way of the natives learning trades, such as being carpenters … People do not want the aborigine in trades.[28]

The commissioners questioned Garnett at length about his views on the capacity and state of readiness of Aboriginals to mange their own affairs, but treated him with courtesy throughout. However, their interrogation of the Aboriginal witnesses often took on the character of a quiz. They seemed intent on trapping the Aboriginals into giving inconsistent answers, revealing ignorance about the prices of stock or lack of detailed thought about their own and their children's futures, or demonstrating poor management of money. The session closed with an outburst from Angus, the chairman of the Royal Commission,

---

26 Alfred Cameron, Henry Lampard, senior, Royal Commission evidence, *SAPP*, no.26, 1913, pp.37–8

27 Alfred Hughes, Tom Adams, Joe Edwards, Royal Commission evidence, *SAPP*, no.26, 1913, pp.112–19.

28 Francis Garnett, Royal Commission evidence, *SAPP*, no.26, 1913, pp.68–71

which is breathtaking in its indifference to the circumstances that had prevailed since European settlement had deprived indigenous people of their land, radically disrupted their culture, and, in the case of the Point Pierce people, closely controlled their lives on a mission:

> You have the whole Commonwealth of Australia open to you just the same as other responsible citizens, and if you have gone beyond being helped by the station, then you should go out into the world and help yourself. I think you people have a wrong idea in your mind regarding this reserve. It was never intended by the Parliament that the station should support you. It was established to assist you into the way of supporting yourselves, and when you have received the necessary training and assistance from the mission it is your duty as well as your privilege to go outside and get employment to maintain yourself and those depending on you. I wish you would realise that.[29]

In other words, Angus was telling these people to show initiative, to exercise independence, to be in control of their own destinies, to be 'just the same as other responsible citizens' – in short, to be part of the public. This is deeply ironical given that government and mission policies, practices and provision to this point had effectively denied the indigenous population all these possibilities, and clearly had never assumed that Aboriginal people were the same as 'other responsible citizens'. Indeed, it had always treated them as a lesser race and a people apart. It is not known how the Point Pierce witnesses reacted to Angus's outburst. But since the whole tenor of their evidence had been concerned with their inability to assume greater control over their lives and futures, and since their requests – not only for land, but also for standard wages and the opportunity to control their own spending – had been treated with scant respect, and in some cases ridiculed, they must surely have found the messages of the commissioners confusing, to say the least.

Another major focus of the Royal Commission was the care and training of half-caste children. The leading witness, Chief Protector South, had much to say on this. He was clear, as he had been since his appointment in 1908, that 'rescuing' half-caste children from the 'blacks' camps' and bringing them up as whites was an urgent government responsibility. He told the Royal Commission that he had not made use of the powers that were provided by the *Aborigines Act, 1911*, and was still relying on the 1895 *State Children Act*. He admitted that the system was not working well. He had 'found difficulty in getting possession of the children in the interior', since the mothers were often reluctant to part with them and the police, who effected the actual 'rescues', often sympathised with the mothers.[30] An additional problem, identified by James Gray, Secretary of the State Children's Council, was 'a disposition on the part of the magistrates to think that an aboriginal child should be brought up in a wurley'.[31] South, while claiming to understand the mothers' feelings, believed that the children's interests must be put first, and that involved removing them from the wurley. He argued his case in the following terms:

---

29 William Angus, chairman, Royal Commission evidence, *SAPP*, no.26, 1913, pp.119

30 WG South, Royal Commission evidence, *SAPP*, no.26, 1913, p.7. By continuing to use the *State Children Act* he was relying on being able to mount a case of destitution or neglect in the case of all children 'rescued'.

31 James Gray, Royal Commission evidence, *SAPP*, no.26, 1913, p.120

The mother is usually a black woman living in comparative savagery and the child is the off-spring of a white man, and I think it is a pity that that child should be brought up amongst the natives. I think that those children, especially the girls, should be taken away from the blacks' camps, and brought up as white children. Some people say that they will go back to the blacks' camp, but I say they never will do that, because they will not know a blacks' camp. If you take a child, practically white, from the centre of Australia, and bring it down here and train it, it will not go back, because it will not know anything about it.[32]

Gray sided with South and against the magistrates. Acknowledging that it was not easy to get half-castes fostered because of the 'great prejudice against colour' in the community, he advocated taking them from their mothers at birth, claiming that even a week in the wurley was 'bad for them' and a year, 'fatal'.[33] Also supporting the early 'rescue' of half-castes' was EC Stirling, Professor of Physiology at the University of Adelaide. He told the Royal Commission that 'the sooner you allow the half-castes and those natives who have a greater admixture of white blood in them to merge in the general population the better'. With a cool pragmatism, he advocated taking the children while they were young, but not as infants: 'when they are a couple of years they do not require so much attention' but they are still 'young enough to be attractive' and therefore likely to be more easily fostered out.[34]

The Royal Commission also gave considerable attention to the other major aspect of 'the half-caste problem', namely the care and training of mixed-race mission children, after they had graduated from the mission schools. They too needed 'rescue', in this case from an aimless, idle and dependent life. There was widespread agreement among the witnesses to the Royal Commission, including the indigenous people themselves, that the children needed post-school training to fit them for life in the wider community, and most thought this needed to take place away from the missions, and would therefore involve boarding out. The appropriate training was universally assumed to be trade apprenticeships for the boys and domestic service for the girls. There was rarely any detailed discussion about how this might occur or what arrangements might be needed to make it work; there was none at all about other futures. Apparently 'trades' and domestic service, along with farm work, exhausted the possibilities open to and likely to be made something of by Aboriginals. Non-Aboriginals tended to argue for such training on two grounds: it was a matter of justice for children who were partly or almost white, and it was a practical solution to the injustice of expecting the non-Aboriginal population to support a race of 'loafers'.[35] The Aboriginals who presented themselves to the Royal Commission argued for the training of their children in terms of providing them with 'the opportunity of betterment', and most

---

32 WG South, Royal Commission evidence, *SAPP*, no.26, 1913, p.7

33 James Gray, Royal Commission evidence, *SAPP*, no.26, 1913, p.121. The system was not working as Gray would have liked. He tabled information regarding the 18 'State Children' of Aboriginal descent who were currently under the care of his department. The ages at which they had been committed ranged from two months to 15 years, with only seven of the 18 having been removed from their families by the age of four. See Progress Report of the Royal Commission on the Aborigines together with Minutes of Proceedings, Evidence and Appendices, *SAPP*, no. 26, 1913, Appendix A, p.126.

34 EC Stirling, Royal Commission evidence, *SAPP*, no.26, 1913, p.124

35 WG South, Royal Commission evidence, *SAPP*, no.26, 1913, p.12

suggested that this might start at between 12 and 14 years of age. However, one of them, Matthew Kropinyeri, of Point McLeay, exhibited considerable prescience regarding other non-Aboriginal agenda driving the proposals. 'On no account' did he want the children to grow up in idleness on the mission, and he certainly wanted them to be trained as 'useful and independent members of society'. But he was alert to other possible outcomes:

> In regard to the taking in hand of our children by the State to learn trades etc., our people would gladly embrace the opportunity of betterment for our children, but to be subjected to complete alienation from our children is, to say the least, an unqualified act of injustice, and no parent worthy of the name would either yield to or urge such a measure.[36]

There were two dissenting views from the general consensus about the training of half-castes. One was from Janet Matthews, the founder of the by-then defunct mission at Manunka, who believed they 'should be kept away from white people as much as possible', in order to avoid interracial attachments which she clearly found morally repugnant.[37] More significant, since they were representative of an influential strand of missionary thinking, were the views of Pastor CA Wiebusch, Superintendent of the Lutheran mission at Koonibba. He was convinced that the Koonibba half-castes of all ages should be maintained at the mission:

> We have about 12700 acres of land at the mission station, and as this class of people do best under some sort of supervision I have not been able to alter my purpose in what I am doing, namely, in giving them employment at the mission and making a home for them. It is when they are away from the mission station that the mischief generally occurs. If they leave the mission and go to the towns they have every opportunity to frequent the hotels, and the mischief is done there. If we can employ them at the mission station and supervise them and give them sufficient wages and a good home, and teach them and care for them spiritually, I think they are best off at such an institution as ours.

If the numbers grew, the mission would simply find more supervisors and put more of its land under crop.[38] Such optimism reflected the relatively sound financial position of the mission and its favourable population–land balance. But it also reflected a profoundly paternalistic attitude which, its unquestioned integrity and good intentions notwithstanding, was based on racist judgements[39] about the Aboriginals' moral capacities, and

---

36 Matthew Kropinyeri, Royal Commission evidence, *SAPP*, no.26, 1913, p.37

37 Janet Matthews, Royal Commission evidence, *SAPP*, no.26. 1913, pp.57–8

38 CA Wiebusch, Royal Commission evidence, *SAPP*, no.26. 1913, pp.47–8

39 I use the words 'paternalistic' and 'racist' advisedly, and not merely as convenient labels. Paternalism refers to decision-making and management by one party on behalf of another who is assumed not to be capable of managing and deciding for itself. Paternalism, while claiming to act in the best interests of those towards whom it is directed, involves an inherent power imbalance and an assumption of radically different levels of competence between the two parties. Racism refers to the use of 'race' or racial characteristics as the fundamental variable to explain differences between groups of people, or to explain consistent features of one group's behaviour or social position. Use of the category 'race' – rather than, say, historical

a failure to envisage or desire for them a future other than one dependent on and defined by the closed world of the mission.[40] For Wiebusch, his charges were people deserving care and compassion. But they were not part of the public and apparently did not have a claim to the choices and freedoms or even the rates of pay that the rest of the public enjoyed.[41]

In relation to this construction of Aboriginals as people without the same rights and needs as the rest of the population, the evidence of two witnesses at the second round of Royal Commission hearings is of interest. Wolfgang Reidel, superintendent of the struggling Lutheran mission at Killalpaninna in the remote north of the state, continued Wiebusch's paternalistic theme. He defined the purposes of his mission in entirely religious terms: 'Our chief aim is to make the natives Christian men and women, to give them support, and generally to raise them to a higher mental and moral level'. In his terms, of course, this was a gift of ultimate value. It was also making a virtue of necessity, since, in fact, there was little else of a more mundane and immediate nature that the mission could offer. It could not pay its workers at rates that applied outside the mission: 'If we put everyone on regular wages, we would fail soon'. It could not provide a future for children, but Reidel nevertheless argued against removing them even though that 'would doubtless be the means of improving them mentally and raising them to a higher level'. And while claiming that he would 'like to see them made honorable and respected citizens', he admitted that 'working as we are in such dry and isolated country, our efforts may not be so successful as they otherwise would'. Even in these difficult circumstances he did not support government takeover. Apparently, the Killalpaninna Aboriginals were to forfeit temporal advantages in favour of the eternal.[42]

The other witness to provide distinctive testimony was Daisy Bates. Her reputation as maverick anthropologist and welfare worker among the Aboriginals was to grow considerably in subsequent years, but she was already well known for her care of remote and threatened indigenous groups, her ethnographic insights and recording of cultural data.[43]

opportunity, social and political structures or economic conditions – as an explanatory variable, leads to judgements that focus on immutable characteristics of persons rather than on modifiable circumstances. Such judgments are 'racist' and are frequently associated with discriminatory and prejudiced attitudes and practices.

40 Wiebusch claimed that Aboriginals did not work hard unless under supervision, were not as morally strong as non-Aboriginals, and would not succeed in the company of other Aboriginals away from the influence of the mission, CA Wiebusch, Royal Commission evidence, *SAPP*, no.26. 1913, p.48.

41 Further evidence of this is provided by the later testimony of the Koonibba farm manager. JW Rudolph, Royal Commission evidence, *SAPP*, no.21, 1916, pp.6–7. For a later view of Koonibba's capacity to deal with growing numbers, see below, pp.152–3.

42 Wolfgang Reidel, Royal Commission evidence, *SAPP*, no.21, 1916, pp.17–19. Reidel's evidence confirmed what had been reported from Killalpaninna in recent years. See Report of Protector of Aborigines, 1908, 1909, 1911, *SA Aborigines Department Report 1902–3 – 1936–7*. For an account of Reidel's work as superintendent of Killalpaninna, and in particular the mission's practices in relation to payment of the Diyari for their work, see Stevens, *White Man's Dreaming*, pp.174–90.

43 For a summary assessment of Bates's life and achievements see RVS Wright, 'Bates, Daisy May (1983–1951)', in Bede Nairn and Geoffrey Serle (eds), *Australian Dictionary of Biography*, vol.7, 1891–1939, Melbourne University Press, Carlton, Victoria, 1979, pp.208–9

At the time of her appearance before the Royal Commission Bates was living with the Mining people at Eucla on the southern edge of the Nullarbor Plain in an area where the destructive forces of 'civilisation' were soon to encroach further as the construction of the east–west railway proceeded. She believed that the Aboriginals would be better off left alone, but since this was not possible she would continue to 'patrol the country' in order to protect them. When questioned about her purpose, she said:

> I think I have just adopted them. It seems to me they are my own poor relations. I am not missionising. I make my own life amongst them and they cannot help being moral when I am in the camp.

She expected the 'full-bloods' and the 'half-castes' who were already 'tubercular', as a large percentage of the people at Eucla were, to die out and the remainder to disappear through absorption into the general population. She sought a government appointment as Honorary Protector and financial support so that she could continue to 'help settle their quarrels and help protect them from their own people and the whites'.[44] The government chose not to support her, but her plea for protection of the Aboriginals via isolation remained an important strand in the debate on indigenous futures for many years to come.

In relation to health, the royal commissioners had only one major concern, and they questioned many of the witnesses about it. This was the one health issue specifically dealt with in the *Aborigines Act, 1911*: venereal disease. The commissioners appeared unconcerned about reports of tuberculosis, or about minimal provision of health services[45], and were clearly unaware of the complex health implications of the constrained material circumstances of Aboriginal lives and of the menial futures envisaged for them. About the contagion of venereal disease, however, and its threat to the health of the wider community, they were much exercised.

South shared their concern and recommended the establishment of a lock hospital – it 'need only be of galvanized iron and whitewashed' – on Wardang Island in Spencer Gulf, offshore from Point Pierce mission station, from which he presumed the patients could not escape.[46] Others, including Garnett and Henry Lipson Hancock, General Manager of Wallaroo and Moonta Mining and Smelting Company and a member of the Board of Trustees of Point Pierce mission, were less convinced of the need for a lock hospital for Aboriginals. Hancock certainly did not want one on Wardang Island, although Garnett thought that would be an ideal site and would require only a small staff and 'an occasional

---

44 Daisy Bates, Royal Commission evidence, *SAPP*, no.21, 1916, pp.30–5

45 It was not just Bates who mentioned tuberculosis. South indicated that it had 'got among them to a slight extent at Point McLeay and also at most other places'. He mentioned that there were medical men who could be called on to treat sick Aboriginals in various localities, and that public hospitals would admit them, though 'of course private hospitals would not', WG South, Royal Commission evidence, *SAPP*, no.26, 1913, pp.2–3. Wiebusch indicated a diminishing of medical services at Koonibba: the doctor no longer made a monthly visit, and so he looked after health matters himself, or in more serious cases, called the doctor or took patients to him. CA Wiebusch, Royal Commission evidence, *SAPP*, no.26, 1913, p.50

46 WG South, Royal Commission evidence, *SAPP*, no.26, 1913, p.3

visit from a medical officer'.[47] Professor Stirling's comments revealed the public's fears about the issue: the perceived threat to the community of venereal disease was magnified by its existence within the Aboriginal population. Doctors, he said, were concerned only with disease, and 'the colour of the patient does not enter into it', but nurses and other patients felt a 'certain repugnance . . . to have among them a blackfellow with a loathsome disease'.[48] This echoed the statement made by Wiebusch in his report to the Aboriginals Department in 1911, in which the fear of a double contagion – moral as well as physical – was apparent:

> Everyone who has the future welfare especially of our white young men on the West Coast, and the welfare of the natives, at heart does earnestly hope our lawmakers will realise that something must be done as speedily as possible for the better protection of the natives and half-castes to prevent the spreading of this loathsome disease and to check the increase of half-castes.[49]

This fear of contagion and the desire to control the distinctive 'other' who is deemed responsible for its spread, is a recurring *motif* in public health history. Rowley has argued that it is also common within colonial situations where protective and restrictive legislation has been normalised as an appropriate administrative mechanism. In such situations 'the tendency to impute to the person of different appearance those characteristics which arouse fear or shame in the prejudiced group' reflects a 'mentality which moves towards apartheid situations.'[50]

The commissioners reported in two stages, submitting a substantial progress report on 2 October 1913 and a smaller final report on 27 September 1916.[51] Given all the effort that went into the commission's lengthy and arduous investigations and the hopes riding on the outcome, the reports are remarkable in failing to reveal much that was not already known, and their recommendations can best be described as slight.

The progress report began by characterising government support for missions as generous. It provided an account of how the £5738 17s 11d vote for 1911–12, which included a special emergency grant to the AFA to support its 'languishing' work at Point McLeay, had been spent to support the state's 4000 'aborigines' and 820 'half-castes'. It noted that this budget supported a staff of two in the Aboriginals Department, as well as the Inspector of Police at Port Augusta who acted as a protector, and suggested that a larger

---

47 HL Hancock, Royal Commission evidence, *SAPP*, no.26, 1913, p.62; Francis Garnett, Royal Commission evidence, *SAPP*, no.26, 1913, pp.71–2

48 EC Stirling, Royal Commission evidence, *SAPP*, no.26, 1913, p.124

49 Report of Protector of Aborigines, 1911, *SA Aborigines Department Report 1902–3 – 1936–7*. This continued to be a matter of concern. See for example the views of the Inspector of Police from Port Augusta, Report of Chief Protector of Aboriginals, *SAPP*, no.29, 1936, p.80.

50 CD Rowley, *Outcasts in White Australia: Aboriginal Policy and Practice – volume 11*, Australian National University Press, Canberra, 1971, pp.59–60

51 Progress Report of the Royal Commission on the Aborigines together with Minutes of Proceedings, Evidence and Appendices, *SAPP*, no. 26, 1913; Final Report of the Royal Commission on the Aborigines together with Minutes of Proceedings, Evidence and Appendices, *SAPP*, no. 21, 1916

staff was needed. However, it undertook no exploration of the values or assumptions that underlay this level of expenditure, and offered no comparisons by which to judge its 'generosity'.[52] The report rehearsed the well-known story of insufficient land, dependence on charity and enforced idleness at Point McLeay and self-sufficiency and commercial success at Point Pierce. It pointed out, however, that this success was 'not due to the work of the aboriginal population' but to that of non-Aboriginal share-farmers who farmed on Aboriginal reserve land. The specific recommendations of the Royal Commissioners stemmed from their conclusion that, while the need 'to protect the native inhabitants' had diminished over the years,

> the problem is now one of assisting and training the native so that he may become a useful member of the community, dependent not upon charity but upon his own efforts.

They asserted, rather than demonstrated, that this could best be achieved through more direct government control.[53]

The leading recommendation was that, from March 1914, the mission stations at Point Pierce and Point McLeay be taken over by the government and administered by the Aboriginals Department. Secondly, the report recommended that the Aboriginals Department be controlled by a board of six members, comprising the Chairman of the State Children's Council, the Director of Agriculture, the Chairmen of the Point Pierce and Point McLeay Local Committees, and two others nominated by the government, and that the current Chief Protector of Aboriginals be the Secretary and Chief Executive Officer of the board. Five-member Point Pierce and Point McLeay Local Committees, all non-Aboriginals, would be appointed by the governor, would manage the stations and be responsible to the board.

In addition to these major recommendations about administrative changes, there were a number of other recommendations. Share-farming by non-Aboriginals at Point Pierce should be abolished and 'the most deserving aborigines and half-castes' be given the work and the requisite equipment. Further, the new board should 'make an experiment of settling one or two of the best-trained men on each station on a small farm not exceeding 300 acres of arable land'. The report noted that these developments were already provided for under the *Aborigines Act, 1911*. The government should continue to support the AFA and 'the various churches attending to the spiritual needs of the people' at Point Pierce and Point McLeay. Able-bodied mixed-race residents of those stations could continue to

---

52 The parliamentary debate which preceded the establishment of the Royal Commission was, on occasion, somewhat less complacent about this. For example, Thomas Smeaton claimed that the government and people had not 'completed their duty when they subscribed about £4000 to support about 4000 people', and the Commissioner of Public Works was quick to interject, when someone else reported that 89 Aboriginals had been employed to put in a crop of 800 acres at Point Pierce, that this was 'two men's work'. These were passing references only, however, and neither parliament nor the Royal Commission engaged with the inequalities that underlay these data. *SAPD*, House of Assembly, 6 November 1912, p.861; 11 December 1912, p.1303.

53 Progress Report of the Royal Commission on the Aborigines together with Minutes of Proceedings, Evidence and Appendices, *SAPP*, no. 26, 1913, pp.v–vii

consider them as their homes 'for the present', but the report recommended that they be 'compelled to go into outside employment wherever possible', and that an inspector be appointed to arrange such employment and to maintain surveillance over its conditions. This inspector – clearly envisaged as a person of energy – would also:

> report from time to time on the conditions of all institutions at which aborigines were living, the out-back blacks, the neglected and destitute children, and have charge of the distribution of stores and blankets throughout the districts of the State where such is considered necessary.

The report recommended the establishment of a 'sub-station ... preferably in new un-developed land near the Murray' to alleviate the problems arising from land shortage at Point McLeay, the placing of a police officer at Port Victoria, to offer 'greater protection' for Yorke Peninsula Aboriginals, greater disciplinary powers for the new local committees at Point Pierce and Point McLeay, and, as far as was possible, the separation of the 'full-bloods' from the half-castes.

In relation to the question of training for survival in the general community the report rehearsed old formulae, recommending, without any indication of how the recommendations might be implemented, that:

> endeavours be made to establish means of training boys in carpentry, building, blacksmithing, plumbing, saddlery, as well as in general farm work; and girls in sewing, dressmaking, house-hold duties and laundry work, with a view to making them fit for outside situations, and that such training be made compulsory at each institution.

The report endorsed the current system of 'saving destitute aboriginal children' in con-junction with the State Children's Department and in addition recommended that the newly constituted board have the power:

> to take control of any children at the age of ten years whose environment is not conducive to their welfare, and at the desire of the parents, of any other children, and place them where the Board deems best in the interests of the children.

Finally, there were several recommendations that indicated the strongly paternalistic character of the report and reflected its underlying assumption that Aboriginal people were unable to take charge of their own lives and, like children, or adults lacking in self-discipline and responsibility, needed considerable control and guidance. For example, it was recommended that the local committees governing the missions have increased powers to maintain control, good order and discipline on the reserves; that a system of bank accounts be established, under the Board's control, 'to train the natives in habits of thrift and care'; and that the earnings of Aboriginals living on reserves be 'apportioned amongst or for the benefit of aborigines'.[54]

The final report of the Royal Commission was submitted in October 1916 and dealt

---

54 ibid., pp.viii–x

with several issues not canvassed in the progress report. The commissioners had by then visited the Lutheran missions at Koonibba and Killalpaninna, and although they believed that 'the blacks' lived under better conditions at these missions than they would 'if left to their own resources', they recommended direct government control, as had by then been effected at Point McLeay and Point Pearce.[55] They claimed that it was the duty of the government to assume this responsibility, since 'the care of the aborigines is a national matter'.[56] This view, which was merely asserted rather than explained or argued for in the report, was to be heard more and more often, and from many different quarters, over the next decades. The final report made brief mention of the 500 or so 'natives outside the mission stations' in the far north of the state. Presumably the duty of the government extended to them too, but the report suggested no policy beyond the establishment of a couple more depots for the distribution of blankets and rations.

The final report dealt specifically with some health issues. Since the evidence on the prevalence of venereal diseases among Aboriginals was contested, it did not recommend the establishment of a lock hospital. What it did recommend was a system of health care that treated 'mission natives' differently from 'outside blacks', and treated both differently from the non-Aboriginal population. Significantly, the provision of health care for Aboriginals was seen as a public responsibility and not a private matter: it was to be arranged through the Central Board of Health in the case of missions, and through the police and Aborigines Department inspectors in all other cases. Such a system clearly indicated that Aboriginal people were assumed to constitute a risk to the health of the rest of the public. On that ground, they were to be provided for in ways that involved no choice on their part but required their submission to high levels of control.

Implementing reform is usually much more difficult than talking about it. The recommendations of the Royal Commission led to only limited action and some of the matters that had engaged the witnesses and commissioners came to nothing or remained merely the subject of continuing discussion.

Among the easiest reforms to achieve was the government takeover of the Point Pearce and Point McLeay mission stations, which occurred on 1 September 1915 and 1 January 1916, respectively.[57] As already noted, this development had been anticipated for some time and was not opposed by the mission authorities. Indeed, they had come to see it as a way out of the difficulties and challenges associated with land shortage, chronic under-employment, inadequate government grants and the complex educational and training needs of the rapidly increasing and often discontent 'half-caste' population. Their willingness to hand over control of the missions to the government is not to suggest that the situation was a straightforward one for the missionaries or for mission

---

55 From the time of the government takeover, the name of the Yorke Peninsula station was consistently spelled 'Pearce'. I adopt that spelling from here on.

56 Final Report of the Royal Commission on the Aborigines together with Minutes of Proceedings, Evidence and Appendices. *SAPP*, no. 21. 1916, p.iv

57 Raynes, 'A Little Flour', p.39; AFA Committee minutes, 8 December 1915, AFA Minute Books, SRG 139/2, vol. iv

residents. The mission administrations acknowledged their inability to run their estab-lishments in a way that afforded the Aboriginal residents the economic and industrial rights that applied in the broader community. However, they were by no means clear about whether it was incumbent on them to do so, or whether they were in fact engaged in charitable activity that operated on different principles.[58] In addition, even though the terms of the government takeover allowed for the former mission authorities to continue their spiritual work at the stations, they worried about the effectiveness of this. The AFA officers were quick to report on the 'decline in tone', 'immorality', loss of 'sympathy, kind-ness, and care' and 'drift away from the standard previously maintained' that followed their relinquishing of control at Point McLeay. They also continued, much as they had always done, to seek to provide for the material needs of the Aboriginals, especially the older 'wurley natives', and regularly to alert the minister to his duties in this regard.[59]

At Point Pearce, as we have already seen, the Aboriginal population had welcomed the prospect of government takeover and expected economic benefits to accrue from it. However, the recommendations regarding an end to share-farming and the allocation of land, on a trial basis, to some Aboriginals were not implemented. The new order proved less than satisfactory in other ways as well. In February 1919, 43 of the residents signed a petition asking the AFA to take over mission work at Point Pearce, claiming that since the government had assumed control

> morally and spiritually this mission is a complete wreck, and having no Christian friends in this
> district to help us, we, in our lost and helpless condition, send to you this Macedonian cry, come
> over and help us.[60]

Although the mission at Koonibba had received less scrutiny by the royal commis-sioners than had Point McLeay and Point Pearce, and their report had not recommended its takeover, the government was interested in extending its control there as well. This met with resistance from the Lutheran church and there was no support for it from the Koonibba residents. The Lutheran synod believed that the government and the Chief Protector were 'against … our mission', and saw the failure of parliamentary bills regarding the takeover as evidence that 'God frustrated these efforts'. To secure their position they tried, unsuccessfully, to buy the Koonibba land, but were able to negotiate another 21-year lease when their original lease expired in 1918.[61] The Lutheran mission at Killalpaninna, always a struggling venture, fared less well. The synod had closed the mission in 1915,

58 See for example, a letter written by AFA committee members, C Taplin and W Dalton, reporting on a visit to Point
    McLeay, 14 October 1912, AFA Minute Books, SRG 139/2, vol. iv

59 AFA Executive Committee minutes, 2 November 1916; Annual Report, 4 July 1917, AFA Minute Books, SRG 139/2, vol. iv

60 AFA Committee minutes, 10 March 1919, AFA Minute Books, SRG 139/2, vol. iv. The biblical allusion is to Paul's vision
    of a plea, from Macedonia, for his missionary services. (Acts 16:9). It was not true that the Point Pearce people had no local
    Christian friends, but the involvement of the local churches was somewhat unpredictable, and several years later the AFA
    noted that strong 'denominational sentiment' stood in the way of the establishment of an interdenominational missionary
    organisation, AFA Committee minutes, 8 May 1924, AFA Minute Books, SRG139/2, vol.iv.

61 Evangelical Lutheran Synod in Australia, South Australian District, Inc., *Synod Report*, 1921, pp.61–2

having sold the plant and stock and transferred the lease into private Lutheran hands on condition that the new owners continue unofficial missionary work. In 1917, as part of war-time security measures that targeted activities and institutions associated with Germans, the government closed the Killalpaninna school.[62] In that year the Chief Protector noted that the former mission was

> now only a depot for the issue of rations etc for the old and infirm, and the cost of those during the year amounted to only $61, whereas they used to cost the department on an average $135 annually.[63]

In 1919 the government resumed the synod's lease of the Kopperamanna Aboriginal reserve, which had been part of 'mission land' since 1867 and necessary for its pastoral activities, on the grounds of non-compliance with the terms of the lease.[64]

Having assumed control of Point McLeay and Point Pearce, the government failed to act on the Royal Commission's recommendation about a central board of control to administer Aboriginal affairs. Instead, in January 1918, on the initiative of the Hon. John Bice, Commissioner of Public Works and ministerial head of the Aboriginals Department, a seven-member Advisory Council of Aborigines was established by regulations under the *Aborigines Act, 1911*, to provide the minister with a source of 'unofficial' advice to complement advice from the Chief Protector. The Advisory Council was charged with making recommendations 'upon any matter connected with the protection, control, training, or education of, or otherwise affecting the interests of, the aboriginal and half-caste inhabitants of the State', and 'generally' to advise him 'as to the best means of carrying into effect the objects of the Aborigines Act, 1911'.[65] Bice chose the members from among the leadership of the AFA and others closely connected with its work. This reflected not only the AFA's prominence and standing in Aboriginal affairs, but also the government's continuing focus on Point McLeay, despite its claims to be concerned with the indigenous population of the entire state.[66]

A third area of action, which demonstrated that it was easier to extend control over Aboriginal people than to provide for their 'advancement' or to enlarge their life choices, was the enactment of a series of regulations to implement the control functions of the *Aborigines Act*. The first of these, which took effect from 10 May 1917, gave super-

---

62 *SAGG*, 28 June 1917, p.1107

63 Chief Protector's Report, *SAPP*, no.29, 1917, p.5; Stevens, *White Man's Dreaming*, pp.199–201

64 *SAGG*, 9 January 1919, p.80

65 *SAGG*, 24 January 1918, p.141

66 The original members of the Advisory Council of Aborigines were the Hon. John Lewis, MLC; Thomas Wilson Fleming, SM, chairman of the AFA and appointed chairman of the Advisory Council; the Rev. John Henry Sexton, secretary of the AFA, and appointed secretary of the Advisory Council; Walter Hutley, JP, former teacher at Point McLeay; Charles Eaton Taplin, JP, member of the AFA committee and son of the founder of the Point McLeay mission; and the Rev. Archdeacon WJ Bussell and Peter Wood, JP, both closely connected with the Aboriginals of the Point McLeay area, *SAGG*, 31 January 1918, p.182. See also John H Sexton, 'An Historical Review of the Work of the Advisory Council of Aborigines', GRG 52/105A/1939.

intendents of Aboriginal institutions considerable power over all residents, and outlined a daily regimen which was distinctly custodial in character:

> All aboriginals or half-castes employed within any aboriginal institution shall rise not later than 6.45am on each day from the first day of October to the thirty-first day of March (both days inclusive), and not later than 7.15am on each day from the first day of April to the thirtieth day of September (both days inclusive). The working hours for aboriginals and half-castes within any aboriginal institution during the period beginning on the first day of April and ending on the thirtieth day of September shall be from 8am to 5pm. Throughout the year there shall be an interval of one hour in the middle of the day for dinner, and on Saturdays there shall be a half-holiday, work being discontinued at 1pm. Provided that the hours for work prescribed in this article may in case of emergency be extended in the discretion of the Superintendent of such institution.

The regulations also empowered the Chief Protector to expel from Aboriginal institutions any persons whom he deemed to be 'habitually disorderly, lazy, disobedient, insolent, intemperate or immoral', or whose presence he judged to be 'inimical to the maintenance of discipline or good order', or who were found to be guilty of such offences as intoxication, 'immoral or disgraceful conduct', use of 'profane, blasphemous, obscene, abusive, or insulting language', insubordination, possession of firearms or alcohol, not attempting to obtain employment outside the institution, or being 'dirty and untidy'. Additional offences, gazetted in 1919, included failing to close gates when entering or leaving the institution, loitering anywhere on the institution while church services or meetings were in progress and playing 'any game in any street or road' in an institution without prior permission of the superintendent. In 1919, these and all previously gazetted regulations were extended to reserves as well as institutions.[67]

These new developments constituted potential for extension of government control deep into the domestic sphere of the lives of at least those Aboriginal people who lived in institutional settings. They meant that the government – whose power was embodied in the persons of the Chief Protector and the station superintendents – could exert direct influence in areas regarded as private by non-Aboriginal Australians. Together with the already established powers and practices relating to the 'rescue' of children from their indigenous parentage and cultural heritage, and with patterns and levels of material provision which had, in many cases, built a profound dependence on the state and severely restricted opportunities and choices, they strengthened the construction of Aboriginals as not part of the public. They were a separate group with some claims on the rest of the community by virtue of their prior possession of the country, but with no opportunities to determine their own lives and futures. Their lives and futures were determined by others who, whatever levels of decency and kindness they displayed, or whatever claims to justice and democracy they made, did not acknowledge that Aboriginals had complex needs and aspirations – material, familial, emotional, educational, vocational – in common with the rest of the population.

---

67 Raynes, 'A Little Flour', pp.40–1; SAGG, 10 May 1917, pp.742–3, 21 August 1919, p.383

Included in this was a failure to acknowledge within the Aboriginal population the diversity of capacity and expectation that was taken for granted within non-Aboriginal society. Not only did Aboriginal people not need such good food, or such comfortable houses, or such high wages, or such freedom in their domestic arrangements as non-Aboriginal people needed, but they all had the same needs and desires as each other. They belonged to an undifferentiated underclass whose potential could be fulfilled and ambition exhausted by the chance to farm, be a pastoral station rouseabout, learn a trade or become a domestic servant. This construction communicated itself to the Aboriginal people themselves. The evidence of indigenous witnesses before the Royal Commission, as well as the nature of the requests that Aboriginal people made, from time to time, to mission authorities and the Chief Protector, may be taken as an indication that they had to a considerable extent shaped their sense of themselves and of what they could reasonably expect in conformity with the model adopted by non-Aboriginals.

In theory – as well as in the recommendations of the Royal Commission and the ongoing ruminations of the AFA and the new Advisory Council on Aborigines – non-Aboriginal views of Aboriginal futures included their development, at least in the case of 'half-castes', into 'useful members of society'. This transformation was assumed to depend on basic education followed by vocational training. However, the programs and services meant to achieve this did not eventuate. Indeed, the government's administration of Point McLeay and Point Pearce was at odds with its expressed developmental and assimilationist goals. By closing the children's dormitories and sending the children back to their parents, the government was encouraging the continuation of the cultural influence which it had for many years argued was inimical to 'progress' and to a 'white' future for mixed-race children. Alarmed at this development, the AFA at its annual general meeting in 1919 called for the establishment of children's homes at the two former missions. Such calls were repeated in subsequent years, but although plans for a home at Point McLeay were approved by the Advisory Council in 1922, no action ensued. There was no progress on other fronts either. On a visit to Point McLeay in 1921, officers of the AFA noted the good work being done by Philip Rigney, David Unaipon and others in the church, but reported that government staff were being retrenched because of 'the exhaustion of the Aborigines' vote', [that is, the budget allocation from the state government] and that old and frail Aboriginals were not being adequately cared for. AFA records from this period indicate the continuation of all the old problems of poor housing, overcrowding, idleness, compromised health and shortage of funds. Chief Protector South's earlier confidence that government control would solve these problems was shattered by the reality of continuing parsimony, prevarication and *ad hoc* arrangements.

In these circumstances, Aboriginal well-being remained fragile. This can be demonstrated in relation to the provision of health care. Reports of the Chief Protector and reports of the Central and Local Boards of Health for this period reveal a good deal about what was considered acceptable provision for the indigenous population. Minimal standards were clearly the norm: anything was better than nothing, and indeed was presented as though it was a reason for applause and gratitude.

For example, Chief Protector South reported in 1919 that death rates were high, apparently as a result of an influenza outbreak in the far north. An isolation camp had been set up in the vicinity of Oodnadatta, and 'no expense [had] been spared in combating the disease', although no medical practitioner had yet been sent through the Far North and North-Western districts to examine, treat and report on the health of the natives. Aboriginals much closer to Adelaide also suffered from want of medical attention. The Point McLeay superintendent thanked the Chief Protector for the 'splendid supply of medicines' and for his 'untiring efforts in getting our people admitted to the Adelaide Hospital', but admitted that 'the absence of a medical man is felt very much here'.[68] Things were more difficult at Koonibba, from where Superintendent Hoff reported that death rates from 'a severe form of influenza which developed into pneumonia' were high and 'it was at times difficult to obtain medical advice, especially since the telephone connection is not as yet taken in hand, although mentioned'.[69] An epidemic of typhoid at Point Pearce in May 1923 highlighted the chronic inadequacy of government provision. Superintendent Garnett suggested that the school be turned into an isolation hospital and that two nurses be hired to deal with the crisis, but had no funds to effect this. The government acted in the short term to avert the health threat to the rest of population, but more permanent provision of the most basic health services rested on the willingness of the AFA to juggle their priorities and scarce resources. In 1924, after their missionary had resigned, they decided to replace him with a nurse and to use his house as a hospital, and subsequently to seek support from elsewhere for their missionary activity.[70]

Minutes of the Central Board of Health for the 1920s indicate that because of a shortage of staff it was often unable to perform its basic roles satisfactorily. They also reveal one well-established pattern for dealing with this deficiency: the Central Board and also a number of Local Boards of Health, although charged with the responsibility for protecting the health of the public, were often reluctant to act on indigenous health concerns. Instead, they regularly referred them to other departments and agencies, thus effectively defining them as other than public health concerns, and the indigenous population as not part of the public.[71].

Chief Protector South's report of 1921 provides a summary illustration of the uncritical complacency that followed from accepting that the indigenous sub-population was not part of the public and therefore had lesser needs and less serious claims on common goods:

> The health of the aborigines throughout the State during the year has been fairly good, and
> their requirements have been well attended to by the depot keepers, who have cheerfully
> given their services free of charge. The numerous medical officers and hospital authorities and
> attendants have all given the native patients every care within their power. Blankets, clothing
> and medical comforts have been liberally supplied to those entitled to same in all parts of the

---

68 Report of Chief Protector of Aboriginals, *SAPP*, no.29, 1919, pp.107–10

69 Report of Chief Protector of Aboriginals, *SAPP*, no.29, 1923, p.137

70 AFA, Committee minutes, 18 May, 19 July 1923; 8 May, 31 July, 19 November 1924, AFA Minute Books, SRG 139/2, vol.v.

71 Central Board of Health, Minutes, 1920–30, GRG 8/19

State, *but care has been exercised to keep down expenditure as far as possible. The enormous increase in prices of all commodities has made it most difficult to make the departmental vote cover the necessary expenditure* [my emphasis].[72]

These reports – and the examples could be multiplied – point to the precariousness of the situation: the normal circumstances and provisions were not sufficient to do more than hold a very basic line; they were certainly not up to protecting the Aboriginals from crises. The government had repeatedly claimed that it wanted to provide 'advancement' to the 'rising' mixed-race population, as well as protection to the 'dying race' of 'full-bloods'. However, having strengthened its legislative capacity to do this, it demonstrated a consistent lack of seriousness about providing the means to make it happen.

At its annual general meeting of 1925, the AFA pronounced the government negligent. There were still no children's homes. No effective action had been taken in relation to training and employment. European share-farmers were still working the land at Point Pearce. In short, 'the easier method of drift had been adopted, with disastrous results', and young Aboriginal people were continuing to spend their lives in idleness.[73] Earlier the AFA had noted not only the government's failure to provide the opportunities it claimed to be committed to, but also a social context which made the transition from mission to the general community an intimidating one. There was a failure to provide 'openings' for the 'half-castes', who were supposed to be making this journey, and so they clung to the missions, 'partly because of the loneliness and isolation they feel in society, and partly because only there can they realize that they are members of a community'.[74] It is difficult to see how Aboriginal people could do other than fail the tests they were set. The government imposed expectations, but supplied no resources adequate to meet them, and in the meantime continued to organise indigenous lives in ways that produced dependence. The Advisory Council quickly proved to be an ineffectual tool of policy development. Perhaps not surprisingly, given its makeup, it sounded like an echo of the AFA, and, in its own judgement and that of others, was not taken seriously by any ministers after Bice. Within government, the Chief Protector of Aboriginals continued to be the only source of advice, to be listened to or not, as ministers saw fit.[75]

In the meantime, attempts to strengthen the legislative capacity of the government to 'rescue' children from Aboriginal influence continued. An Aborigines (Half-Caste Children) Bill, which sought the placing of 'half-castes' under the control of the State Children's Council without having them declared neglected under the *State Children Act*, was introduced into parliament in 1921. This bill lapsed, but the Aborigines (Training of

---

72 Report of Chief Protector of Aboriginals, *SAPP*, no.29, 1921, p.109

73 AFA, Annual Report, *Advertiser*, 18 February 1925

74 AFA, Annual Report, *Register*, 2 February 1922

75 Sexton, 'An Historical Review'. The issue of the minister having access to 'official' and 'unofficial' advice was complicated by the decision to make Francis Garnett a member of the Advisory Council when he took over as Chief Protector following South's death in May 1923.

Children) Bill, introduced in 1923, fared better.[76] It allowed the Chief Protector to remove 'half-caste' children at any age and maintain them in any state children's institution up to the age of 18 if, in the view of the Protector and State Children's Council, they were neglected. In addition, it allowed for the removal and institutionalistion of any Aboriginal or 'half-caste' children who had attained 14 years and successfully completed primary schooling. Chief Protector Garnett, who had been appointed as South's successor on 23 July 1923, and had immediately aligned himself with South's clearly established policy of assimilation *via* control and training, was strongly supportive of the bill:

> I consider the most urgent problem to be dealt with in our work for the Aborigines is the better control and training of the rising generation … A Bill dealing with this important matter, trans-ferring aboriginal children at the age of fourteen years to the care of the State Children's Department, will be dealt with by the present session of Parliament. This much-needed legis-lation, if passed, will mean a big advance in our methods of dealing with the aborigines, and should result in our fitting the young to become self-supporting members of the community and an asset to the State.[77]

The bill was assented to on 14 November 1923, but an early attempt by Garnett to use the act to remove a child from its mother at Point McLeay aroused such criticism that it became a dead letter. Three Point McLeay men, Leonard Campbell, Willy Rankine and John Stanley, travelled to Adelaide to present the governor and members of the govern-ment with a petition that challenged the government to recognise the claims of maternal love. Unable to gain an audience with the governor, the men provided the *Register* news-paper with an interview, in which they said that although they wanted their children to 'get on' and 'be useful', they were fearful of losing them. They were asserting their natural rights as parents but also rejecting the notion that their children, by virtue of their 'race', belonged to the disadvantaged category of 'state children': 'They are our own children … our children have never been state children, and we don't want them to be'.[78]

We cannot know what the reaction of parents of Koonibba children would have been if Garnett had tested the new act there. However, the Mission Board, while aware of the 'danger' that Koonibba children might find themselves in non-Lutheran homes, welcomed the act in terms of what it might contribute to their mission's viability. It would 'result in draining Koonibba of its surplus population to some extent'. This would be a good thing, since 'it should be clear to Synod that we as a church could not definitely keep all the natives … without jeopardizing the very existence of our Mission'.[79] The existence of

76 Raynes, 'A Little Flour', pp.41–4

77 Report of Chief Protector of Aboriginals, *SAPP*, no.29, 1923, p.133

78 *Register*, 21 December 1923, p.9. The article, headed 'Three dusky deputies', is extremely patronising. It indicates that the interviewer tried to deflect the Point McLeay men from their purpose by focusing on the past and insulted them by using pidgin English and by suggesting that they would prefer to 'go walk about' rather than work. Campbell, in reply, hinted at the real issue in relation to employment: 'We like to work if we get a fair wage'.

79 *Report of the Proceedings of the Synodical Convention of the Evangelical Lutheran Synod in Australia, South Australian District, Inc., 1924*, pp.40–1, **See** above, pp.139–40

the mission, it seems, was of more account than what the act might mean for the children towards whom it was directed.

The fact that the *Aborigines (Training of Children) Act* became a dead letter did not mean that the policy of removal and training met a similar end: governments simply pursued it under the *State Children Act* and regulations under the *Aborigines Act, 1911*. What is significant about all this is that the government's training, 'advancement' and assimilation agenda for indigenous people involved the use of mechanisms which, in the case of non-indigenous people, were used only in cases of family dislocation, neglect, abuse and delinquency. Although training and employment opportunities for non-indigenous South Australians were of course mediated by class and social standing, they were not routinely associated with the submission to custodial control which it was thought appropriate and necessary to require of Aboriginals.[80]

A second wave of missionary activity continued to support this government agenda alongside an agenda of its own. Several new ventures, mostly poorly resourced 'faith missions' supported by the non-denominational evangelical United Aborigines Mission (UAM), were established in this period, some in remote areas that the government largely ignored and others on the outskirts of white settlements where dispossessed and marginalised Aboriginal people had become fringe dwellers. The frankly evangelistic impulse of these missions went hand in hand with a humanitarian response to evidence of neglect, physical suffering, cultural and moral decline and the perceived likelihood of imminent racial extinction. Over time, modest official support of and involvement with these missions developed as a matter of expediency, while governments continued to prevaricate, and academic debates about how to deal with the 'native problem' gathered momentum. The first UAM mission in South Australia was established in Oodnadatta in 1924, and was followed by missions at Swan Reach (1925), Quorn (1927), Nepabunna (1929), Ooldea (1933) and Finniss Springs (1939). The Open Brethren established the Umeewarra mission on the outskirts of Port Augusta in 1937, the same year in which the Presbyterian church, goaded into action by Dr Charles Duguid, established a very different kind of mission at Ernabella in the Musgrave Ranges in the far north-west of the state. The most substantial and influential of the UAM's enterprises in South Australia were Colebrook Home, an 'orphanage' and training home that was an outcome of its work at Oodnadatta, and the mission established among the Adnyamathanha people at Nepabunna in the Northern Finders Ranges.

Between 1926 and 1981, Colebrook Home for Aboriginal Children (later Colebrook Training Home) supported the government's agenda of assimilation and rescue. It was established first in the far north at Oodnadatta, moved to Quorn in 1927, and then to Eden Hills, a southern suburb of Adelaide, in 1943. In 1973, the UAM handed over control of the institution to the state government. By the time it closed in 1981 more than 350 children had been in its care. Between 1926 and 1952 Colebrook Home was run by

---

80 Of course, when non-indigenous children were placed in institutional or other forms of out-of-home care, they, like indigenous children in care, were likely to suffer various forms of abuse and neglect. See Senate Community Affairs Reference Committee, *Forgotten Australians: a report on Australians who experienced institutional or out-of-home care as children*, Commonwealth of Australia, Canberra, 2004.

two UAM missionaries, Sisters Ruby Hyde and Delia Rutter. Such consistency of staffing was unusual and contributed significantly to a process of institutional identification which, for many residents, persisted and supported them after they left Colebrook.[81]

The UAM saw Colebrook Home as rescuing 'half-caste' children from the 'depths of ignorance, superstition and vice' that characterised Aboriginal life. The mothers 'knew nothing but camp life and could not speak English. What chance had the children under such conditions?' They simply 'ran wild with their native mother[s]'. The 'bush men' who were the fathers of these children valued what the home could do in implanting the 'nice ways' and 'good moral training' that would aid their 'merging' into white society. Thus, the Aboriginal mothers were without agency, mere objects of the agenda and policy goals of others, the non-Aboriginal fathers were allowed to abrogate their responsibilities, and the children became 'little inmates' in an institution where they would be 'gently governed' and trained 'for a place in the community here, and in the Kingdom of Heaven hereafter'.[82]

Government and community attitudes towards Colebrook home during the 1920s and 1930s were ambivalent.[83] In the wake of hostile reactions to attempts to implement the 1923 *Aborigines (Training of Children) Act*, Chief Protector Garnett was wary of taking children without their mothers' consent. He resisted UAM requests to move the home further south. He was concerned about probable additional expense for the government and the exacerbation of the 'half-caste' problem, and also doubted the likelihood of the 'ultimate absorption' of Colebrook residents as 'self-supporting citizens'. Indeed, in 1932, after receiving complaints from residents and the Local Board of Health in Quorn about the moral and health risks associated with the presence of Colebrook children in the local school, he recommended that the home be moved from Quorn back to its original site in Oodnadatta and that, where possible, the children be returned to their parents. He was 'becoming more and more convinced that you cannot make a black, white', and continued to argue for a curtailment of Colebrook's activities, even after a government investigation of the home gave it a favourable report and declared allegations against it to be unfounded and racist.[84]

If Garnett had lost some of his assimilationist nerve, others had not. The Advisory Council was sympathetic to the Colebrook experiment and the Aborigines Department acknowledged it as 'an inexpensive way of testing' the idea that 'half-caste children removed completely from the environment of aboriginals' camps would lose their abo-

---

81 Despite the profound grief and loss associated with being taken from their families, and the many hardships and restriction of opportunity and choice associated with institutional life, former Colebrook residents frequently attest to the qualities and commitment of Hyde and Rutter and to their own ongoing self-identification as 'Colebrook kids'. See, for example, Harris, *One Blood*, pp.563–4; Mattingley and Hampton, *Survival in Our Own Land*, pp.213–19.

82 VE Turner, *Pearls from the Deep: the story of Colebrook Home for Aboriginal Children, Quorn, South Australia*, United Aborigines' Mission, Adelaide, [nd] 1936.

83 I rely here on Jane M Jacobs, Caroline Laurence and Faith Thomas, '"Pearls from the Deep": Re-evaluating the early history of Colebrook Home for Aboriginal children', in Tony Swain and Deborah Bird Rose, *Aboriginal Australians and Christian Missions: ethnographic and historical studies*, Australian Association for the Study of Religions, Bedford Park, South Australia, 1988, pp.140–55.

84 Jacobs, Laurence and Thomas, '"Pearls from the Deep"', pp.149, 151

riginal longings and habitats and become more Europeanised'.[85] All of this revealed the ambiguity and half-heartedness of the government's position: it claimed to believe in assimilation, but its own institutions continued to be segregationist in character; it accused the UAM and Colebrook Home of having no practical program of absorption and self-support, but shied away from making financial commitment to this itself; it continued to talk of providing training and employment opportunities for young people in government institutions, but these did not eventuate.

This half-heartedness was exacerbated by the difficult economic circumstances of the 1930s. The Great Depression threw underlying attitudes towards Aboriginals into stark relief. As Garnett declared in his 1932 report, 'not until most of the unemployed white population is absorbed in occupations will there be an opportunity of doing very much for the natives'. In 1934 he reported that the Koonibba mission's solution to its economic problems had been to sell the whole of their farming operations to two non-indigenous share-farmers. That this was said to make 'practically no difference to Koonibba as a 'home' for all West Coast natives' says much about government and mission disregard for the benefits, in terms of income and self-esteem, of the 'natives' having a stake in their own economic enterprise. The Chief Protector's 1935 report indicated that the Aboriginals Department's 'usual routine work' of supplying rations and medical assistance was neither keeping the Aboriginals healthy, nor contributing to their independence. Health as always, was poor. As well as 'outbreaks of cold and other common ailments', he mentioned whooping cough, influenza, septic sores and a 'strong tendency towards tuberculosis and diabetes'. In addition:

> The continued drought in the far north and general unemployment throughout the more settled parts of the State have made it impossible to curtail in any way the services rendered to the Aboriginals; in fact the native, both full-blood and half-caste is now more dependent upon the assistance of the Department than ever before.[86]

The UAM did not suffer from any failure of will, despite the hard times and its modest financial endowment. At Colebrook, the assimilationist program of 'civilising' and 'Christianising' children was energetically pursued. After the move to Eden Hills, some were encouraged to undertake secondary education within the general community and, once they reached the age of sixteen years, were supported while they established themselves in the workforce.[87] Within a few years of establishing its work at Oodnadatta, the UAM extended its missionary activities to other sites in South Australia, including the northern Flinders Ranges, home of the Adnyamathanha.

The Adnyamathanha had been in contact with non-indigenous influences since the

---

85 ibid., pp.147, 149

86 Report of Chief Protector of Aboriginals, *SAPP*, no. 29, 1932, p.38; *SAPP*, no.29, 1934, p.41; *SAPP*, no.29, 1935, pp.41–2

87 This system was highly regimented and paternalistic, offered only limited choice, and showed no respect for Aboriginal culture or identity, but some indigenous people who lived through it and remain critical of it, acknowledge that it had some positive aspects. See, for example, Margaret Forte, *Flight of an Eagle: the dreaming of Ruby Hammond*, Wakefield Press, Adelaide, 1995, pp.72–7, 187–9. See below, pp.200–1.

1850s. The pioneering period of pastoral expansion had been marked by conflict, by disruption of the ochre trade which linked the Adnyamathanha with the Diyari and other peoples from further north, by population decline and by loss of land and food and water supplies. To deal with the impact of these changes, government ration depots and a police presence were established in the northern Flinders Ranges from the early 1850s. By the 1880s, a means of peaceful coexistence had been reached, with the indigenous people camping near pastoral stations, which were sources of work, food, and water and were also, in some cases, sites of spiritual significance. Their dependence on the pastoralists and the ration depots varied with the season and with work opportunities. Periodic drought and economic downturns highlighted their inability to compete on equal terms with non-indigenous people, but in good times, many of the able-bodied obtained full employment, and government rations provided for the old, sick and frail. This did not come at the cost of cultural disintegration. Despite many challenges and strategic accommodations to settler culture, the Adnyamathanha maintained a strong communal identity. They remained on their land, although not in control of it, keeping alive their language, law and ceremonial life, thwarting government attempts to remove their children for schooling, and bringing them up within their own culture.[88]

In the late 1920s, however, their fortunes were at a low ebb because of continuing pressure on their camping places, prolonged drought and the greatly reduced employment opportunities associated with the early days of the Great Depression. Choosing not to be dependent fringe dwellers in any of the surrounding towns, the Adnyamathanha responded to their difficulties by moving to an area within their traditional lands known as Ram Paddock Gate. There they established a settlement, 'were careful not to be a burden on any of the pastoral stations' and 'maintained their communal cohesion, community pride and independence'.[89] However, by 1929, when UAM missionaries joined them there, they were facing starvation. The missionaries were able to avert the immediate crisis by organising government rations. Over the next months, in the face of hostility on the part of the lessees of Ram Paddock Gate to the idea of a permanent mission station, negotiated with the lessees of nearby Balcanoona Station for control of an area of land at Nepabunna. The special conditions of this arrangement included an agreement that, if the UAM left, the land was to revert to the lessees.

Although starting a mission from scratch had not been its intention, the UAM remained in charge of the mission at Nepabunna from its establishment in 1931 until 1973, when, at the request of the Adnyamathanha, it was taken over by the government.[90] While the UAM's control of the Nepabunna land brought it unexpected power and control over the lives of the Adnyamathanha, it did not lead to the kind of institutionalisation that existed at Poonindie and at Koonibba. The UAM did not establish the community at Nepabunna; nor

---

88 Brock, *Outback Ghettos*, chapter 8. Brock characterises the post-contact/pre-mission experience of the Adnyamathanha as 'survival without instutionalisation', and sees it as an example of Spicer's argument that post-contact experiences need not be 'an uninterrupted, inevitable progression from autonomy to cultural disintegration and dependence'. Brock, *Outback Ghettos*, p.122, and see above, pp.93–4.

89 ibid., p.138

90 ibid., pp.140–1. See also Harris, *One Blood*, pp.564–8, and Mattingley and Hampton, *Survival in Our Own Land*, pp.227–34.

did it attempt to make it self-supporting through employment and the creation of a closed and artificial mission economy.[91] While paternalistic and lacking in respect for the Adnyamathanha's traditions, beliefs and language, the missionaries did not exploit them economically. In fact, especially in the early days, they earned their respect by acting as advocates and supporters of their rights in the community. The 'Christianising' agenda of the mission was forthright and caused some tensions among the Adnyamathanha and between them and the missionaries, but it was not linked with a 'civilising' agenda, since a significant level of assimilation to non-Indigenous patterns of life and work had already been established.[92]

In Brock's view, the UAM's main contribution to the Adnyamathanha was that it sustained them at a particularly vulnerable point in their history.[93] The mission provided them with stability and security not experienced since the invasion of their land by pastoralists. It gave them a base from which to take advantage of new economic opportunities which emerged in the 1940s, with the extension of roads and the railway and the establishment of coal-mining at Leigh Creek. It is true that isolation, unproductive land and poor water supply, and the UAM's lack of resources, which was reflected in its failure to employ trained teachers or provide schooling except on an intermittent basis, as well as in the absence of health care, meant that conditions at Nepabunna, even by mission standards, were poor.[94] Material impoverishment was also maintained by the government's continuing treatment of indigenous people as not part of the public, graphically reflected in the significant differences between the sustenance relief, or 'dole' given to unemployed non-indigenous Australians during the Great Depression and the rations provided for aged, infirm and sick Aboriginals. These rations, sometimes referred to during this period as the 'black dole', consisted merely of sugar, flour, tea and tobacco, whereas the 'white dole', niggardly though it was, consisted of bread, butter, sugar, meat, jam, milk, cheese, tea and soap. As Harris has observed, apparently Aboriginals 'could do without protein as long as they got a smoke'.[95] It is true also that the Adnyamathanha, like other indigenous South Australians, suffered from racial prejudice and discrimination in the community. For example, while their labour was welcome in the mines at Leigh Creek, they were not welcome as tenants of the houses built by the Electricity Trust of South Australia in the new Leigh Creek township.[96] Despite all these difficulties, however, they continued to exercise a significant level of control over their own lives. The mission, by enabling them to maintain their links with their land, contributed to the survival of their identity as a distinctive cultural and language group.

---

91 This was not simply making virtue of necessity, given the depressed economic conditions of the time and the limitations of the site. It also reflected the UAM's characteristic style of mission.

92 Brock, *Outback Ghettos*, pp.143, 148, 158, 161–2

93 ibid., p.162

94 ibid., pp.144–5

95 Harris, *One Blood*, p.576. See also Margaret Ann Franklin, *Black and White Australians: an interracial history 1788–1975*, Heinemann, South Yarra, Victoria, 1976, pp.92–4. Franklin claims that although Aboriginals who had been employed at award rates before the Great Depression were legally entitled to the 'white dole', 'administrators usually forgot this'.

96 Brock, *Outback Ghettos*, p.144

These brief case studies of Colebrook Home and Nepabunna Mission provide a glimpse of the complexity of mission experience and its impact on indigenous people in the period covered by this chapter, and of the connections between missionary activity and government agenda. It is a story full of contradictions. Missions, especially when they operated as 'outback ghettos' in the way Brock has described, were capable of providing security and opportunity within narrow boundaries and of leaving some aspects of indigenous culture intact while allowing Aboriginals to decide their own levels of assimilation. However, few were able to separate their program of 'Christianisation' and 'civilisation' from the denigration and undermining of indigenous culture and the racist judgements about indigenous futures that prevailed in the wider community. In addition, many were wedded to a program of institutionalisation of children which fractured families and sowed the seeds of a later harvest of grief, loss, distrust, despair and dysfunction radically at odds with their stated goals of 'rescue' and promotion of well-being. Harris, in an overview of reserves, missions and institutionalisation during this period, in South Australia and elsewhere in Australia, gives voice to many Aboriginal people who were brought up under this system. Although not opposed to missionary activity, he argues that much of it 'sprang not from the gospel of Christ, but from racism'. It was 'admirable' in his view to teach Aboriginals the Christian message of love and hope, but it was:

> another thing entirely to link this ... to harsh discipline and narrow and trivial moral rules, to preach a gospel distinctly lacking in grace and to lead children to believe that a loving God destined them to a life of servitude and inferiority.[97]

This distorted view of what 'a loving God' had in mind for them meshed neatly with the interests of governments that were at best paternalistic and at worst negligent and with the views of a public not inclined to see Aboriginals as being much like them. Aboriginal 'advancement' was not high on any public agenda: if it were to occur it had to be in ways that did not involve governments or taxpayers in expense beyond a historically endorsed minimum, and did not unsettle views of Aboriginals as 'other' and inferior. This is chillingly captured in the words of Mrs Garnett, wife of Francis Garnett, then Superintendent at Point Pierce, before the Royal Commission in 1913:

> The great need in dealing with the girls at the mission is that they be placed out to domestic service as they reach a suitable age ... Personally I feel strongly that ... compulsory systematic placing of them out is necessary. Some of them are fitted to take situations at a small sum just as they are. It would be an expensive thing to train them for cooking and dressmaking. I think that would be putting the government to needless expense, because there is such a demand for them as raw material. They can all wash dishes and scrub floors.[98]

---

97 Harris, *One Blood*, pp.568–602

98 Mrs Francis Garnett, Royal Commission evidence, *SAPP* no.26, 1913, p.75; cited in Harris, *One Blood*, p.592

Meanwhile, by the early years of the twentieth century, beyond the missions, government institutions, pastoral stations and the Aboriginals Department, the 'Aboriginal problem' had become the focus of increasing attention of another kind – scientific, medical, anthropological and humanitarian. This contributed to growing interest in the possibility of Aboriginal survival or even assimilation and in policies that would promote these ends, although it did not extinguish the widely held view that Aboriginals were incapable of civilisation and therefore doomed to extinction.

Serious scholarly and humanitarian interest in the indigenous population had been apparent before this period, of course. Russell McGregor suggests that two main views about Aboriginals were held by non-Aboriginals during the nineteenth century and the early decades of the twentieth, and that they waxed and waned in relation to the intellectual currents and preoccupations, and the political and economic concerns of the time.[99] Both these views were linked to prevailing scientific ideas about human evolution, but took from these different emphases. The first, strongly influenced by Enlightenment ideas, and especially Rousseau's concept of the 'noble savage', held that Aboriginals, although arrested in a primitive stage of development, 'possessed a capacity for reason and progress' in common with the rest of humanity and would therefore, 'in the environment of civilisation, become civilised'. By contrast, the second view, characterised as hard primitivism, saw Aboriginals as 'so fundamentally different from Europeans that they could never attain the status of civilisation'. During the nineteenth century, the latter view, bolstered by scientific interest in the origins and evolution of humankind, as well as in racial differences, gained ascendancy, and by its end, 'evolutionary theory had consolidated an image of innately primitive Aborigines', who, 'unable to adapt to the circumstances of civilisation . . . would be exterminated by its progress'.[100]

Thus the indigenous population of Australia, at least those of the 'full-blood', were deemed to be 'doomed'. Such thinking was complex, evolving and often contradictory, but by the late nineteenth century had gathered sufficient coherence and sufficient scholarly support to be spoken of as 'doomed race theory'. At the same time, a lay version of it had taken hold in the public imagination. While the evidence of their eyes suggested to settlers that, as European settlement advanced, the indigenous population diminished, there were only limited 'hard demographic data' available to confirm this. McGregor suggests that doomed race thinking 'drew its major sustenance' from other sources:

> More than anything else it was a manifestation of ultimate pessimism in Aboriginal abilities. As the Enlightenment vision of universal human progress faded, as attempts to civilise and convert failed, and as racial attitudes hardened, it came to be considered that the best that could be done for the Aboriginals was to protect them from overt injustice and brutality.[101]

---

99 See McGregor, *Imagined Destinies*, for a detailed account.

100 McGregor, 'Protest and Progress', pp.558–9. While McGregor maintains that the broad themes of the debate remained constant, they were elaborated by a bewildering array of variations, which, in *Imagined Destinies*, he lucidly analyses. For further insightful analysis of this complex topic, see Warwick Anderson, *The Cultivation of Whiteness: science, health and racial destiny in Australia*, Melbourne University Press, Melbourne, 2002, especially chapters seven and eight.

101 McGregor, *Imagined Destinies*, pp.16–18

Missions, as we have seen, acted as official and unofficial agents of government and were partners in its civilising and pacifying role, often seeing their efforts as protecting Aboriginals from the demoralising effects of contact with the worst of white society. While their religious motivation implied hope for change, the general context for their activity was infused with doomed race thinking. Missionaries, like others, regarded Aboriginal people as primitive, and in some cases, barbaric, and did not expect 'to find among [them] ideas of any intellectual or spiritual depth'.[102] However, they were perhaps less inclined than were many scientists and anthropologists to embrace biological determinism which posited the immutability of racial types, being more sympathetic to historical and environmental arguments that stressed the importance of material, social and cultural factors in the evolution of societies. Such arguments held out hope for the civilising of even very primitive peoples.[103] While there were scientists, anthropologists and missionaries in both camps, many of them quite capable of shifting their ground and of holding inconsistent views, one thing is clear: all variations on the doomed race theme served to underpin the policies and practices of protection and segregation adopted in the Australian colonies from the late nineteenth century. Some encouraged tutelage in order to hasten progress towards 'civilisation' and accommodation to 'mainstream' culture, even while doubting its attainability; others called merely for the provision of comforts as the inevitable end approached. By the 1920s and 1930s, however, the hard primitivism and attendant fatalism of the evolutionists and their ascendancy in public debate was under challenge from several directions:

> as the evolutionary anthropological paradigm broke down, as cracks began to appear in the edifice of racial science and as the humanitarian lobby group became more and more vocal ... there was a revival of the enlightenment view that progress in civilisation may be attained by all humanity, regardless of race.[104]

The contribution of South Australian medical scientists and anthropologists to this shift was important and complex. From the 1920s, building on the pioneering work of Professor Edward Stirling, physiologist, ethnologist, parliamentarian and Director of the South Australian Museum, systematic study of physical anthropology was fostered by an interdisciplinary group of medical scientists and anthropologists connected with the South Australian Museum and the University of Adelaide. They focused attention on the physiology, racial origins and health of the indigenous population.[105] A Board for

---

102 Harris, *One Blood*, p.539

103 McGregor, *Imagined Destinies*. pp.24, 61. McGregor traces the relationship between and influence of these two lines of argument throughout his book. On pp.24 and 61 he illustrates them specifically by reference to evolutionary theorist Alfred Russell Wallace, and Jesuit missionary Donald MacKillop, respectively.

104 McGregor, 'Protest and Progress', p.559

105 For useful discussion of these developments and of the leading contributors to anthropology in South Australia in the 1920s and 1930s, see PG Jones, 'South Australian Anthropological history: the Board for Anthropological Research and its early expeditions', *Records of the South Australian Museum*, vol.20, May 1987, pp.71–92. See also Anderson, *The Cultivation of Whiteness*, pp.195–206.

Anthropological Research, established in 1926, encouraged expeditions and field studies in Central Australia and the remote north of South Australia,[106] and its members, most notably Professors Frederic Wood Jones and John Burton Cleland and Dr Thomas Draper Campbell, were active contributors to international anthropological scholarship. The board represented a conservative stream in anthropological thinking: it had not embraced the increasingly influential social and functional orientation that predominated in anthropological circles in Sydney and Melbourne.[107] It was still clearly preoccupied with the decline of the indigenous population and reinforced doomed race ideas in popular opinion.[108] Nevertheless, its expeditions encouraged positive and sympathetic views of still-tribalised 'natives' and gathered support for the establishment of inviolable reserves for their protection. Over time some of its prominent members contributed tentatively to the undermining of the doomed race view, arguing that extinction, though probable, was not inevitable, and that survival was a possibility, given appropriate protective action by governments.[109]

These were significant shifts, although to a later generation which has distanced itself from evolutionary race science they may appear timid, involving movement of the one-step-forward-two-steps-back variety. Evolutionary theory gradually became less salient in the explanations offered by biologists, medical scientists and anthropologists for the differences between 'races'. Indeed, the notion of 'race' itself came under question, both from advances in biology and from the ugly and destabilising manifestations of race science that emerged in Europe in the 1930s. In this context, Huxley and Haddon's We Europeans, with its condemnation of the 'vast pseudo science of "racial biology"', and its argument about 'the relative unimportance ... of purely biological factors as opposed to social problems in the broadest sense' in explaining differences between human groups, was an influential challenge to the evolutionary paradigm.[110] By emphasising the primary importance of culture and environment – by arguing, in other words, that people are products of history and opportunity, rather than of fixed genetic inheritance – such thinking challenged 'doomed race' fatalism, and pointed to the possibility of change and 'advancement' via social and political intervention.

However, shifts discernible with the long vision of history are not always so apparent

---

106 Early expeditions mounted by the Board, with the financial backing of the Rockefeller Foundation, included Alice Springs and Macumba, 1927, Koonibba, 1928, Hermannsburg, 1929, Macdonald Downs, 1930, Cockatoo Creek, 1931, Mt Liebig, 1932, and Ernabella, 1933. See JB Cleland, 'The Natives of the North-West of South Australia', *Medical Journal of Australia*, 30 June 1934, pp.848–53.

107 For a discussion of developments in anthropology in Australia in the 1920s and 1930s and Adelaide's place in this, see McGregor, *Imagined Destinies*, pp.102–7.

108 Jones, 'South Australian Anthropological History', pp.76–7

109 See, for example, Frederic Wood Jones, in an address to the Australasian Association for the advancement of Science, 1926, cited in McGregor, *Imagined Destinies*, pp.113–14; J Burton Cleland, 'Disease amongst the Australian Aborigines', Part 1, *Journal of Tropical Medicine and Hygiene*, vol.xxxi, no.5, 1 March 1928, pp.53–9.

110 Julian S Huxley and AC Haddon, *We Europeans: a survey of 'racial' problems*, Jonathan Cape, London, 1936, pp.7–8. For a discussion of the tension between racial and environmental arguments, and their connections, in Australia, to questions of white survival which formed part of the context in which questions of indigenous survival were considered, see Anderson, *The Cultivation of Whiteness*, chapter six.

at the time. In any case they are never complete or clear-cut. McGregor suggests that if the notion that Aboriginals were captive to a fixed racial primitivity was beginning to appear 'a little shaky' by the 1930s, this was 'only a beginning'. Although social anthropologists and others might be 'turning away from racial explanations, they certainly had not entirely turned their backs.'[111] The historical record repeatedly demonstrates this lack of clarity and conviction. Conceptual complexities and contradictions remained and appeared in official, professional and lay views.[112] This is neatly demonstrated in relation to health in a major, five-part series of articles by Cleland on 'Disease Amongst the Australian Aborigines', published in the *Journal of Tropical Medicine and Hygiene* between March and December 1928.[113] While much of Cleland's attention was focused on details of individual clinical cases – he openly confessed his interest as academic, not therapeutic or humane – the prevalence of tuberculosis among the indigenous population encouraged him to consider whether this reflected environmental or racial factors. Employing a common line of argument about susceptibility to the disease among Europeans of 'tuberculous stock', he concluded that Aboriginals, as a race, were of this stock:

> I am certainly inclined to think that the native is in general racially more susceptible to tuberculous infection than the average European, but is not, perhaps, more susceptible than those Europeans who come of what is spoken of as a tuberculous stock ... there are certain races, and amongst Europeans there are certain families in which there is an inherited tendency to succumb to tuberculous infection from a dose of bacilli that can be readily overcome by the racially more resistant individuals.[114]

Cleland was clearly not turning his back on categories of race and heredity as explanations for health differences between different populations, even though strong evidence existed to support an environmental explanation of susceptibility to tuberculosis. In the case of 'certain races' as well as 'certain families', what he construed as an 'inherited tendency to succumb to tuberculous infection', was really the result of political choices which condemned some populations to material deprivation and poor nutrition.

While Cleland's favouring of heredity over environment as an explanation of susceptibility to tuberculosis reflected the culture of his profession, in others the frustrations of experience reversed the direction of the general trend in thinking and allowed them to employ contradictory explanatory categories. Chief Protector South's early optimism about assimilation and subsequent resignation to the unlikelihood of making 'a black, white', and

---

111 McGregor, *Imagined Destinies*, p.107

112 This has already been demonstrated, for example, in the variety and contradictory nature of views expressed in reports of protectors and missionaries, parliamentary debates, and evidence before Royal Commissions.

113 J Burton Cleland, 'Disease Amongst the Australian Aborigines', *Journal of Tropical Medicine and Hygiene*, vol. xxxi, nos. 5–6, 11–18, 20–4, 1 March, 15 March, 1 June, 15 June, 2 July, 16 July, 1 August, 15 August, 1 September, 15 September, 15 October, 1 November, 15 November, 1 December, 15 December 1928.

114 Cleland, 'Disease Amongst Australian Aborigines', *Journal of Tropical Medicine and Hygiene*, 1 March 1928, pp.54–6. This article was also noteworthy in providing an early example of the 'thrifty gene' hypothesis, which Basedow, and, much earlier, Eyre, had reported, ibid., p.57.

missionary Hoff's conclusion that, God's goodness and the missionaries' efforts at Koonibba notwithstanding, 'you simply cannot make a silk purse out of a sow's ear', are examples of such reversals.[115] Thus experience and practical difficulties were capable of invoking in people working in the field a kind of lay, atheoretical racial prejudice which was at odds with their own efforts at 'civilising', as well as with prevailing or emerging theoretical positions. Scientists and anthropologists might be reassured, by their strengthening conviction that Aboriginals were racially homogeneous and of Caucasian stock, that cultural assimilation and biological absorption were possible.[116] Often lay people were not so reassured; Aboriginal 'culture', they feared, would not allow it. A compelling example of such thinking appeared in a report addressed by the Rev. JH Sexton, long-term office-bearer and activist in the AFA and member of the Advisory Council of Aborigines, to the Advisory Council in January 1938. He argued that even though the assimilation of mixed-race people would present no 'biological' difficulty, 'as the colour very quickly breeds out with each new infusion of white blood', there were other problems:

> morally and socially the difficulties are immense. Whatever our feelings are towards these people, those of us who know cannot be other than greatly alarmed at the moral abuses to which they fall. Chastity is a virtue which the majority do not appreciate and honesty and truthfulness are handled very lightly. How many white people are there, even amongst those who clamor for social equality and full citizen rights for these mixed bloods, who would accept them into their homes, their recreations or their religious congregations on an equal social footing to themselves ... the majority of mixed bloods must be controlled and protected by some government department.[117]

Thus, for Sexton, assimilation was unworkable on two grounds: Aboriginal unfitness, 'morally and socially', and non-Aboriginal lack of will. The second was an honest and accurate assessment of the prevailing situation with which Sexton had had much opportunity to become acquainted. Through his work in the AFA and on the Advisory Council of Aborigines he knew, for example, of the objections of non-Aboriginal women to sharing accommodation with Aboriginal women at the Queen's Home prior to their confinements. He knew that at Port Augusta non-Aboriginal parents objected to Aboriginal children being in school and that it was deemed a 'happy solution' to have them removed to the verandah in the mornings and sent home in the afternoons. And he knew that similar 'trouble' was repeated in many other places.[118] Sexton's first claim, however, about assimilation being unworkable was actually a racist argument masquerading,

---

115 See above, p.154. Hoff's remark was included in his report from Koonibba, quoted in report of Chief Protector of Aboriginals, *SAPP*, no. 29, 1926, p.54.

116 For discussion of the development of this assimilationist thinking, especially in connection with JB Cleland, see Anderson, *The Cultivation of Whiteness*, pp.200–6.

117 JH Sexton, Report on Definition of Aboriginals, attached to submission to the Advisory Council of Aborigines, 31 January 1938, Miscellaneous Papers of the Advisory Council of Aborigines, Correspondence, 1932–1938, GRG52/15

118 AFA Committee minutes, 29 March 1926, 22 July 1926, 3 October 1934, 3 March 1937, AFA Minute Books, SRG 139/2, vols v, vi: Advisory Council of Aborigines, Minutes, 5 October 1934, GRG 52/12/2

albeit unconsciously, as a cultural one: on what other grounds apart from the assumption of fixed racial types could moral and social 'difficulties' be deemed immutable? Sexton's views were the more remarkable since they referred to the mixed-race populations of Point Pearce and Point McLeay, recipients of decades of effort on the part of the AFA aimed at social and moral change.

If, in the 1920s and 1930s, scientific and anthropological opinion was contributing tentatively to the demise of doomed race thinking, the strongest faith and loudest voice in relation to indigenous survival and social inclusion was coming from the humanitarian lobby. This contributed significantly to the context in which Australian governments moved towards assimilationist policies and practices.[119]

A notable expression of organised humanitarian concern originating in South Australia was the 1927 petition to the House of Representatives on 'A Model Aboriginal State'.[120] This petition claimed that, despite the clear duty incumbent upon the colonists to care for the indigenous population, the spread of non-indigenous settlement meant that the original inhabitants were 'mostly fast dying out'. Rejecting arguments about Aboriginals' inferior capacity it asserted that it was not too late to put things right. This would involve not only treating Aboriginals as equals and assisting their accommodation to new conditions, but also returning land to them so that they could live 'free from white encroachment'. Hence the petitioners recommended the establishment of 'a model Aboriginal State', which would have representation in federal parliament, would be managed by an Aboriginal tribunal and from which non-Aboriginals, 'except Federal government officials, and authorized missionaries, teachers and agricultural instructors' would be banned. No Aboriginals would be forced to be part of it, but there was a suggestion of tightening of current practice in order to remove 'hangers on to the fringe of civilization' as far as possible from 'contaminating contacts'.[121]

The petition originated in Adelaide where, in 1926, Colonel JC Genders, disaffected former member of the AFA, had formed an Aborigines Protection League.[122] Committee members of the league included Dr Herbert Basedow[123] and Dr William Ramsay Smith[124],

---

119 Humanitarian concern was not unlinked to developments in science and anthropology of course. See Henry Reynolds, *This Whispering in Our Hearts*, Allen and Unwin, Sydney, 1998, chapter X1 for a discussion of these links, and of other major drivers of reform.

120 I draw here on Michael Roe's analysis of the petition and its reception: Michael Roe, 'A Model Aboriginal State', in *Aboriginal History*, vol.10, 1986, pp.40–4. See also McGregor, *Imagined Destinies*, pp.119–20.

121 Roe, 'A Model Aboriginal State', pp.41–2

122 Genders introduced the topic of establishing a 'Black State' at a committee meeting of the AFA in January 1925. The committee shelved the idea at that meeting, but in March 1925 declared that they had 'fully considered' it and found it 'fantastic', 'impracticable' and unlikely to make a 'real contribution to the Aboriginal problem', AFA, Committee minutes, 29 January 1925; 31 March 1925, AFA Minute Books, SRG 139/2, vol.v

123 Ian Harmstorf, 'Basedow, Herbert (1881–1933)', in Bede Nairn and Geoffrey Serle (eds), *Australian Dictionary of Biography, vol.7*, Melbourne University Press, Carlton, Victoria, 1979, pp.202–3

124 See above, p.4.

both of whom were influential in scientific and anthropological circles and had had long-term, public involvement in Aboriginal issues; Ngarrindjeri leader, David Unaipon[125]; prominent feminist activist, Constance Ternent Cooke[126]; and church leaders. Most of the 7113 signatories were 'ordinary folk' from the Adelaide suburbs.[127] The petition did not propose a politically viable line of action, but parliamentary debate on it led to the appointment of JW Bleakley, Chief Protector of Aboriginals in Queensland, to report to the Commonwealth Parliament on Aboriginal matters in central and northern Australia.[128] In his report, submitted in 1928, Bleakley scorned the idea of an Aboriginal state, insisting that 'the natives' had never evinced, nor were likely to, the understanding of democracy or the capacity for federation and mutual government that the petition pre-supposed.[129] However, he had clear recommendations for government action in relation to four groups of Aboriginals whom he identified. The remaining 'nomadic tribes' should be made secure from privation, not unnecessarily interfered with, but their young educated 'to desire better social conditions and the settled industrious life'. The 'uplift' of the 'semi-civilized' who lived in towns or on stations should be sought through the fos-tering of more humane public attitudes, fair pay and improved social conditions, the sup-pression of moral abuses and 'energetic medical measures, in the interest of the health of the community'. Those living in Aboriginal institutions needed to be better resourced, closely supervised and provided with vocational education. Finally, 'half-castes' should be 'rescued' from Aboriginal settlements, prevented, via the application of protective regu-lations, from breeding further 'crossbreeds', and especially in the case of those in whom 'white blood' preponderated, educated with the goal of entering the workforce and being 'absorbed' into the wider community.[130]

This familiar program did not cut any ice with Genders or the Aborigines Protection League. A paper published in 1929 declared the League 'strongly opposed to this rescue business' and reaffirmed its plea for Aboriginals to be 'given a chance to work out [their] own destiny'.[131] In April of that year, Genders and Constance Cooke represented the League at a one-day conference convened by the Commonwealth Minister of State for Home Affairs, the Hon. CLA Abbott, and attended by 33 representatives of missions, philanthropic and activist societies, and the pastoral industry. Genders and Cooke moved that traditional lands be restored, in perpetuity, to 'all nomadic tribes still with their tribal

---

125 See above, pp.134–5.

126 See Reynolds, *This Whispering in Our Hearts*, chap XI, and Margaret Macillwain, 'South Australian Aborigines Protection Board (1939–62) and governance through 'scientific' expertise: A genealogy of protection and assimilation', PhD thesis, University of Adelaide, 2005.

127 Roe, 'A Model Aboriginal State', pp.42–3

128 JW Bleakley, 'The Aboriginals and Half-Castes of Central and Northern Australia', *Commonwealth Parliamentary Papers*, 1929, vol.2, no.21, pp.1159–226, cited in Roe, 'A Model Aboriginal State', p.44

129 Roe, 'A Model Aboriginal State', p.44

130 Bleakley Report, *Commonwealth Parliamentary Papers*, 1929, vol.2, no.21, pp.1197–8, (pp.39–40 of report)

131 Aborigines Protection League, *Australian Aboriginals: A statement by the Aborigines Protection league explaining its basic principles and proposals and discussing statements in the Public Press and recent reports and recommendations*, Aborigines Protection League, Adelaide, 1929

governments'. Genders noted that the pastoralists were concerned about how this would affect their claims to land and that, although some of the missionaries supported some kind of recompense to the Aboriginals, subject to 'the economic position of the white settlers', none lobbied for the restoration of their land. The minister was unequivocal: he declared Genders 'a little ahead of [his] time' and the land question one which 'did not concern him or affect his department', whose duty was 'to secure the Aboriginals from privation, protect their hunting grounds wherever possible, and relieve sickness and destitution' and to 'advance their moral and material welfare'. Genders rejected this as charity. In his view 'the main task of government [was] to do equal justice to all British citizens, regardless of class, creed, race or colour'.[132] The discussion and outcomes of this small, low-key and inconsequential conference foreshadowed decades of future debates, government prevarication and widespread public acceptance of the privileging of non-indigenous economic freedoms and aspirations at the expense of indigenous concerns and claims. They identified Aboriginals quite clearly as people who were neither in charge of their own destiny, nor part of the Australian public.

Despite Genders' disillusionment with it, it was the AFA that provided the most sustained focus for non-indigenous humanitarian activism in relation to indigenous people in South Australia in the 1920s and 1930s. Relieved of day-to-day responsibility for its former mission at Point McLeay, it increasingly turned its attention to larger questions: it lobbied state and federal governments in relation to indigenous policy; it kept alert to incursions on reserves and to the impact of European development, including maverick missionary activity, on the lives of remote and still 'tribalised' Aboriginals; it corresponded with the British Anti-Slavery and Aborigines' Protection Society which was actively lobbying for a better deal for Australian Aboriginals; and it provided a platform for the views of the National Missionary Council and other prominent spokespersons for the Aboriginal 'cause'.[133] Through several publications which reflected humanitarian, anthropological and missionary views, the AFA helped develop a context that favoured assimilation for 'half-castes' and urged more effective protection for 'full-bloods'.

One of the most significant of these publications was *The Aborigines: a Commonwealth problem and responsibility*, of which 2000 copies were printed in 1934.[134] The purpose of this document was to explain and publicise the policy endorsed by the National Missionary Council of Australia in 1933. Arguing that the states were too poorly resourced to meet their legal obligations to the indigenous population, this policy called for the

---

132 Aborigines Protection League, *Report of Hon. Secretary, JC Genders to State Executive on the Bleakley Report Conference, convened by the Minister of State for Home Affairs of the Commonwealth, held Melbourne, 12 April 1929*, Aborigines Protection League, Adelaide, 1929 (no page numbers).

133 This orientation is clearly demonstrated in AFA minutes for this period. For further details of links between Australian activists and the British Anti-slavery and Aborigines' Protection Society, see also Reynolds, *This Whispering in Our Hearts*, chapter ix. The National Missionary Council represented a wide range of Australian missionary societies with missions in Australia and overseas. At its 1937 conference, representatives of 16 such societies were present.

134 Aborigines' Friends' Association Inc, *The Aborigines: a Commonwealth problem and responsibility*, issued for educational purposes under the editorial supervision of the Rev. JH Sexton, Hon. Secretary of the AFA Inc, Adelaide, 1934. All the AFA's publications in this period relied on the commitment and energy of the long-serving Sexton.

Commonwealth to assume control of indigenous affairs, and administer them through a separate government department advised by a board with educational, medical, missionary and anthropological expertise. The core of the proposals was that separate legislation was needed for 'full-bloods' still living a traditional life, and for 'half-castes'. Traditional 'full-bloods' were to be protected on 'inviolable' reserves that paid attention to traditional territory and language groups. These reserves should be adequately provided with food and water and be serviced by government or missionary institutions which would provide religious education and vocational training and establish economic activity. Different provisions were needed to allow 'half-castes' 'ultimate incorporation into full citizenship'. The Missionary Council formula, well-rehearsed, although vague, suggested training opportunities to develop habits of industry, followed by supervised employment. The AFA went further: it supported the 'new conception' of breeding 'half-castes' white. Rejecting the older view that 'the half-caste embodied only the vices of his white and black progenitors', it argued:

> The time … has arrived to give him special consideration … For he is not really an Aboriginal. He is the white man's child … He should be removed from the status of an Aboriginal so that he may feel a closer affinity to the white race.

This radical process of breeding out the colour and of cultural re-identification, in addition to the more mundane one of training and education, was 'essential if he is to take his rightful place in the community'.

Other recommendations indicated the complexity of the colonial legacy. They were concerned with the need for greater government subsidies for missions, control of conflicts between Aboriginals and pastoralists, a prohibition on Aboriginals being in areas in the vicinity of mining camps and railway lines where they were deemed especially vulnerable to degradation[135] and protection of Aboriginal women from both unscrupulous non-Aboriginals and oppressive traditional practices. In addition, the need for better health care was highlighted. This was something that had never been attended to adequately, and there was an 'urgent need' for a government-sponsored travelling medical service in 'widely-scattered areas' of the state. There was also an ongoing need for rations, since many older Aboriginals 'after years of fine service on stations and elsewhere, find it difficult to obtain the necessities of life'. Finally the AFA introduced a note of caution that is highly significant in the light of subsequent debates about the nature of 'Aboriginality' and about who is and who is not a 'real Aboriginal'. They were concerned that the new focus on 'half-castes' might penalise the 'full-bloods'. This had to be avoided, for 'the old full-blooded black is the real romantic picture of the Australian landscape. Around him, really all interest centres'.[136] Ironically, according to this line of thinking, this group, so long

---

135 This issue had long concerned the AFA and the Chief Protector of Aboriginals. The presence of missionaries at Ooldea and Tarcoola which tended to encourage the gathering of Aboriginals in the vicinity of the Transcontinental Railway was a particular concern. See for example, AFA Committee minutes, 11 July 1929, 4 October 1933; Report of Chief Protector of Aboriginals, *SAPP*, no.29, 1916, 1918, 1924; Mattingley and Hampton, *Survival in Our Own Land*, pp.235–7.

136 Aborigines' Friends' Association Inc., *The Aborigines: a Commonwealth problem and responsibility*, pp.2–10

thought to be doomed, needed to be preserved, while the less romantic mixed-race people were to disappear by a process of genetic and cultural whitening.

In its publication, *Aboriginal Problems: articles by various writers*, the AFA used prominent spokespersons to pursue these policy objectives further.[137] The Rev. Dr AP Elkin, Professor of Anthropology at the University of Sydney, argued the case for reserves that recognised spiritual and linguistic ties and encouraged indigenous confidence and hope for the future, as well as for anthropological training of non-indigenous administrators and more sociologically and linguistically informed missionary work. Professor JB Cleland, chair of the Board of Anthropological Research, University of Adelaide, reinforced the recommendation for a travelling medical service. Dr A Grenfell Price, Master of St Mark's College, University of Adelaide, focused on '[p]reserving the Aboriginal Race' through the provision of inviolable reserves, the 'infiltration' of 'white' women into the north of Australia, a program of 'breeding the Aboriginal white', through the marriage of Aboriginal women with non-Aboriginal men.[138] He also urged continued support of missions which did good work and did not cost much. Mr WT Lawrie, Head Teacher of the Point McLeay School, argued the case for modification of school curricula to meet indigenous learning needs and vocational training for a limited range of rural occupations. He held no great hopes for indigenous achievement: 'I would not care to suggest that we can produce tradesmen able to work independently', but 'for farm and station purposes they would be exceedingly useful'.[139] The last article, 'An Aboriginal Pleads for his Own Race', was written by David Unaipon who was identified, without reference to occupation or achievements, as a 'Full-Blooded Member of the Narrinyeri Tribe'. He argued that non-indigenous Australians had a duty to guide Aboriginals 'until they can stand alone in the new world', and until 'a new civilised race could be built up'. His vision of assimilation was expressed in terms of adaptation, and the opportunity to contribute to society, within narrow boundaries:

> It might take two generations, perhaps more, but eventually we would be able to take our stand among the civilised peoples. Already the Aborigine has shown he can fit in with the white civilisation. In the early days he helped the squatter and he made a fine stock rider and station hand. Educate him properly, treat him properly, and he will show his value.[140]

As these articles show, 'Aboriginal problems' were construed in a variety of ways and addressed with varying levels of insight. However, the proposed solutions, despite their apparent lack of cohesion, all indicated that indigenous peoples' futures were not a matter

---

137 Aborigines' Friends' Association Inc., *Aboriginal Problems: articles by various writers*, issued for educational purposes by the AFA Inc., Adelaide, nd [c.1934]

138 ibid., p.15. Price was confident that this would be effective, since 'Blood tests appear to show that the Aborigine is akin to the white man. There are no records of throw backs'. Like most other proponents of programs to breed out colour, he made no mention of what was to become of Aboriginal men, who had no part in the scheme. He also appeared unaware of how unpalatable his suggestions would seem to many Australians.

139 ibid., pp.15–6

140 ibid., p.16

for their own deciding and involved incorporation, although not on free and equal terms, into the non-indigenous world.

Several years later, the report of a National Missionary Council conference endorsed many of the arguments and recommendations made in the AFA publications, although it developed a different position on the future of 'half-castes'. The need for training, education, employment, care and services of various kinds was not disputed, but the goal of incorporation into non-indigenous society, especially through intermarriage, was rejected. In its place the council recommended separation:

> If the half-caste population can be assisted to develop self-reliant family and community life under benevolent supervision, it is possible that in the future a distinct new race will be developed ... We feel that the wisest policy for the future of the half-castes is to provide self-contained communities for them in which they will be removed from the inferiority which their ostracism from white communities produces.

In a departure from many other analyses of this period, the report specifically named 'colour prejudice' and poverty among 'the main difficulties from which Half-castes suffer'. Yet its proposal for the future, rather than confronting these sources of 'ostracism' in order to deal with them and thus open up more possibilities and choices, accepted them as givens which meant that separation was the only viable option. Not everyone at the conference agreed with the separate futures proposal. Sexton, representing the AFA, pleaded for the gradual incorporation of 'half-castes' into the general community, taking care to preserve what was best in indigenous culture. Elkin, representing the Australian Board of Missions, went somewhat further in suggesting that segregation and incorporation were not the only options: 'nothing less than ... training, guiding, winning the Aboriginal people to become a self-respecting, distinctive but real and integral part of the Australian Community' was an appropriate objective.[141]

Thus, in the 1920s and 1930s, the humanitarian and missionary lobby, together with differing schools of anthropological and scientific thought presented the Australian Government and people with a complex, often contradictory agenda for dealing with the 'Aboriginal problem'. But for all its complexity and contradictions, there were two strong threads that held it together and gave it some coherence. One was the implicit notion that the indigenous people themselves had little or nothing to contribute to the agenda; the other was the explicit argument that the solution to the problem involved some kind of protection for the dying race of 'full-bloods', and some kind of assimilation of the rising mixed-race people.

Concern and action about these matters was not solely the province of non-indigenous people of course. There was indigenous activism in this period also, although in an organised form, this was more significant in New South Wales and Victoria than in

---

141 *Australian National Missionary Conference 1937, Report*, Conference Continuation Committee in association with the National Missionary Council of Australia, Sydney, 1937

South Australia. However, from the early years of the twentieth century reports from missions and government institutions reveal instances of the preparedness of South Australian Aboriginals to express discontent and make material or other demands. This assertiveness was most frequently reported from the perspective of non-indigenous missionaries or government officials and reveals their discomfort with it. For example, members of the AFA committee after a visit to Point McLeay in 1912 reported that 'the Natives knew too much', that 'their attitude' was 'too familiar', and that staff were not exercising 'that control which is necessary in dealing with Natives'.[142] At Killalpaninna just before the First World War, missionary Reidel was regretting, as inappropriate, the change in 'tone' that led to the Aboriginals being 'cocky' and demanding wages.[143] The Lutheran Mission Board acknowledged in the early 1920s that it was time to replace the 'original patriarchal supervision and control' at Koonibba with 'more practical steps to train our natives to be more self-sufficient' and justified this in terms of gospel recommendation and economic and administrative necessity. However, a later assessment suggested that this shift was also to do with 'the natives' being 'no longer quite so tractable'.[144]

Given the consistent claim of government and missions that their goal was to make Aboriginal people into self-reliant, responsible members of the community, there is remarkably little evidence of rejoicing at signs that these goals were being met. Aboriginal people appeared vividly, as we have seen, as named, assertive, dignified individuals when giving evidence to official inquiries or complaining against discriminatory legislation. But in the records of the Chief Protector, the Advisory Council, and the AFA and other mission societies, they remain, for the most part, shadowy, nameless and undifferentiated from one another. This is clearly shown by reading the prolific records of the AFA. The AFA's long, continuous and undoubtedly genuine commitment to the 'welfare of Aboriginal people' has an abstract quality about it that seems not to involve engagement with actual individuals. In fact, individual Aboriginal people appear only minimally within the AFA records. They do so in two main ways. From time to time groups from Point McLeay and Point Pearce communicated lists of grievances or asked for the opportunity to discuss concerns. While such petitioners are named and their requests recorded, indications of how they were dealt with are often missing, and it is difficult to discern whether they were taken very seriously. The second way in which individual Aboriginals appear, albeit sometimes anonymously, is in relation to small, specific requests for money, to buy some rabbit traps, or a nurse's uniform, or to help with acquiring a house, or to meet the expenses of visiting Adelaide. The AFA does not appear tight-fisted – it usually came up with some money – but there is no apparent reflection on what these isolated requests said about the limited opportunity, choice or room to move in the

---

142 AFA Committee minutes, 14 October 1912, AFA Minute Books, SRG 139/2, vol.IV. These comments were contained
     in a letter addressed to the President of the AFA by committee members C Taplin and W Dalton.

143 Stevens, *White Man's Dreaming*, pp.187–9

144 Evangelical Lutheran Synod in Australia, South Australian District Inc., *Synod Report, 1922*, p.70; E Harms and C Hoff
     (eds), *Koonibba: a record of 50 years work among the Australian Aboriginals by the Evangelical Lutheran Church of
     Australia 1901–1951*, Adelaide, 1951, p.9

lives of indigenous people, or about the paucity of government planning and provision.[145] In addition, the records reveal little sense of satisfaction or pleasure in the achievements of either individuals or of groups. There are no positive reports about the numbers earning their own living or completing certain levels of schooling, or about individuals exercising effective leadership. Even David Unaipon, the shining star of Point McLeay, appears mostly as a supplicant, seeking financial support for his various creative schemes. There is nothing that suggests partnership between the AFA and the people it purported to serve.

In this context, two examples of organised, intentional and public indigenous activism, one involving Point Pearce people and the other Point McLeay people, are worthy of note. As we have already seen, the Point Pearce people had, over a number of years, been assertive in relation to the administration of the station and had voiced their unhappiness with the government's failure to provide them with training or with control over some of their land.[146] In 1935, RM Wanganeen and 97 other residents of Point Pearce petitioned the government. Claiming to speak for all Aboriginal inhabitants of the state, they indicated a level of initiative, political awareness, and shared aspirations for their future that government and missionary pronouncements usually ignored:

Petition of the Aboriginals (sic) inhabitants of South Australia
to His Majesty (sic) Government of South Australia

The humble petition of the undersigned aboriginals [sic] inhabitants of South Australia respectfully showeth

That the small remnants of the tribes who occupied the State when the white race came to South Australia have a strong moral claim to proper treatment from the white race. That race today is occupying our lands and in return we are forced to accept charity.

Under their rule nearly the whole of our race has disappeared, and those of us who survive, resent to be treated as paupers or outcasts.

We demand fair treatment.

We respectfully ask

1. That in order to deal adequately with the aboriginal and Halfcast [sic] problem a Board of management be appointed consisting of suitable representative [sic] of the various interests involved.

2. That to represent the needs of our race grant us power to propose a member in the person

---

145 AFA Committee minutes, 30 July 1925, 28 July 1927, 21 May 1931, AFA Minute Books, SRG139/2, vol.v. The paucity of government provision is exemplified especially clearly in the case of the 'young married half-caste' who asked the Chief Protector for some rabbit traps. The Chief Protector asked the AFA to provide them to avoid the setting of a precedent which might cause financial embarrassment to the Aboriginals Department (21 May 1931).

146 The discontent of the Point Pearce people was apparent, as we have already discussed, in their testimony before the 1913–16 Royal Commission. Reports of the Chief Protector of Aboriginals during the 1930s refer to ongoing tensions and difficulties at Point Pearce and indicate something of the attitudes and behaviour of the staff that contributed to indigenous discontent. See, for example, Report of Chief Protector of Aboriginals, *SAPP*, no.29, 1932, p.39; *SAPP*, no.29, 1935, p.43; *SAPP*, no.29, 1937, p.48.

of or own blood to be employed by the Government as a member of the Board, so that we may have a voice in deciding the future of the race.

3. That the white race which is charged both by the direct command of those who established these colonies and also by every moral obligation which can bind an honest nation shall make a proper effort to redeem us from the degrading condition under which we are at present forced to live or to give us the opportunity to redeem ourselves so that we will cease to be a burden on the taxpayers of the State.[147]

In a letter accompanying this petition, Wanganeen suggested that as this matter was of 'National interest' it 'behove[d] every citizen to aid my less fortunate brethren', and sought the government's 'urgent assistance'. A reply from the premier's office assured him that the matter was 'receiving attention'. And there it rested.[148]

Point Pearce people were not the only ones to seek official action at this time to redress various wrongs. At its meeting of 1 June 1938, the AFA committee received a petition that Point McLeay residents had sent to the Advisory Council of Aborigines. The Advisory Council, despite its status as the body providing independent advice to the Aboriginals Department, passed it on to the AFA. Signed by H Rankine, senior, A Cameron, G Rigney and J Harradine, it was a mixture of nostalgia for the 'good old days' of AFA administration of the station and proposals for a more independent future. It repeated decades-old requests for a dormitory system, training, land, and opportunity to earn their own living. It asked for access to river water via an irrigation scheme. Revealing a lack of basic material comforts and safeguards of health, it asked for reliable domestic water supplies, improved sanitary arrangements and houses of 'not fewer than two rooms'. And it asked for a system of administration that involved less surveillance by police, 'whom the natives consider are prejudiced against them'.[149] The minutes do not record how this petition was regarded by the AFA, and there is no mention of it in the minutes of subsequent meetings. It seems that, as with the Point Pearce petition, it was received and there the matter rested. In the long run, action depended on political will and that was in short supply. Governments simply did not devote significant financial or human resources to indigenous affairs. Constance Cooke had argued in 1930 that it was a 'hopeful sign' that there

---

147 This hand-written petition with 98 signatures attached was sent on 13 November 1935 with an accompanying letter from RM Wanganeen to the Premier, the Attorney-General, the Commissioner of Public Works, the Minister for Agriculture and members of parliament for Yorke Peninsula. Correspondence received by the office of the Commissioner of Public Works, GRG 23/1/317/1935.

148 In a reply from the secretary to the premier, Wanganeen was assured that 'the matter [was] receiving attention'. Internal correspondence reveals the nature of that attention. The recommendation, dated 25 November 1935, of the Chief Protector, MT McLean, from whom the Commissioner of Public Works sought an opinion, was as follows: 'The question of appointing a board to control and administer the Aboriginals Department has already been placed before the Hon. the Minister by a deputation which waited on him some little time ago. Even if the board were decided on I would not recommend the inclusion of an aboriginal among its members.' The final annotation on the file, dated 5 December 1935 is by the Premier: 'Hold for the present'. Correspondence received by the office of the Commissioner of Public Works, GRG 23/1/317/1935.

149 AFA Committee minutes, 1 June 1938, AFA Minute Books, SRG 139/2, vol.vi

was 'an earnest minority' who recognised that 'we have a problem'. However, solving it depended on the response of the appropriate government minister and the reality was that:

> Native affairs is only one of the Minister's many duties, and it is exceptional for a minister to find time to deeply interest himself in the problems that have been created through the contact of two such different civilisations.[150]

Thus, by the end of the 1930s Aboriginals occupied various restricted and marginal sites within the public life, economic structures, imagination and future hopes of other South Australians. The 'dying race' of 'pure bloods' was no longer dying, it seemed, although in many cases their culture and their well-being remained under severe threat, leading to debate about the possibility of protection on inviolable reserves. The 'rising people' of mixed race were proliferating, but not becoming whiter by degrees and still in need of training and education to develop their capacity for responsible community membership. Except for the people of the remote north-west, they had all lost their land. They were all likely to be poor by the standards of the rest of the community, and official records and unofficial observations regularly attested to their poor health. If they were employed within the western economy it was in low-paid, low-skilled and low-status occupations, often on seasonal or casual terms. If they lived on cattle stations, missions or government institutions, it was under conditions marked by high levels of control which denied them status as independent persons. If they lived in Adelaide or in country towns, it was in the poorer areas, on the physical and social margins, struggling against heavy-handed official surveillance, outright discrimination or deeply ingrained doubts – which harboured both racial and cultural fears – about their capacity for assimilation. These doubts and fears were tellingly revealed in continuing attempts to keep indigenous people who usually resided on missions and government institutions out of Adelaide. This, as we have already seen, was a perennial preoccupation: it had tested the patience and ingenuity of Matthew Moorhouse in the 1840s and 1850s. It appeared that little had changed: Aboriginals were coming to Adelaide without permission, were readily obtaining alcohol, and in some cases pursuing 'immoral purposes', and associating themselves with 'places of ill-repute'. Even those who lived permanently in the city were regarded as a problem, and the Adelaide City Council was 'tak[ing] steps' to remove them to country towns.[151]

Debates about the future of Aboriginals, and activism that aimed to promote their cause, also occupied restricted space. The boundaries were set by the historic parameters of the race debate in Australia, and implied by the various notions of assimilation that were emerging as solutions to the 'problem' of the 'rising population' of mixed-race people. As we have seen, this restricted discourse applied not just to non-indigenous thinking and

---

150 Constance M Ternent Cooke, 'The Status of Aboriginal Women in Australia', (1930), in Graham Jenkin (ed.), *Between the Wars: documents relating to Aboriginal affairs, 1919–1939*, South Australian College of Advanced Education, Magill, South Australia, 1989, pp.101–15.

151 AFA Committee minutes, 28 February 1928, 5 November 1930, 24 March 1931, 1 May 1935, 1 September 1937, AFA Minute Books, SRG139/2, vols v, vi

action: when indigenous activists entered the political arena in the 1920s and 1930s, they too operated within these parameters. What Wanganeen and his fellow petitioners, and the group representing the Point McLeay people were asking for amounted to an opportunity for assimilation. They sought an opportunity to be outcasts no longer, but to be incorporated into the normal civic structures that kept other citizens from degradation. This amounted, in the words of the Point Pearce document, to 'fair' and 'proper treatment'. Far from making a case for recognition of particular rights on the basis of 'Aboriginality' or for the opportunity to maintain any kind of separate or distinctive existence, they were subscribing to what McGregor calls an 'ideology of incorporation'.[152] Some later commentators, influenced by a radically altered historical context, have decried this as evidence that Aboriginal activists of the 1930s must have been 'mere dupes of a dominant ideology', and on the basis of this judgment, have accorded their thinking little respect or discursive space. However, as McGregor suggests, this discounts indigenous agency and is ahistorical in its understanding of 'ideologies of liberation'. These, he argues:

> like regimes of oppression (or hegemony), are contingent upon historical circumstance. There are no eternal doctrines of liberation, merely argumentative strategies which have force at particular times, in particular circumstances.

Whatever judgements were made about it later, for Aboriginal activists in the 1930s, 'after 150 years of . . . exclusion from white society, an ideology of incorporation was both radical and liberationist'.[153]

Where was all this leading? New legislation, reflecting the emerging assimilationist discourse, supported by new scientific and anthropological understandings that undermined older certitudes about 'race' and evolutionary determinism, and encouraged by a sharpened humanitarian conscience, was soon to make significant changes to the lives and futures of the indigenous population. The next chapter explores whether these changes amounted to the 'incorporation' of Aboriginals within the broader Australian community, thus allowing them, after a century of dispossession, to become part of the public.

---

152 McGregor, 'Protest and Progress', p.560. While focusing on New South Wales and Victorian activism, and especially the work of John Patten and William Ferguson of the Aborigines Progressive Association, and William Cooper of the Australian Aborigines' League, this article has broader application.

153 ibid., pp.559–560, and footnote 28, p.560

Chapter 6

1939–1962:
Assimilation – 'Breeding Out'
or 'Socialising In'

From a practical and from a humanitarian aspect, the development of a 'colour problem' in Australia cannot be tolerated for a moment. The detribalized native and the half-caste in some way must be gradually absorbed into the white community.　　　　**JB Cleland 1938**[1]

It may well be assumed that with the present-day improved living conditions, closer supervision by the departmental officers, missionaries and police officers, in addition to more readily available medical attention, the aboriginal population, both full and mixed-bloods, will naturally increase. The Board is aware of this fact and are [sic] anxious to improve the lot of all aboriginals, particularly by means of education, vocational training, and better housing, in order that these people can be better fitted to eventually take their place in the community independent of government assistance.　　　　**Aborigines Protection Board 1954**[2]

... a great number of our aborigines simply have no desire to be assimilated, but understandably would rather lead a life of their own choice. Forced assimilation is simply not practicable nor possible and can only end in tragedy for the aborigine concerned ... every effort must be made to create a desire on the part of the aborigine for his ultimate assimilation.　　　　**Aborigines Protection Board 1960**[3]

In 1941 the Aborigines' Friends' Association (AFA), committed to 'watch over the interests of the aboriginal inhabitants of the Commonwealth of Australia – and particularly of the state of South Australia and the Northern Territory – and promote their spiritual and temporal well-being in any way that circumstances may suggest', expressed its concerns about the new generation of Aboriginal people and South Australia's new government policy of assimilation. Whereas the traditional Aboriginals were an 'attractive race because of their simple, frank ways, their happy temperament and their contentment with a few

---

1　JB Cleland, 'Some aspects of the problem of the Australian Aboriginal and his descendants in South Australia', notes submitted to the Royal Anthropological Institute, 1938, GRG 52/10/3/1938

2　Aborigines Protection Board, Annual Report, 1954, *SAPP*, no.20, 1954

3　Aborigines Protection Board, Annual Report, 1960, *SAPP*, no.20, 1960

simple things in life', now '. . . a new generation has arisen through miscegenation, and has brought with it more difficult problems than when the authorities were dealing with a purely primitive race'. It appeared to the AFA that the situation was degenerating. The first generation of half-castes 'were much superior to the present strain', while 'the progeny of the present-day half-castes lack viability and strength and if their stamina is not improved they will become a burden rather than an asset to Australia'. Given this, they saw 'Dangers Lurking in the New Act' and questioned especially the 'wisdom' of the exemption provisions that allowed for 'removing natives from the protection of the Aborigines Act in order to bring them into citizenship'. However, assimilation seemed inevitable and therefore had to be embraced. After the war was over, 'a place for the aborigines' had to be found 'in the new order':

> [They] should no longer be left in the backwash of our civilization, but should be taken in hand and be properly educated and trained for citizenship, for they must sooner or later take some place in a civilized community'.

It was no longer reasonable to imagine that they could be left alone 'with their outmoded social order'. And by embracing assimilation, Australia would be able to 'roll away the reproach made abroad that Australia is quietly acquiescing in the passing of the aborigines to racial degeneracy and death'.[4]

This distinctly ambivalent statement by the AFA, made shortly after the passage of legislation that owed much to its advocacy and commitment, is indicative of the complex mixture of hope and fear, expectation and doubt, admiration and denigration, compassion and indifference, shame and national pride that characterised non-indigenous attitudes towards the indigenous population. The government of South Australia, in response to the scientific, anthropological and humanitarian developments discussed in the previous chapter, and to the persistence of the 'Aboriginal problem', and in particular the growing numbers of mixed-race people, had moved towards a policy of assimilation during the second half of the 1930s. In 1934, it had passed the *Aborigines (Consolidation) Act* which repealed both the *Aborigines Act, 1911* and the *Aborigines (Training of Children) Act, 1923*, while consolidating much of their content and import.[5] In 1936, however, before this act had come into force, the government introduced an amending bill which sought to replace the Advisory Council of Aborigines with an Aborigines Protection Board, a move that had the support of the Advisory Council, the AFA and 161 indigenous petitioners. The bill generated considerable parliamentary debate, which focused more on problems with the current administration of Aboriginal affairs than on the welfare and future of the indigenous population. In particular, there were concerns about the wisdom of the bill's proposal to make the Chief Protector, who was the administrative head of the Aborigines Department, the chairman of the Protection Board.[6] While much of the debate was concerned with the perceived shortcomings of individuals in the Aborigines Department

---

4 AFA, *Annual Report*, 1941, pp.3–12

5 *Aborigines (Consolidation) Act*, no 2154 of 1934

6 For a brief summary of the debates on the 1936 bill, see Raynes, *'A Little Flour'*, pp.48–9.

and on the Advisory Council, Baden Pattinson, member for Yorke Peninsula, understood that the problems of effective administration within the Aborigines Department reflected the broader issues of policy drift and lack of government commitment:

> Instead of [their welfare being directed by] a well-defined and continuous policy the natives have been allowed either to roam at large or have been huddled into these mission stations where they have been allowed to vegetate. Instead of finding some scope for their undoubted abilities they have been kept largely in enforced idleness with the natural consequences following the want of employment. With the changes of Government and policy which have taken place from time to time naturally this department is one of the last which a busy Commissioner of Public Works takes any trouble to become acquainted with, and therefore we find a lack of continuous effort and policy.[7]

The 1936 bill lapsed, but a subsequent Aborigines Act Amendment Bill, introduced in August 1939, addressed the administration issues, enunciated a clear policy direction, and was assented to on 28 November 1939, having aroused little parliamentary dissent.[8] The detail of the act reflected recommendations that had been repeatedly canvassed by National Missionary Council and the AFA in the late 1930s, and which the AFA had regularly communicated to federal and state parliamentarians.[9] The assimilationist ideology of the act, although later to be widely regarded as abhorrent in its denigration of the values of indigenous culture and identity, was in fact strongly influenced by humanitarian concerns and reflected the ideology of many 1930s Aboriginal activists. For them, the alternative was continuing dependence or an enforced return to or maintenance of primitivity, which they saw as a dead end and as a denial of rights. They wanted to be taught to live in the modern age, as modern Australians. As members of the Aborigines Progressive Association put it, 'We want to be absorbed into the Nation of Australia, and thus to survive in the land of our forefathers, on equal terms'.[10] The Point Pearce people wanted 'fair treatment' and a chance to escape 'the degrading condition under which we are at present forced to live'.[11] Aboriginal organisations all saw the attainment of 'civilisation' through education and training as the prerequisite for 'citizenship', and the process of assimilation as the route to the desired end of an equal and respected place in Australian society. The only apparent alternative was the 'leave them alone' policy adopted by governments and reinforced, in the

---

7 Baden Pattinson, *SAPD*, House of Assembly, 2 November 1936, p.2419

8 *Aborigines Act Amendment Act*, no. 14 of 1939. Also referred to as the *Aborigines Act, 1934–1939, Acts of Parliament of South Australia, 1939*, Government Printer, Adelaide, 1940

9 For example, at its annual general meeting in June 1938, the AFA considered resolutions from the 1937 National Missionary Conference and made a series of recommendations for a new act that closely resembled the one that was eventually passed. It dealt with the definition of Aboriginality, education aimed at integration, citizenship based on 'character and fitness', and not on 'degrees of colour', and a system of exemption from the act for approved Aboriginals, AFA Committee minutes, Annual Report, 1 June 1938, AFA Minute Books, SRG 139/2, vol. 6.

10 John Patten and William Ferguson, Aborigines Progressive Association (NSW), 1937, in McGregor, 'Progress and Protest', p.555.

11 RM Wanganeen and 97 other signatories, GRG 23/1/37/1935

view of the AFA, by 'scientific men who [were] unwilling to supersede the primitive systems of the aborigines by something better', and anthropologists who wanted 'the native to remain static if possible, in the midst of an advancing civilisation'. The AFA pronounced these approaches as 'unprogressive and disastrous', and argued that 'the only way to prolong the life of the aborigines is to give them a cleaner, healthier and more intelligent life', removed from 'tribal methods' which 'carry the seeds of decay'. Those who were 'worthy of a better status should be exempted from aboriginal laws, and brought under the laws governing the general community'.[12] Such thinking clearly underlined the view of indigenous Australians as not part of the public. For other Australians, being guaranteed a free and equal place within 'the Nation of Australia' and 'the general community' was consequent on birth, not on proving their worth or their degree of 'civilisation'. This hurdle was erected only in relation to descendants of the original inhabitants.

However, the business of being 'absorbed into the nation' was not just about demonstrating a capacity for civilised living; it was also about 'breeding out the colour'. Through programs that McGregor has called 'perverse', the assimilation policy, not just in South Australia but in other states as well, attempted to deal with the evils of miscegenation by encouraging miscegenation and to keep Australia white by encouraging racial impurity. The policy was not eugenic in a formal sense. It was about improving 'the nation's complexion, not its gene pool', and 'sought not to make fitter people, but to make people better fit in'. While from that time there were claims – and these have become more strident in recent years – that the policy was really about extinction and eradication, this was never the whole story: the historical evidence makes it clear that what some have seen as genocidal intent went hand in hand with genuine humanitarian concern.[13]

The Aborigines Act Amendment Act, 1939, was a complex and contradictory mix of new and old. It superimposed assimilationist ideas over an older paradigm of protection and segregation whose assumptions and parameters it did not question. It abolished the position of Chief Protector of Aboriginals and disbanded the Advisory Council of Aborigines. Henceforth, the act was to be administered by an honorary Aborigines Protection Board with executive powers rather than merely an advisory function. It was to be appointed by the Governor and to consist of the minister responsible for Aboriginal affairs and six others, two of whom were to be women.[14] The minister was to be the chairman of the

---

12   AFA Annual Report, 1939, *Advertiser*, 1 March 1939

13   Russell McGregor, '"Breed out the Colour" or the Importance of Being White', *Australian Historical Studies*, vol.33, no.120, October 2002, pp.286–302

14   The inaugural members of the Aborigines Protection Board were Rev. Canon STC Best, Acting Secretary of the Australian Board of Missions; Prof. JB Cleland, who was the Vice-Chairman, and given the frequent absence of the Minister, the effective chairman; Mr LJ Cook, a senior bureaucrat from the Department of Agriculture and a trained experimental agriculturalist; Mrs Constance Cooke, prominent advocate of women's and Aboriginal rights, foundation member of the Aborigines Protection League and member of the Advisory Council of Aborigines since 1929; Dr Charles Duguid, medical practitioner and founder of the Presbyterian Mission at Ernabella; and Mrs Alice Johnston, who was, like Cooke, a nominee of the League of Women Voters to the Advisory Council on Aborigines.

Board and the permanent head of the department its secretary. While the Board was new in both composition and powers[15], its duties mirrored those previously undertaken by the Chief Protector of Aboriginals and reflected long-held views of the indigenous population as a people apart, with social and economic needs different from and lesser than those of other South Australians. The act constructed them either as mendicants, or as people needing to be controlled or trained, or, in the case of 'full-blood' or traditional Aborigines, to be protected. The level of services directed towards them related not to their needs or rights, but to an unspecified, but limited capacity of government to provide. Thus the Board was to control and promote the welfare of Aborigines by deciding on how the money at its disposal was to be used, by distributing rations, by providing, 'as far as practicable' for the needs of sick and aged Aborigines, by providing, 'when possible' for the custody, maintenance and education of Aboriginal children, by managing all reserves, and by exercising 'a general supervision and care over all matters affecting the welfare of the aborigines, and to protect them against injustice, imposition, and fraud'. All members of the Board were Protectors of Aborigines and the legal guardians of all Aboriginal children until the age of 21, regardless of whether they had living parents or other relatives.[16]

As had been the case in the past, it was hoped that new administrative arrangements would of themselves deliver benefits to Aboriginal people. For example, LG Riches, member for Stuart, speaking in favour of the bill, suggested that the creation of the Aborigines Protection Board would give the Aborigines Department, which until then had had no clout, a tiny budget, and reflected the 'general belief that aborigines should take second place', the opportunity to exert more influence on government. In the absence of any evidence that this underlying situation had changed, it seemed that a good deal of faith was being placed in the capacity of the new Aborigines Protection Board to reform or override it. The naivety of this faith was eloquently expressed in the contribution of TC Stott to the parliamentary debate about the proposed administrative changes. Displaying a complete disregard for the troubled history of the land- and resource-poor institution at Point McLeay he thought that the board would

> probably provide ways and means, especially at Point McLeay, for the native population to grow vegetables and cereals and teach them to take more interest in work so that they may ultimately become self-reliant.[17]

The parliamentary proceedings provide no evidence of the more sophisticated understanding of the Aborigines Department's administrative difficulties that appeared in a memorandum presented to the government by the Royal Anthropological Institute in 1938. This memorandum, designed 'to call attention to certain matters of fact in a disinterested attempt to help governments in a difficult task', pointed out that:

---

15 For a detailed analysis of the notions of expertise underlying the composition and functioning of this board, and their impact on modes of governance, see Margaret Macilwain, 'Aborigines Protection Board (1939–1962) and governance through 'scientific' expertise: a genealogy of protection and assimilation', PhD, University of Adelaide, 2005.

16 *Aborigines Act Amendment Act*, no 14 of 1939.

17 TC Stott, *SAPD*, House of Assembly, 19 September 1939, p.879

the training of those persons who are in charge of the protection … of natives in the actual
tribal area, their general level of education, their salaries, working conditions, and their chances
of an attractive career in aboriginal affairs, are not equal to the qualifications demanded of and
conditions given to officers with similar work to do in Melanesia, Papua and Africa.

The reality was that many local administrators in Aboriginal affairs were working beyond
their competence, and the whole enterprise was poorly financed.[18] These were not simple
matters that could be rectified by the replacement of one central administrative structure
with another, but those debating the Aborigines Act Amendment Bill in 1939 did not confront such challenges.

Section 5 of the act dealt with the vexed question of the definition of 'aborigine'. It
expanded the definition to include all persons of Aboriginal descent without reference to
degrees of colour or quotients of blood. The Hon. M McIntosh, member for Albert and
the minister in charge of the Aborigines Department, in proposing the bill, acknowledged
that this was a difficult issue. He told a moving anecdote that doubtless reflected the
experience of many Aboriginal people:

> I can remember an occasion in my district when a man, obviously of aboriginal descent,
> approached me. He asked me what I thought he was and I inquired what he was driving at. He
> wanted to be told whether or not I thought he was an aborigine, and I told him that I
> thought he was a half-caste. He then stated that if he went into an hotel for a drink he was told
> that he could not be served because he was an aborigine, but if he communicated with
> Adelaide and asked for any of the privileges available to aborigines he was informed that he was
> not one. He wanted to know just where he stood.[19]

The new inclusive definition made it clear where he and others like him stood: they were
'aborigines'. This definitional change made for administrative clarity and efficiency and
there was little parliamentary dissent about it. However, CJD Smith, member for Victoria,
betraying a common prejudice that to be defined as Aboriginal was to be defined as inferior, and assuming that it meant being segregated into compounds and camps, was concerned that the new definition would return 'half-castes' and 'quarter-castes' and 'lesser
bloods' – some of whom were fine people! – 'to the cess pits from which, to their eternal
credit, they [had] emerged'. 'Why should they be dragged back into the mire?' he asked.
They should be given their birthright, that is, the portion of their blood that was 'white'
should prevent them from being classified as Aboriginal.[20] His views were echoed in the
Legislative Council by the Hon. FA Halleday, who believed that being identified as
Aboriginal was stigmatising, and that octoroons were white enough to be allowed to decide
for themselves if they wanted to be so identified.[21] However, by erecting a system whereby

---

18 'Memorandum on the condition of the Australian Aborigines: statement drawn up for the Royal Anthropological
    Institute by its Committee on Applied Anthropology', 1938, pp.5–6, GRG 52/37
19 Hon. M McIntosh, *SAPD*, House of Assembly, 8 August 1939, p.467
20 CJD Smith, *SAPD*, House of Assembly, 7 September 1939, p.847
21 Hon. FA Halleday, *SAPD*, Legislative Council, 24 October 1939, p.1422

persons of Aboriginal descent could be exempted from their legal status as Aboriginals, and be regarded as far as the law was concerned as 'whites', the new law reinforced the notion that assimilation was about capacity for 'civilisation', not about blood.

The system of granting exemptions from the *Aborigines Act Amendment Act, 1939* to selected Aboriginals was one of the cornerstones of South Australia's assimilation policy. It reflected new thinking that was competing with, although not ousting, older segregationist views. Section 14 of the act allowed that:

> In any case where the board is of the opinion that any aborigine by reason of his character and standard of intelligence and development should be exempted from the provisions of the Act, the board may, by notice in writing, declare that the aborigine shall cease to be an aborigine for the purposes of this Act. Any such declaration may be made by the board whether or not an application is made by the person to whom the declaration refers.

Exemptions were of two kinds: unconditional exemptions which were by definition non-revocable and limited exemptions which could either be revoked or made unconditional at the board's discretion at any time during a three-year probationary period.[22] Here then was a clear message about how Aboriginals could become part of the public: they simply had to demonstrate the character, intelligence and standard of development of 'civilised', that is non-Aboriginal, Australians. No longer deemed to be barred from such attainment by virtue of their racial inheritance, they could get there by effort and will.

Subsequently much maligned by indigenous and non-indigenous critics for its denigration of Aboriginality and its unquestioned assumption of the value of cultural absorption, the thinking behind the exemption system was implicit in the position of many indigenous activists. For example, as McGregor has demonstrated, it was central to the political agenda of eastern states indigenous activists associated with the Aborigines Progressive Association, the Australian Aborigines' League and the 1938 Day of Mourning. They argued that the unequal position of Aboriginals within Australia was the result not of innate racial differences, but 'a matter of education and opportunity'. In their discussions with governments over enfranchisement and eligibility for social security payments their plea was, 'let the determination be, not color, [sic] but capacity'.[23] Under the exemption system, judgements of the Aborigines Protection Board about capacity overrode any based on colour.

The exemption system received a mixed reception from indigenous people when it was in force. Some welcomed it, often because they perceived it to be a pathway to enhanced social and economic opportunities for themselves and their children. Others thought the price to be paid in separation from kin and banishment from reserves was too high in relation to the perceived benefits. Many, even if they sought exemption, resented the surveillance and the need for identification that were part of the system. In addition,

---

22 *Aborigines Act Amendment Act*, no. 14 of 1939, section 14. Similar systems of exemption were established in New South Wales, by the *Aborigines Protection (Amendment) Act, 1943*, and in Western Australia by the *Native (Citizenship Rights) Act, 1944*. See Human Rights and Equal Opportunity Commission, *Bringing Them Home*, pp.599–648.

23 McGregor, *Imagined Destinies*, pp.254–8. See also, McGregor, 'Protest and Progress', pp.557–8.

many misunderstood what the system was about. Not surprisingly, they were unable to untangle the conundrum of having ceased to be an Aboriginal for the purposes of the law while unmistakably continuing to be one in terms of ethnicity, appearance, cultural and familial attachment and in the estimate of others.[24] Far from perceiving the system as an opportunity to experience legal equality with non-indigenous Australians, some saw it as discriminatory and as yet another example of non-indigenous high-handedness that singled them out unfairly. They resented its erosion of their 'protected' status as Aboriginals, a status they preferred, despite its intrinsically discriminatory nature and in-adequate provisions, to the apparently inexplicable and insulting status of 'ceasing to be an aborigine' for the purposes of the act. Finally, they found that exemption from their former legal status as Aboriginals was one thing; acceptance and opportunity within the non-Aboriginal community was another thing altogether. In short, if exemption was meant to be a tool of assimilation and inclusion within the life and culture of the general community, for many it simply did not work.

Strongly articulated negative reactions to the exemption system are a familiar part of indigenous memoirs of the period. Much commented on is the requirement that exempted Aboriginals carry at all times certificates of exemption, often referred to as 'dog tags' or 'dog licences'. The reason for this requirement was on one level straightforward, inoffensive and practical. No one could identify, simply by looking, whether an Aboriginal was exempted or not: legal status made no difference to outward appearance. Therefore a form of identification was needed, making it possible for police, other government officials and members of the public to know – in a way that appearance did not – whether the person they were dealing with was, according to the law, an Aboriginal. In practical terms, this mattered, because in relation to, for example, education, receiving government benefits, living on reserves or in Aboriginal institutions, drinking alcohol, and 'consorting' with non-Aboriginal persons, the laws were different for Aboriginal and non-Aboriginal persons. However, for many Aboriginal people these pragmatic considerations carried no weight. They experienced the system as confusing, discriminatory and demeaning, and resented it strongly.[25]

Recorded reactions of Aboriginal people to the exemption system also make it clear that while they sought a 'fair go' and the right to be 'citizens' in their own land – in short, equality with non-Aboriginals and acceptance as part of the public – they also claimed their right to continue to be 'Aboriginal'. While their notion of being 'Aboriginal' appears un-developed and only minimally politicised when compared with the claims made by sub-sequent generations to a distinctive identity, culture and political role, the seeds of these later understandings were nevertheless apparent in statements of people exempted under

---

24 This confusion, and the resentment that accompanied it, is powerfully evoked in Brodie, *My Side of the Bridge*, chapters 6 and 7.

25 See, for example, Mattingley and Hampton, *Survival in Our Own Land*, pp.48–52; Brodie, *My Side of the Bridge*, chapters 6 and 7; Margaret Forte, *Flight of an Eagle: the dreaming of Ruby Hammond*, Wakefield Press, Adelaide, 1996, pp.52–5; Doris May Graham and Cecil Wallace Graham, *As We Have Known It: 1911 to the present*, South Australian College of Advanced Education, Adelaide, 1987, pp.60–1. For a different view, though still involving rejection of the exemption system, see Nancy Barnes, *Munyi's Daughter: a spirited Brumby*, Seaview Press, Adelaide, 2000.

the 1939 act. For example, Veronica Brodie, a woman of Kaurna and Ngarrindjeri descent, who 'became white' when she married an exempted man, recalled:

> I looked at my dark skin, and I thought to myself, who are these people? How could they tell me that I'd become white if I married this man? ... But being made white didn't make much difference to the way I felt. I said to the Board, 'What are you making me white for? The colour don't rub off.' I still felt Aboriginal, and I still mixed with my own people ...[26]

Similarly, Cyril Coaby, an Alawa (Northern Territory) man who as a youth lived at Koonibba, valued his identity as an Aboriginal more than the opportunities that exemption offered:

> I never held a permit [exemption certificate]. I didn't like the wording, 'Cease to be an Aboriginal'. Although I wanted the alcohol, which I could get easily through having an exemption, I think my pride was stronger than my need for alcohol. No way in the world would I give up my Aboriginality for anything. I considered it an insult to my mother.[27]

Brodie and Coaby were ahead of government and community thinking, however. The notion that 'Aboriginality' as a distinctive cultural and political phenomenon could be part of Australia's future, or that it could be seriously desired and sought after had few adherents in this period. The accepted wisdom was the view, reinforced by Commonwealth–State Native Welfare Conferences from 1937 and reflected in several state laws that 'the destiny of the natives of aboriginal origin, but not of the full blood, lies in their ultimate absorption by the people of the Commonwealth'.[28] The third Native Welfare Conference, meeting in 1951, formally adopted a policy of assimilation, and the Commonwealth Minister for Territories, Paul Hasluck, reported to the federal parliament that this meant 'in practical terms, that, in the course of time, it is expected that all persons of aboriginal blood or mixed blood in Australia will live like white Australians do'. It has been argued that Hasluck saw assimilation as 'a policy of opportunity' concerned with gradual 'cultural adjustment' and a chance for 'the aboriginal' to 'shape his own life'. However, over time it became a policy of absorption, which made it clear that there was only one acceptable 'shape' for the lives of descendants of the original inhabitants:

> All Aborigines and part-Aborigines are expected eventually to attain the same manner of living as other Australians and to live as members of a single Australian community, enjoying the same rights and privileges, accepting the same responsibilities, observing the same customs and influenced by the same beliefs, hopes and loyalties as other Australians.[29]

---

26 Brodie, *My Side of the Bridge*, pp.89–91

27 Mattingley and Hampton, *Survival In Our Own Land*, p.51

28 Human Rights and Equal Opportunity Commission, *Bringing Them Home*, p.32

29 Statement adopted by the 1961 Commonwealth/States Native Welfare Conference. Richard Broome, *Aboriginal Australians: black response to white dominance, 1788–1994*, 2nd edn, Allen and Unwin, Sydney, 1994, pp.171–3

This statement, frequently quoted as both the essence of what was meant by assimilation and the goal of assimilation policies, makes a seductive surface appeal to non-indigenous notions of democracy and equality. Its plausibility and reasonableness readily commend it to 'ordinary', 'decent' Australians. But it is dismissive of the possibility that indigenous people may see themselves as distinctive, and may, even while 'enjoying the same rights and privileges', and 'accepting the same responsibilities' as other Australians, nevertheless be responsive to some different customs, beliefs, hopes and loyalties. In dismissing this possibility it effectively presumes that there is only one way to be part of the Australian public and mistakes a 'single community' for a monolithic one. Over the decades since this statement was made Aboriginal people have frequently challenged this view. They have demonstrated – and asked non-Aboriginal people to accept – that there are many ways of 'being Australian' and 'being Aboriginal', ways which are characterised by varying degrees of assimilation to the cultural mainstream.[30] While access to rights and acceptance of responsibilities may not be negotiable within a society laying claim to being just and democratic, flexibility in relation to customs, beliefs and ways of doing things may be central to that claim. Assimilation, is not, as suggested by the much-quoted statement of 1961, prescriptive and indivisible: on the contrary, it can accommodate choice and variety. As indigenous insistence on this has become stronger and more sophisticated, it has bred fear and resentment among non-indigenous people who mistake distinctiveness for privilege; it has also complicated understandings of what it means to be part of the public.[31]

Although the 1939 act made no mention of this, there was a widespread if not comfortably accommodated understanding that assimilation of persons of Aboriginal descent into the general community could be achieved through intermarriage as well as through the behavioural shaping-up that could lead to exemption from one's legal status as an Aboriginal. Such an outcome was not unconnected to the system of exemption, since the demonstration of the characteristics of 'civilised' living that was necessary to earn an exemption was also the most likely way to demonstrate suitability as a partner in marriage with a non-Aboriginal. In any case, the section of the act which made it illegal for non-Aboriginal men to 'consort' with Aboriginal women meant that liaisons between the racial groups involved only those Aboriginals who been exempted.[32] Certainly there was some expectation that children of exempted persons, especially girls, growing up within the general community and conforming to its values and standards, would 'marry out'. Thereby Aboriginal blood, as well as Aboriginal ways, would, in time, disappear. As Cleland put it, what was needed was a scheme of:

---

30 This is not to say that Aboriginals have been the only contributors to understandings and debate about cultural diversity. However, it is fair to suggest that their views and claims have been widely seen as the most problematic and as potentially divisive.

31 For further discussion of this point see below, pp.277.

32 Section 34a of the *Aborigines Act, 1934–1939*, states that 'Any male person, other than an aborigine, who, not being lawfully married to the female aborigine ... (a) habitually consorts with a female aborigine; or (b) keeps a female aborigine as his mistress; or (c) has carnal knowledge of a female aborigine, shall be guilty of an offence against this Act.

settling young married half-castes in country centres, finding suitable employment for them, if necessary and until established, in part at government expense, and arranging for their children to be brought up at the local school and thus grow up under favourable European circumstances with a prospect of the lighter-coloured among them, from the point of view of marriage, passing as European.[33]

However, although such thinking was implicit in the act, it was too contentious to be made explicit. As already noted, intermarriage and 'interbreeding', especially if they involved Aboriginal men and non-Aboriginal women, were feared by many in an Australia obsessed with 'whiteness' and responsive to deeply entrenched ideas of social status. Yet they kept occurring, thereby ensuring the persistence of a problem whose solution seemed inevitably to involve embracing the very thing that was feared. The 1939 act was no less contradictory and no more open and constructive about this than the Bleakley Report had been a decade earlier. Bleakley had urged the 'discountenance' of intermarriage, and the checking 'in every way possible' of the breeding of half-castes, yet also called on governments to 'give half-castes proving to be superior a chance to better themselves', and to 'separate the quadroon and octoroon types at an early age, from the aboriginal, and give special training for future reception into the white races'.[34] He again argued this position, against some opposing views, at the inaugural Native Welfare Conference in 1937: assimilation should not occur through 'breeding out', but through 'socialising in'.[35] But these two processes were less easily separated in real life than in rhetoric. As coy and uncomfortable as laws, scientists, politicians and the general public might be about it, assimilation was, at least in part, about 'breeding out the colour'.

Reflecting the old protection model, other sections of the 1939 act provided for the maintenance of Aboriginal institutions and reserves and continued the historic practice of paying most attention to the comparatively small numbers of Aboriginals who lived in government-controlled settings, while largely ignoring those who lived elsewhere. Aboriginal institutions were to be run according to government regulations, and restrictions on the movement of Aboriginals to or from such places were specified in the act. The act dealt also with the perennial problems of education, training and the 'rescue' of children deemed to be neglected. Aboriginal children, like other South Australian children, were bound by the provisions of the *Education Act, 1915–1935*, which made education compulsory up to the age of fourteen years. In addition, the *Aborigines Act Amendment Act* empowered the Aborigines Protection Board to commit Aboriginals, up to the age of 18 years, or, in the case of females, 21 years, to institutions controlled by the Children's Welfare and Public Relief Board to be dealt with as if they were neglected children, according to the terms of the *Maintenance Act, 1926.*[36] Children confined under the

33 Cleland, 'Some aspects of the problem of the Australian Aboriginal', p.6

34 Bleakley, 'The Aboriginals and Half-Castes of Central and Northern Australia', p.1198

35 Rosalind Kidd, *The Way We Civilise: Aboriginal affairs – the untold story,* University of Queensland Press, St Lucia, 1997, pp.141–2

36 According to the *Maintenance Act, no.1780 of 1926,* a 'neglected' child was one who begged, wandered about, had no settled abode, associated with prostitutes, vagrants or habitual drunkards, had an unfit guardian, was illegitimate and whose mother was dead or unfit, was under 14 years old and not in school, or frequented public houses.

Maintenance Act (and sections 37–40 of the *Aborigines Act* also gave the Board wide powers to have Aboriginal children so confined) became 'state children' and could be apprenticed or placed out to foster care. Thus in the name of assimilation the 1939 act added legislative muscle to the long-standing practices of removing Aboriginal children, especially those of mixed race, from their families and culture, claiming this as an act of 'rescue' that would deliver social, economic and, in some cases, spiritual benefits. If these measures were designed to assimilate Aboriginal children into the wider community, it seems that the route chosen – segregation and institutional control – was highly unlikely to lead to the desired end. On institutions and reserves all Aboriginal children between 14 and 16 years were required to be in employment or to be in school, and if they were not, their parents would be deemed guilty of an offence against the act. Here, perhaps, the assimilation message was clearer: idleness and lack of engagement in the education system or in employment was not acceptable, and if Aboriginal people did not take the initiative themselves, the state would take it for them. However, the act, like previous legislation, said nothing about actually providing the education and employment, or the living wage on which opportunities for genuine economic and social assimilation rested.

The law's preoccupation with surveillance and control of Aboriginal people was further exemplified in the sections of the act pertaining to Aboriginal camps and prohibited areas, and to health. The board was empowered to remove Aboriginals who were camped close to towns, or found 'loitering' within them, and the Governor could proclaim towns and other areas prohibited to Aboriginal people unless 'lawful employment' gave them reason to be there.[37] In relation to health, the preoccupation of the act lay with the control of infectious diseases. As has so often been the case throughout history, the chief mechanism was the control of diseased persons, or those suspected of being diseased, rather than seeking to deal with the root causes of infection. The act provided for the authorisation of any legally qualified medical practitioner to enter any premises where Aboriginal people were located, to medically examine any Aboriginal 'in such manner as the practitioner deems necessary' and, calling on the police if necessary, to remove infected Aboriginals to any lock hospital for detention and treatment. Any Aboriginal who resisted any part of this procedure would be deemed to be committing an offence. Clearly, it was a very limited assimilation that the act embraced, and one defined entirely according to non-indigenous terms.

What did the 1939 act and the assimilation policy which it enshrined amount to for indigenous South Australians? The minutes and annual reports of the Aborigines Protection Board, which met as frequently as fortnightly throughout much of its life, provide a broad, and in some cases, an intimate view of the situation; parliamentary debates, mission records and the recorded memories of some Aboriginals provide other perspectives.

At the first meeting of the Board in February 1940, the chairman, the Hon. M McIntosh, defined its purposes in simple charity terms: the Aboriginals, 'these unfortunate

---

37 *Aborigines Act Amendment Act, no. 14 of 1939*, sections 6, 28, 29, 42

people', were 'a very serious problem' and the Board's efforts were to be directed at doing 'something practical' to help them. Over the next 22 years the Board did indeed engage in much practical activity and demonstrated a somewhat greater capacity for policy development and responsiveness to changing circumstances than McIntosh's banal inaugural remarks might have suggested. The records of its activities reveal that its major preoccupations were the implementation of the exemption system, encouragement of indigenous people off the missions and into jobs and housing in country centres, the care and training of 'neglected' mixed-race children, health, or at least the quality and quantity of the health care provided for Aboriginal people, living standards prevailing in missions and institutions, indigenous access to the 'mainstream' welfare system and, less consistently, economic exploitation of Aboriginals, especially on the mining and pastoral frontiers. This agenda, which reflected the increasingly complex and varied relationship of the indigenous population with the state, was pursued in a context of considerable state government complacency, despite increased expenditure, growing federal government involvement, continuing negative community attitudes, and a persistent failure to provide genuine opportunities for education, training and employment, except in a handful of cases. It also reflected confusion about whether services were a privilege or a right, and whether assimilation was a process of granting entitlements from which social absorption of Aboriginals might be expected to result, or a process of Aboriginals' 'measuring up', and thereby earning acceptance and entitlements.

At a special meeting convened on 18 May 1956, the Board approved a revised policy aimed at achieving 'the objective of total assimilation'. Together with recommendations about child protection made at a meeting held on 3 February 1956 and revisited at the May meeting, this policy tells us much. Without question, it reflected a genuinely humane desire to improve social and economic opportunities and the material circumstances of Aboriginals' lives. However, its vision of 'total assimilation' was in fact very limited. It was pursued in a context constrained by the ongoing influence on policy of restricted historical constructions of indigenous people and their futures, by persistent 'buck-passing' between government departments in relation to difficult aspects of Aboriginal affairs, and by a failure to involve Aboriginal people in planning or decision-making about any of this.[38] The following sections trace, in turn, the Board's attempts to implement 'total assimilation' through its focus on exemption, health, welfare, and rescue of children.

The exemption system was a key strategy for realising the goals of the assimilation policy. Its administration was an ongoing task of the Aborigines Protection Board and a significant part of its meeting time was spent considering applications for exemptions from the act. Reporting on the year ending 30 June 1946, the Board noted that 32 Aboriginals had been granted unconditional exemption, including 26 who had satisfactorily completed three years of exemption on probation. Fifty-five others had been exempted on probation. On the other hand, four had had their exemptions revoked because of misuse of alcohol and 15 new applications had not been entertained 'as it was considered improbable that the applicants could be successfully absorbed in the general community'. This brought to 330 the numbers exempted over the past six years. Of these, 225 'appeared satisfactory' to the

---

38 Aborigines Protection Board, Minutes of Special Meeting, 18 May 1956, GRG 52/16, See below, Appendix 5.

Board, 67 remained on probation, and 38 had been 'brought under the control of the Board'. This was judged to be an 'eminently satisfactory result' which indicated that 'a considerable proportion of the native population in the settled areas is capable of enjoying the privileges and accepting the responsibility of citizenship'.[39]

Behind this bland reporting lay stories of great poignancy. It is not clear how many indigenous South Australians sought, obtained or had imposed upon them the supposed boon of acceptance into the general community via the mechanism of exemption from their legal status as Aboriginals, nor what this amounted to in material and emotional terms.[40] But what is clear is that the exemption system gave to the handful of well-intentioned non-Aboriginal people who constituted the Aborigines Protection Board enormous power over individual Aboriginals and families and the right to sit in judgement on the intimate details of their domestic lives. For example, on 3 August 1955 the Board found in favour of one family who

> ... were well thought of, and were conducting themselves in a proper manner. [The adult male], who was a returned soldier, has been allocated a War Service Settlement Block about twenty miles from [regional centre] and continues to live a useful and decent life. The family are staunch Methodists, taking an active part in church matters and are accepted generally as useful citizens in the community.

Such evidence of potential for assimilation was rewarded with an unconditional exemption. However, another application processed at that same meeting was turned down since the applicant

> has no permanent home, no furniture, and little clothing, no permanent employment, is not clean and tidy and has been convicted on a number of occasions for breach of the Licensing Act.[41]

Perhaps he could have taken advice from another applicant, a 'well educated and intelligent young man', who several weeks later was granted an exemption on the testimony of his land lady, who found him 'exceptionally clean in personal habits', and said he had 'not caused any trouble or worry during the twelve months he [had] been living with her'.[42] Non-indigenous notions of what it meant to be a 'decent' and 'responsible' member of the community' meant that indigenous people had to negotiate many moral hurdles on the road to assimilation via exemption. It must have been difficult for them

---

39 Aborigines Protection Board, Report, 1946, *SAPP*, no.20, 1946

40 Reports of the Aborigines Protection Board from time to time include annual summaries of the numbers of exemptions granted and revoked. Files of the Aborigines Department, GRG 52/19 and GRG 52/20, contain duplicate copies of certificates of unconditional and limited exemption for the period 1941–54. While these provide an incomplete picture, since exemptions were not discontinued until new legislation was passed in 1962, they indicate that the numbers exempted must have been in excess of 550 persons from all over the state but with the greatest concentrations in the city and suburbs of Adelaide.

41 Aborigines Protection Board, Minutes, 3 August 1955, p.69, GRG 52/16/2

42 Aborigines Protection Board, Minutes, 31 August 1955, p.80, GRG 52/16/2

to anticipate them all. For example, early in 1956 the Board reported on an applicant for exemption who was

> a reasonably clean type of aborigine, and dresses very tidily, but unfortunately … resides with [a woman] his *de facto* wife, with whom he has lived for the last eight years in a shack constructed of masonite, cornsacks and a corrugated iron roof'.[43]

It is not clear whether it was his fidelity to his *de facto* wife or the building materials of his house which caused the greater moral offence. In any case, he did not make the grade.

One recurring problem related to the exemption system involved alcohol. The Protection Board minutes and reports contain frequent references to exempt Aboriginals drinking to excess, as well as associating with non-exempt Aboriginals and illegally supplying them with intoxicating liquor. This was doubtless a common and easily detectable breach of the law, but it is also telling evidence of several significant and ongoing issues. Most obviously it was a sign of the hold that alcohol had over many Aboriginal people. However, it also reflected the difficulties experienced by Aboriginals who sought to reconcile what the non-Aboriginal community demanded as signs of suitability for assimilation with their connections and obligations to their own people. These difficulties were exacerbated by the poor reception that 'exempted' Aboriginals received from the wider community into which their new status was meant to give them entrée. The Protection Board was well aware of this, as its 1948 report indicates:

> In view of the general tendency to regard the aborigines as a separate race of people, and also the reluctance displayed by members of the general community to receive exempted persons on basis of social equality, the continued association of exempted persons with aborigines is not surprising, indeed the gregarious instinct renders such a condition of affairs inevitable. The result is that the development and progress of the exemptee towards citizenship is definitely hindered if not entirely precluded.

The Board regretted that, in this unhelpful social context, some Aboriginals, previously judged to be of 'exemplary character … deteriorated seriously when granted complete freedom from control and supervision chiefly because of excessive drinking'. As a solution they suggested a 'supervised intermediate stage', which would involve settling family groups of exemptees in 'a number of small village settlements', where they would live 'under conditions calculated to prepare them for full citizenship'. This, they believed, would be 'an incentive to those capable of advancement'.[44] Thus, within the space of a paragraph, the challenges of assimilation evoked a segregationist solution that ignored the contribution of general community expectations and behaviour to the problem and constructed it once more as being about indigenous capacity.

Not surprisingly, the 'supervised intermediate stage' did not eventuate and the problems identified in 1948 persisted. In 1951 the Aborigines Protection Board reported

---

43 Aborigines Protection Board, Minutes, 11 January 1956, p.112, GRG 52/16/2
44 Aborigines Protection Board, Annual Report, 1948, *SAPP*, no.20, 1948

that, of the 555 exempted since the inception of the system, 381 had gained unconditional exemption, and that the majority of these were 'undoubtedly making a praiseworthy effort to live independent and useful lives ... accepting the responsibilities and enjoying the privileges of full citizenship'. The 'progress' of a minority, however, was still being retarded by their non-acceptance in the general community, their 'inability to break finally with old associations', and excessive indulgence in alcohol.[45] By 1954, the Board had 'little doubt that many applications are made for the sole purpose of permitting the native to obtain intoxicating liquor', and it repeatedly noted that exempt persons were suppliers of intoxicants to their non-exempt kin and associates.[46] The intractability of these problems doubtless contributed to the Board's sober assessment of the prospects for assimilation. In 1956 it declared itself

> opposed to any attempts to assimilate the native people rapidly as it is felt that to hasten such a policy would surely end with tragic results. It is believed that to prepare the aborigines for assimilation it is likely that at least three or four generations must pass before these people would be absorbed. Since the inception of the State, many aborigines and their families, thrust into white communities or entering them at their own desire, have found it impossible to be absorbed, in fact, as might be expected, they have been ostracized with frequent tragic results.[47]

Here is another example of a phenomenon, already noted, endemic in the history of public health and public policy: the capacity to overlook a mismatch between the way a problem is constructed and the solution that is suggested. In this case, 'white communities' are acknowledged as being at fault, since they have ostracised Aboriginals who have sought to be 'absorbed'. But they are not involved in the proposed solution: it is Aboriginals, not non-Aboriginals, who must be 'prepare[d] for assimilation'. The prediction that this might take a long time – three or four generations – seems to relate to indigenous lack of preparedness, not that of the wider community.

A second strategy of assimilation pursued by the Aborigines Protection Board involved an attempt to improve indigenous health. The Board recognised and was concerned about various health-related problems. These included outbreaks of illness, especially communicable diseases which could constitute a threat to the rest of the community. The provision of medical services was also perceived as an area for action. Perhaps because of Dr Charles Duguid's presence on the Board, plans for improved medical attention featured at its first meeting at which it was agreed to pay doctors an annual fee and an allowance for mileage and medicines to attend to the needs of Aboriginals at 20 different locations.[48]

---

45 Aborigines Protection Board, Annual Report, 1951, *SAPP*, no.20, 1951

46 Aborigines Protection Board, Annual Report, 1954, *SAPP*, no.20, 1954; Minutes, 7 March 1956, p.131; 18 April 1956, p.146; 20 June 1956, p.175; 4 July1956, p.183 etc., GRG 52/16. The Board's concerns were probably well founded. It is apparent from many Aboriginal recollections of the exemption system that it was frequently seen as being primarily about 'drinking rights'.

47 Aborigines Protection Board, Annual Report, 1956, *SAPP*, no.20A, 1956

48 Aborigines Protection Board, Minutes, 27 February 1940, p.1, GRG 52/16. The locations at which the Board provided medical

In 1941 Duguid was working with Dr DRW Cowan, physician in charge of the chest clinic at the Adelaide Hospital and later Director of Tuberculosis Services in South Australia to organise a medical survey of the indigenous population to detect and deal with cases of tuberculosis. The survey extended over several years, examined large numbers of Aboriginal people and happily found few cases of the disease.[49] In 1948 the Board reported on an outbreak of infantile paralysis at Point McLeay and a 'very serious epidemic' of measles which spread rapidly from Oodnadatta to a number of settlements and pastoral holdings in the north-west of the state, resulting in many deaths. Duguid travelled to the worst affected areas and, alongside the Flying Doctor Service, nurses, police and station proprietors, 'spent many anxious and arduous days ministering to those in need'. This honorary involvement of Duguid and the fact that the cost of medical supplies as well as the transport and fares of all involved in combating this emergency was met by the Aborigines Department rather than coming from the health budget suggests that maintaining the health of the indigenous population was not a 'mainstream' concern.[50] Certainly, Aboriginal people or issues related to their health rarely rated a mention in *Good Health for South Australia*, the bulletin issued regularly by the South Australian Department of Public Health.[51]

As already noted, outbreaks of infectious disease within the indigenous community which threatened to spill out in to the general community were most likely to galvanise health authorities into action. However, there was little evidence of this worrying either the Department of Public Health or the Aborigines Protection Board at this time. The Board reported regularly on how few cases of tuberculosis their surveys found, and in 1959, the state Director of Tuberculosis, Dr Philip Woodruff, reporting on ten years of the National Tuberculosis Campaign, confirmed that there was no greater prevalence of tuberculosis among the Aboriginal population than the non-Aboriginal, although those 'living as Europeans', exhibited a 'slightly greater liability to disease' than those living under 'semi-tribal conditions'.[52] There were probably several conclusions to be drawn from this about the impact of the material environment on health, especially in the light of earlier claims that the indigenous population was constitutionally deficient in relation to chest complaints. But neither Woodruff nor the Protection Board pursued them. The Board claimed that other diseases also were being held in check. In 1960 it reported that 'prompt action'

---

attention were Adelaide Hospital, Swan Reach, Mannum, Sedan, Tailem Bend, Wellington, Meningie, Point McLeay, Quorn, Baroota, Port Germein, Whyalla, Iron Knob, Blackford, Kingston, Ceduna, Koonibba, Oodnadatta, Maree and Farina.

49 Aborigines Protection Board, Minutes, 9 April 1941, p.93, 23 April 1941, p.96, 22 October 1941, p.130, GRG 52/16; Annual Report, 1942, *SAPP*, no.20, 1942; 1944, *SAPP*, no.20, 1944

50 Aborigines Protection Board, Annual Report, 1948, *SAPP*, no.20, 1948

51 The first issue of *Good Health for South Australia*, which replaced *Public Health Notes*, appeared in January 1932. Issued by the Department of Public Health for distribution to chairmen, members and secretaries of Local Boards of Health and to Officers of Health and Health Inspectors, its aim was 'to provide health workers in the State with information on Public Health and to stimulate enthusiasm in community hygiene'. With periodic name changes, it continued to be published until 1977.

52 PSWoodruff, 'The Campaign against Tuberculosis', *Good Health for South Australia*, no.111, July 1959, pp.34–37

had 'practically eliminated' venereal disease in outback areas and that effective immu-nisation campaigns were providing effective protection against diphtheria, whooping cough, tetanus, influenza and infectious hepatitis.[53]

The Protection Board's 1949 report recognised a different kind of health problem:

> One of the principal causes of ill-health, particularly among children, is the irregular and in-adequate meals provided by some of the mothers, who are incompetent and neglectful. No doubt such children would enjoy better health and be much happier if placed in institutions provided by missionary organizations, and in some cases action along these lines has been taken. The board desires, however, as far as possible, to preserve the family life intact and, with this object in view, the welfare officer, Sister McKenzie, and the nurses and helpers on all aborig-inal stations and missions are busily engaged advising and encouraging the parents to raise the standard of living in their homes.[54]

The Board was on firm ground in linking health to 'standard of living' and good nutrition. And it was following well-established patterns of thinking and practice among health pro-fessionals in assuming that these could be assured by maternal competence and attention, which in turn could be evoked by advice and encouragement. However, while persistently subscribed to, such an approach was flawed and of limited use: living standards are substan-tially determined by factors other than professional advice and individual behaviour and are not amenable to significant improvement without more fundamental social and eco-nomic change.[55] The 1949 report made it clear that the application of a judgemental, advice-giving approach to Aboriginal families was connected to the fact that many of them had increased disposable income available to them from this time. Amendments to the *Commonwealth Social Services Act* had made child endowment payments available to all Australian mothers from 1941, except those categorised as 'nomadic' Aboriginals.[56] This extension to much of the indigenous population of a 'mainstream' entitlement simul-taneously enlarged the scope for official surveillance and interference in their domestic lives. The Aborigines Protection Board was unembarrassed about entering this new site of control:

> While in some homes reasonably good use is made of the family income, it is obvious that in many cases there is an appalling incompetence in the management of money. The endowment

---

53 Aborigines Protection Board, Annual Report, 1960, *SAPP*, no.20, 1960

54 Aborigines Protection Board, Annual Report, 1949, *SAPP*, no.20, 1949

55 Expert advice-giving that focuses on individual behaviour and largely ignores material circumstances has long been a favoured approach to improving health, despite evidence, accumulating from the late nineteenth century, of the impact of social and economic environments and especially of poverty, and more recently, of inequalities *per se*, on health. The advice-giving approach has been particularly strong in relation to infants and young children and in relation to any pat-terns of behaviour and consumption that do not reflect middle-class values and standards. For an analysis of this phe-nomenon see Judith Raftery, '"Mainly a Question of Motherhood": professional advice-giving and infant welfare', *Journal of Australian Studies*, no. 45, June 1995, pp.66–78; Raftery, 'Keeping Healthy in Nineteenth Century Australia'.

56 See below, pp.194

in such cases is brought under the control of the department with a view to ensuring that the children are properly fed and clothed.[57]

The heavy-handed departmental paternalism referred to here impinged in demeaning and threatening ways on families, and especially on mothers, who, while under constant pressure to measure up and act as responsible adult citizens, were in fact treated as children, and accorded neither dignity nor respect.[58] However, like other people on the receiving end of advice and regimens of control, they were capable of exercising judgement and did not always comply. In 1951 the Protection Board reported that some of the mothers at Point McLeay were 'not very cooperative' with the efforts of a nurse to establish a baby clinic, and did 'not appear to realize the importance of adequate and regular meals for the children'.[59]

Increasingly, the Protection Board was preoccupied with other kinds of health-related compliance. By 1954 it was advocating that Aboriginal people who were in regular employment should be contributing to medical and hospital fees.[60] This was the 'normal responsibility of the ordinary citizen', and, as part of the assimilation agenda, Aboriginals should be encouraged to accept it. It was also a matter of justice, since 'with very few exceptions, natives are accepted and treated in hospitals in the same manner as paying white patients'.[61] If this appeared to be a recognition that Aboriginal people had a call on services in the same way as non-Aboriginal people did, subsequent reports cast doubt on this: 'Unfortunately the native does not always realize the privilege of the medical services supplied. He considers it rather as an obligation and is inclined to demand it'. Such uppity thinking and behaviour did not recommend itself to the staff of Aboriginal institutions:

---

57 Aborigines Protection Board, Annual Report, 1949, *SAPP*, no.20. 1949

58 Restricted files of the Aborigines Department for this period contain official evidence of the efforts of identifiable Aboriginal women to access and exercise control over modest amounts of their own money, and of demeaning and hectoring treatment at the hands of departmental and institutional officials. This material, obviously not able to be quoted, adds weight to the publicly recorded memories of Aboriginal people of constant affronts to their sense of self-worth as they struggled to meet the expectations of officialdom.

59 This kind of criticism was commonly made by nursing staff working in the 'mainstream' infant welfare field, especially in relation to poor or working-class mothers. The advice they offered mothers and the regimens they expected them to follow reflected middle-class values and material circumstances. In addition, it was also implicitly 'white' and Anglo-Celtic in its assumptions and was slow to accommodate cultural complexity. See Judith Raftery, 'Saving South Australia's Babies: the Mothers' and Babies' Health Association', in Bernard O'Neil, Judith Raftery and Kerrie Round, (eds), *Playford's South Australia: essays on the history of South Australia, 1933–1968*, Wakefield Press, Adelaide, 1996, pp.275–94, and especially pp.286–8.

60 In fact, many Aboriginal people were not in a position to pay medical or hospital fees and these were frequently waived upon application to the Aborigines Protection Board, which assessed each application on its merits. Full or partial relief from medical and hospital fees was not uncommon at that time among non-indigenous patients, but the mechanism for securing relief was of course quite different. Since many could not afford private health cover, nor meet doctors' bills in full, or within a reasonable time, it was not uncommon for medical practitioners to negotiate special arrangements. See for example, Neville Hicks, 'Cure and Prevention', in Ann Curthoys, AW Martin, Tim Rowse (eds), *Australians: a historical library. Australians from 1939*, Fairfax, Syme, Weldon and Associates, Sydney, 1987, pp.329–31.

61 Aborigines Protection Board, Annual Report, 1954, *SAPP*, no.20, 1954

they expected 'the native' to be submissive and grateful.[62] By 1960, the Protection Board was enrolling indigenous families who had left the missions and reserves and were employed in the general community in medical and hospital insurance schemes, at government expense, and still complaining about their 'demanding' attitudes.[63] Given the complexity and contradictory nature of assimilationist expectations and special provisions, it is hardly surprising that indigenous people were often at a loss to know what was a 'right', what was a 'privilege', and what was required of them.

The Protection Board was greatly concerned by indigenous use of alcohol, as had been government officials, missionaries and many others since the earliest days of colonisation. However, it often referred to this not as a health issue but as an issue of compliance with the law and acceptance of community norms of 'responsible' living. It was of course a health issue of great complexity. Drinking habitually and to excess not only had direct and indirect effects on the physical and mental health of the drinkers and their families, but also fuelled negative community and government attitudes and prejudices that helped to maintain a social and political environment inimical to indigenous well-being. In fact for many non-indigenous Australians, it was taken to demonstrate the indigenous population's inherent unsuitability for inclusion as members of the public.

Besides the exemption system and health-related issues, another matter which occupied the attention of the Aborigines Protection Board was the vexed question of welfare entitlements. Those indigenous people who were exempted from their legal status as Aboriginals were thereby legally entitled to all the rights and privileges of non-indigenous South Australians, including access to Commonwealth social welfare benefits. These were paid to exempt persons from 1942. However, there was no provision in federal law to allow for payment of the full range of benefits to indigenous people in whom Aboriginal blood preponderated, who were still bound by the *Aborigines Act*, and who lived within Aboriginal institutions. The situation was complicated and was a source of discontent and misunderstanding. Aboriginal mothers with a 'preponderance of white blood' had been eligible for the Maternity Allowance since 1912, and from 1942 eligibility for this benefit was extended to all 'full-blood' mothers provided they were not living in state-controlled institutions. In addition, from 1941 Child Endowment was payable to all mothers except Aboriginals leading nomadic lives. From 1945 the Aborigines Protection Board regularly drew attention to anomalies in the eligibility criteria and sought reforms that would make benefits available to all Aboriginal people whom the board certified to be 'living under conditions comparable to the European way of life'.[64] Because of technical and attitudinal issues, the Commonwealth was slow to act[65] and in 1952 the Board decried the situation as

---

62 Aborigines Protection Board, Annual Report, 1955, 1957, 1959, *SAPP*, nos.20, 1955, 1957, 1959

63 Aborigines Protection Board, Annual Report, 1960, *SAPP*, no.20, 1960

64 Aborigines Protection Board, Annual Report, 1945, *SAPP*, no.20, 1945. Those not living in the European manner; that is, those referred to as 'traditional', 'tribalised', 'semi-tribalised' or 'nomadic', were deemed still to be in need of protection, which implied a different kind of government response.

65 For an analysis of this see William De Maria, '"White Welfare: Black Entitlement". The social security access controversy, 1939–59', *Aboriginal History*, vol.10, 1986, pp.25–39.

manifestly unjust, as all aborigines, irrespective of the degree of aboriginal blood, are required to pay income tax, and a considerable number do in fact pay income tax, including social services tax. One section which adversely affects aborigines and causes much discontent is that which precludes a mother in whom there is the slightest preponderance of aboriginal blood receiving the maternity allowance. Aborigines applying for invalid, age and widows pensions are required to leave their homes on aboriginal stations or missions, where they have lived and worked all their lives, and where all their interests lie, and if aboriginal blood preponderates, they must also be exempted from the provisions of the Aborigines Act in order to qualify for the benefit.[66]

If the system was 'manifestly unjust', it was also unclear and it undermined the attempts of South Australian legislation to clarify questions of definition of Aboriginality and access to rights, and to make judgments not on the basis of colour or 'preponderance of blood' but on the basis of capacity. A strong sense of injustice as well as incomprehension is apparent in the efforts of Narungga man, Eddie Sansbury from Point Pearce, to fathom his standing in relation to the law. When told he would have to leave Point Pearce in order to collect the age pension, Sansbury is reported to have asked, 'Why can't I get my pension on the mission? That's what I worked for. That's where I belong. That's my home. Why should I have to leave?'[67]

Eventually, with the passage of the Commonwealth *Social Services Act, no. 57 of 1959*, all Aboriginal people, except those classified as 'primitive' or 'nomadic', qualified for age, invalid and widows pensions, unemployment and sickness benefits, maternity allowance and child endowment. The first payments were made in February 1960. The Aborigines Protection Board reported that there was some initial confusion about the provenance and significance of these payments among people long accustomed to receiving rations from the South Australian Government.[68] It seems likely that such confusion was exacerbated by the way in which the payments were made: they were paid directly to Aboriginals only 'where the Department of Social Services is satisfied that a native's social development is such that he can with advantage handle the pension himself'.[69] In practice, for many Aboriginals, and certainly for those living on missions, reserves and stations, this meant that their money was managed for them.[70] The funds were transferred from the Commonwealth as a block payment to the state Aborigines Department, which instructed superintendents to make a cash payment of 15 shillings a week to those entitled to receive a pension of £4/15/0. The remaining £4 was paid into individual trust accounts, maintained in Adelaide, upon which the superintendents drew to supply bread, butter, meat, firewood, electricity, stores, fruit and vegetables to the value of £2/10/2 a week. Superintendents also had the discretionary authority to issue orders for clothing, blankets, fares and other items against the remaining £1/9/10 per week held in

---

66 Aborigines Protection Board, Annual Report, 1952, *SAPP*, no.20, 1952

67 Recalled by Sansbury's son-in-law, Kaurna elder Lewis O'Brien. Mattingley and Hampton, *Survival In Our Own Land*, p.52

68 Aborigines Protection Board Annual Report, 1960, *SAPP*, no.20, 1960

69 De Maria, 'White Welfare: Black Entitlement', p.27

70 This practice was not confined to South Australia. See Kidd, *The Way We Civilise*, p.166; Broome, *Aboriginal Australians*, p.170.

the trust accounts, 'always providing that a reasonable credit balance [was] maintained'. The Commonwealth considered it 'necessary to control pension moneys', but made it clear that such moneys were the property of the pensioner.[71] Thus Aboriginals continued to be involved in an unequal and demeaning situation, as had previously occurred in relation to maternity benefits and child endowment, in which non-indigenous authority figures exercised coercive and withholding power in situations of immediate, day-to-day control. Actual access to the Commonwealth social welfare benefits to which they were newly entitled was linked to Aboriginals' conformity to an approved lifestyle, just as exemption from their status as Aboriginals was, under state legislation. While poor non-Aboriginals were also frequently subject to and judged wanting by this kind of thinking, the impact on Aboriginal people was magnified and more palpable:

> ... not only did they need to satisfy the statutory requirements ... they also had to make their lifestyle (and by extension their Aboriginal culture) available for assessment. They had to demonstrate to the Department of Social Services that there were no cultural impediments to the proper expenditure of these 'cash benefits'.[72]

It can reasonably be argued that the extension of 'mainstream' welfare entitlement to the indigenous population from 1959 signalled a significant shift in government thinking and provision. It was a major step away from the protection system under which indigenous lives were governed by a separate panoply of laws, and a demonstration of government willingness to assimilate Aboriginal people into 'mainstream' relationships with the state and with other Australians. However, the way in which delivery of the new entitlements was controlled raises questions about how much of a shift had really occurred. Indeed, it suggests that the concept of welfare rights as contingent on citizenship – on belonging to the Australian public – was 'not part of serious political dialogue' in this period.[73] As Rowse argues, the handing over of merely a ' "pocket money" portion' of the government benefits to Aboriginal beneficiaries indicated that a 'prolonged paternalism' was still operating. Further, he identifies the unwillingness of governments to relinquish control over indigenous people's access to cash, despite having legislated their entitlement to benefits, as evidence of

> a tension between two understandings of 'citizenship'. One is primarily juridical, and empha-

---

71 AFA, Annual Report, 1960; Hon. GG Pearson, in response to questions from DA Dunstan, *SAPD*, House of Assembly, 31 March 1960, pp.15–16; 13 April 1960, pp.160–1. Despite Pearson's reassurances, subsequent historical research has shown that money – wages and well as welfare benefits – belonging to Aboriginal people and retained by the government in trust accounts has not always been paid to its owners. See Kidd, *The Way We Civilise*, p.x; Anna Haebich, *Stolen Wages and Consequential Indigenous Poverty: a national issue*, Occasional paper no.17, History Department, University of Melbourne, Melbourne, 2004.

72 De Maria, 'White Welfare: Black entitlement', pp.28–9

73 ibid., pp.28–9

74 Tim Rowse, *White Flour, White Power: from rations to citizenship in Central Australia*, Cambridge University Press, Cambridge, 1998, pp.111–14

sises entitlements; the other is primarily sociological, and stresses trained capacities to behave according to implicit norms of kinship and domestic order.[74]

While these two understandings were in some respects contradictory – for example, a too-niggardly or paternalistic interpretation of the former could thwart the 'trained capacities' goal of the latter – they rested on the common foundation of western values relating to individual responsibility, 'family', and appropriate and inappropriate forms of dependence, interdependence and redistribution of income. The gap between these values, which extolled individual self-sufficiency and the economic autonomy of the family (understood as a man, and his wife and children) and those which underpinned the functional integration and communal culture of Aboriginal societies was wide. This discrepancy in values meant that the extension of welfare benefits – and the payment of cash wages, as this became more widespread – to Aboriginal people, created a new problem for governments and many non-indigenous Australians. It was the problem of deciding 'how much redistribution of goods and earned money, from earners to non-earners, is compatible with the ideal that people should not be parasitic but self-supporting'. Rowse demonstrates that this problem was unresolved at both a conceptual and policy level in the 1950s, as governments, anthropologists, policy-makers and others debated various meanings of assimilation, citizenship and independence.[75] It remains unresolved half a century later, and is manifested as fears and resentments about whether Aboriginal people 'earn' or 'properly' use government benefits, and tensions over the various costs to the nation entailed in support for minority values and alternative social and economic forms. These concerns continue to contribute to hostile public opinion and to failures of nerve about policy that attempts to move beyond paternalism.

A fourth preoccupation of the Aborigines Protection Board was child removal. As we have seen, child removal was not a new practice: despite various legal difficulties it had been pursued by governments of earlier periods under the rubric of 'protection', and it was a fundamental strategy of missionary activity. From the mid-1950s, relying on extended powers under the 1939 *Aborigines Act*, the practice was intensified as part of the assimilation policy. Increasing numbers of Aboriginal children were being 'assimilated' by being removed from their families and communities and placed either in institutional care or, as 'mainstream' critique of institutional care grew, in private foster homes. In 1959, 412 children were so placed – 260 in institutions and 152 in private homes – and by then small numbers were also being formally adopted by non-indigenous families.[76] The Protection Board, the Aborigines Department, the AFA and the institutions and homes involved were remarkably silent about just who these children were, or where they came from. However, they continued to make generalised and unsubstantiated claims that they were being rescued from a life of destitution, neglect, hopelessness and deprivation for

75 ibid., p.116. These issues are explored by Rowse at a theoretical level in chapter 7 of *White Flour, White Power*, and then elaborated in the following three chapters, in the context of Central Australia.

76 Aborigines Protection Board, Annual Report 1959, *SAPP*, no.20, 1959; Raynes, '*A Little Flour*', p.55 For a more substantial discussion of this trend and the context in which it developed, see Anna Haebich, *Broken Circles: fragmenting indigenous families, 1800–2000*, Fremantle Arts Centre Press, Fremantle, 2000, especially pp.533–57.

a new life of opportunity which, at least in the case of the missions, promised eternal as well as temporal benefits. The rescuers were less inclined to evaluate what the strategy of placement – or removal – actually achieved in relation to the assimilation of children into 'mainstream' society, much less what it meant in terms of their emotional well-being and that of their families. The numbers of children 'placed' or removed was reported as if this were in itself evidence of policy goals being met.

From time to time the Aborigines Department felt it necessary to explain and justify its child removal practices. It presented them as being non-coercive and respectful of the rights of indigenous parents. For example, in 1959, CE Bartlett, former Superintendent at Point McLeay, who had succeeded William Penhall as Secretary of the Aborigines Protection Board in 1953, defended the Board against allegations of malpractice and of exceeding its authority:

> It should be clearly understood that the Aborigines Protection Board have no authority to remove aboriginal children from their parents.
>
> In all cases where a parent or parents of a child request that their children be cared for by the Board, the children are placed with foster parents and maintained by the Board.
>
> In other cases, particularly with single girls who have illegitimate children, or with native women, deserted husbands and neglected children, the Department endeavours to persuade the parent to allow for the Board to care for the child and in such circumstances the child is again placed with foster parents. On some occasions the parents do sign a form consenting to the fostering of the child by the Board, or alternatively the parent agrees and signs the usual consent form agreeing to the adoption of the child. In many other cases where parents refused to sign any such agreement the child is placed out for fostering.
>
> In all such cases other than where adoptions are contemplated, the Department must retain the right to remove any child or children from any foster parents for the ultimate benefit of the child concerned. Further, the native parents can remove any child from a foster parent without the authority of the Department or the Board.[77]

This positive portrayal of child removal as a consensual practice undistorted by power imbalances or complicated by human attachment is at odds with later evidence which reveals it as frequently coercive and deeply traumatising. It indicates the extent to which the ideology of assimilation had taken hold within the non-indigenous world. Such a practice could be pursued and defended only if it was believed to constitute genuine 'rescue' or salvation, and this implied a corresponding lack of belief that there was any value in indigenous familial and cultural ties.[78]

While the Aborigines Protection Board paid regular attention to the exemption system, to specific areas of health, to welfare entitlement, and to the removal of Aboriginal children, its focus on the issues underpinning these various problem areas was more haphazard and

---

77 Bartlett to Minister of Works, 20 April 1959, GRG 23/1/1959/52, cited in Raynes, 'A Little Flour', p.55
78 See below, pp.207–8, 211–13

piecemeal. These matters included the ongoing challenges of education and training, employment and housing, areas in which the passage of time and of legislation seemed to add little in the way of new insight or new vision. In fact, despite decades of mantra-like statements about training and opportunities leading to inclusion in the general community, records of government, missions and other interested bodies reveal little evidence of this transition actually occurring and are characterised by continuing low expectations of what Aboriginal people were capable of achieving. Furthermore, they demonstrate a marked tendency for a commitment to assimilation to give way to attitudes and practices of protection, at the first sign of difficulty. It is as if those who fashioned the assimilation policy did not seriously entertain the likelihood that indigenous people were capable of realising its goals. What was operating was a tendency persistent in public health history and in much policy development: normalising the social and economic *status quo*, which renders some populations, in this case Aboriginals, dependent, marginalised and disadvantaged, and seeking only to ameliorate some of the worst effects of this, rather than problematising this situation and seeking more fundamental change.

This tendency is clearly evident in the attitude of the Aborigines Protection Board to education and training. It appeared to have no defined policy: it merely provided guidance and support to what missions and other institutions were doing. For example in 1941, when the Lutheran Synod sought advice about what to do with Aboriginal 'girls' at their mission at Koonibba after they had attained the age of 21, the Board replied that,

> as the girls should be thoroughly trained by the time they reach eighteen years of age, they should let them be placed in suitable homes preferably in the Koonibba district.

Their 'thorough training' was for domestic service: neither the mission nor the Board envisaged any other vocational future for them. On the same occasion the Board revealed another aspect of its narrow expectations about the capacity of indigenous people for training and assimilation to 'white' ways. It advised the Lutheran Synod not to rent cottages to the Koonibba people, since it predicted 'considerable difficulty ... in collecting rent from persons unwilling or unable to pay'. This would in time lead to the residents being 'ejected' and thus 'the work of the Church is hindered'. The implication was clear: the people of Koonibba were still not reliable candidates for assimilation and were to remain as dependants.[79]

At the same meeting at which the Board provided this advice to the Lutheran Synod, it also responded to a request from the General Superintendent of the Home Missions Department of the Methodist Church. This body sought authorisation to bring two unidentified infants from the half-caste institution at Alice Springs 'for training' at the Methodist Babies' Home in the Adelaide suburb of Brighton, 'with a view to their absorption into the white community'. The church would accept full responsibility for them, and in the case of their developing 'any traits that make them a menace to themselves or other people', would arrange for 'their return to the care of the Federal authorities'. The Board agreed, on the grounds that the infants had only 'a slight admixture of

---

79 Aborigines Protection Board, Minutes, 6 August 1941, p.117, GRG 52/16

aboriginal blood', and were therefore presumably good candidates for 'absorption'.[80] Here, as in so many other instances, the meaning of key policy objectives – training, absorption, assimilation – and the content of strategies by which they were pursued remained vague.

Vagueness and restricted vision were apparent even when the Board attempted to address the issues more directly. In 1944, it was considering:

> vocational training for young aborigines of both sexes, particularly in the larger centres of aboriginal population. An investigation is being conducted by officers of the Department of Education, in conjunction with officers of the Aborigines Department, with a view to undertaking a post-war scheme of training boys and young men in plumbing and sheet metal work, saddlery, bootmaking and repairs, carpentry, cement construction etc., and to instruct young girls and women in dressmaking, millinery, cooking, hair dressing etc.[81]

Apart from the reference to the war, this statement could have been made at any time during the previous half-century. And like all such earlier statements, it bore little fruit. In 1947, William Penhall, head of the Aborigines Department and secretary of the Aborigines Protection Board from 1940 until his retirement in 1953, argued that some education of Aboriginal children was wasted since they tended to 'drift back into their old way of life' at its completion. His suggestion that they should be exempted from the act to prevent this drift did not take into account the abundant evidence that it took more than exemption to provide opportunities for employment and social inclusion.

In the same year, AW Christian, the Member for Eyre, referred to the 'pathetic attempts' of poorly resourced missions to provide secondary schooling and vocational education. He strongly urged the government to accept responsibility for this 'or lay itself open to the charge of complete neglect of the obligation we owe to these people'.[82] The government did not rise to Christian's challenge. Small numbers of Aboriginal people, especially young women from the UAM's Colebrook and Tanderra Homes and young men from St Francis House, an Anglican institution at Semaphore in suburban Adelaide, were given the opportunity for secondary education and for further training, for example, in nursing, teaching and in skilled trades.[83] Indigenous young people who were able to take advantage of such opportunities included many who later became influential in

---

80 Aborigines Protection Board, Minutes, 6 August 1941, p.118, GRG 52/16

81 Aborigines Protection Board, Annual Report 1944, *SAPP*, no.20, 1944

82 AW Christian, *SAPD*, House of Assembly, 6 August 1947, pp.226–7, cited in Raynes, 'A Little Flour', p.51

83 Aborigines Protection Board, Annual Report, 1952, *SAPP*, no.20, 1952. For further information on the first Aboriginal nurses in South Australia and the prejudice they encountered, see Joan Durdin, *They Became Nurses: a history of nursing in South Australia, 1836–1980*, Allen and Unwin, Sydney, 1991, pp.158, 166–7 and Barnes, *Munyi's Daughter*, pp.91–3. For an account of St Francis House and its program of education of young men, many of them originally from the Northern Territory, see John P McD Smith, *The Flower in the Desert: a biography of the Rev. Canon PMcD Smith, MBE*, Seaview Press, Adelaide, 1999. Tanderra was a UAM home in the Adelaide suburb of Parkside. It catered for Aboriginal girls who, having successfully completed primary schooling on various missions or reserves, were supported for three years of secondary education in Adelaide. For an account of life at Tanderra, see Brodie, *My Side of the Bridge*, chapter 5.

indigenous organisations and in government employment in South Australia, and several, including Lowitja O'Donoghue and Charles Perkins, who rose to national prominence. These 'success stories' should not be seen as evidence that the government offered anything approaching a serious program of education and training. On the contrary, they reflect significant individual achievements against the odds and in the face of general government and community complacency. Indeed, in 1953, McIntosh, the minister responsible for Aboriginal affairs, appeared to wash his hands of the problem of education of indigenous South Australians. Probably much community opinion was in accord with his:

> There have been one or two cases of half-caste boys coming to Adelaide and entering into apprenticeships, and although they have done well, such cases are rarities, because it is hard to turn a nomad into a stool-sitter in one generation. All that can be done, has been done.[84]

Surely a better explanation for the rarity of indigenous educational success – although it was not as rare as McIntosh suggested – was that the government had ever only applied itself to the issue in a piecemeal and illiberal fashion. In the light of this, the assertion that all that could have been done had been done betrayed a profound lack of faith in the capacity of indigenous people, and a devaluing of their human worth. Missionaries were perhaps less inclined to wash their hands of the 'Aboriginal problem', but their resignation to minimal returns on their labour often betrayed a limited view of indigenous capacity. For example, the Rev. CV Eckermann, Superintendent at Koonibba, reflecting in 1958 on the mission's modest educational achievements, sought explanations in the racial character of the Aboriginals rather than in restricted opportunities or the self-fulfilling prophecies created by the mission ethos:

> we will not have to cater for the highly-specialised callings or professions. It is quite unrealistic to hope for doctors, lawyers, highly-skilled tradesmen, and the like, to arise from the ranks of these folk – not because the intellect or ability is lacking in every case, but because of that frustrating racial characteristic, their passiveness. These folk will not keep their noses to the grindstone steadfastly enough to enter any of the highly-specialised callings.

He concluded that manual, technical and artistic skills were the appropriate focus of indigenous education and that anything else would merely produce frustration.[85]

Faced by state government inaction, and sceptical of what missions could achieve, Penhall pursued the objectives of the 1939 *Aborigines Act* in other ways. He advocated the acceptance by the Commonwealth Government of responsibility for Aboriginal affairs, either directly, or through comprehensive financial support to the states. In 1947, his outline of a strategy that could be pursued if such support was forthcoming, and which would meet some assimilationist objectives, including education, housing and move-

---

84 Hon. M. McIntosh, *SAPD*, House of Assembly, 3 November 1953, p.1267, cited in Raynes, 'A Little Flour', p.53.

85 *Australian Lutheran*, 17 December 1958, pp.427–8. These comments appeared in an article that was part of a long series by Eckermann on Aboriginal missions.

ment from segregated settlements into the general community, was presented at a national conference of state premiers. The basis of the plan was to settle selected mixed-blood couples in country towns where the men could obtain employment as railway fettlers:

> If financial assistance could be given to enable ten or twelve such young couples to be estab-
> lished each year in such a scheme, it would be a great help in absorbing the mixed bloods and
> relieving the problem of excess population on Mission Stations and in other institutions.
> Children of parents absorbed would then grow up in the general community, and would have
> no knowledge of Mission life, which experience has shown to be a definite deterrent to their
> development as citizens. In experimental cases of this kind native children have been accepted
> in the public schools without question, and they have acquired knowledge as readily as the
> average white child attending the school.[86]

Commonwealth support for this modest proposal for the assimilation of Aboriginal people into the lowest economic ranks of the general community was not forthcoming. The South Australian Aborigines Department and the Protection Board nevertheless pursued a version of it by encouraging, through the provision of housing and by allowing the institutions to run down, selected Aboriginal people to leave institutions and settle in the general community. In 1950 the Protection Board reported that 'several families' from Point McLeay had 'removed to various parts of the State and appear[ed] to be able to maintain themselves in the general community'. The Board considered that Point McLeay and Point Pearce were overpopulated. Its policy was to settle young people from there who were regarded as capable of surviving outside the institutions in country towns and provide them with housing and employment. This would serve immediate and long-term assimilationist goals by allowing children to grow up 'without a knowledge of mission life and the disabilities associated therewith'. This was a small-scale project however: in 1951 the Board indicated that three families had left Point McLeay in response to the provision of housing and employment with the Commonwealth Railways. It considered that a second group of Aboriginals whose 'standard of living' was too low for assimilation into the general community might survive in hypothetical 'small villages' in the vicinity of country towns, but the remainder were still to be regarded as 'mission natives'.[87]

In 1951 Penhall expounded this as general policy, rather than merely a response to overcrowding in some centres, and indicated that an element of interdepartmental co-operation could be assumed:

> The policy of the board is to have the aborigines, particularly the mixed bloods, assimilated into
> the general community as they reach the stage in their development where such action is
> possible. As an indication of the method of implementing this policy, I may state that the Board
> is at present negotiating with the Housing Trust with a view to having groups of from two to

---

86 Penhall, to Minister of Works for the Premier, 14 August 1947, GRG 52/1/1947/12, cited in Raynes, 'A Little Flour', p.51.
    There is a striking similarity between this proposal and one made by Cleland in 1938. See above, p.185.

87 Aborigines Protection Board, Annual Report, 1950, 1951, SAPP, no.20, 1950, 1951

four houses erected in appropriate country towns to provide accommodation for families regarded as most likely to succeed in the general community. Work will be provided for them in Government concerns, if desired.[88]

Some movement from centres of Aboriginal population into the general community at this time occurred not in response to policy, of course, but as a result of 'drift' in pursuit of economic opportunity. In the early 1950s the Board noted this in relation to indigenous adults leaving the mission at Nepabunna to seek work on the coalfields at Leigh Creek, on pastoral stations or in the nearby towns of Copley, Beltana and Hawker. Comparable movement was taking place on Eyre Peninsula with many people from Koonibba 'now scattered' and employed in agriculture or with the railways.[89] These developments aroused concern in the Aborigines Department about wages and working conditions for Aboriginals employed within the 'mainstream' economy. Previously the department had sought an amendment to the *Aborigines Act* to empower it to deal with what it identified as serious cases of injustice, and Penhall had advocated unsuccessfully for a minimum wage for Aboriginal pastoral workers. These concerns were still being raised, but not resolved, as increasing numbers of indigenous people sought work in the 1950s.[90]

At this time Aboriginal people were also forced to relocate in order to accommodate developments within the non-indigenous world. In 1951, the Aborigines Department purchased land at Yalata near Fowlers Bay on Eyre Peninsula to enable them to relocate the Ooldea people. The lives of these people had already been significantly disrupted by the construction of the transcontinental railway line, the 'protection' offered by Daisy Bates[91], the missionary endeavours of the UAM, and the degradation of their fragile physical environment. They were now threatened by the imminent testing of atomic weapons at nearby Maralinga. The move from Ooldea to Yalata was more abrupt and traumatic than the government had envisaged because of the sudden closure of the Ooldea mission in June 1952 as a result of an internal dispute within the UAM. At the new settlement at Yalata, several different groups of Aboriginal people were herded together, as has so often happened when Aboriginal interests have been subjugated to the political and economic imperatives of non-indigenous Australia.[92] This enforced removal of the Ooldea people had long-term effects on their well-being and

---

88 Penhall to Mrs BR Wyllie (a researcher seeking information on policy), 19 September 1951, GRG 52/1/1951/30, cited in Raynes, 'A Little Flour', p.53

89 Aborigines Protection Board, Annual Report, 1952,1954, SAPP, no.20, 1952, 1954

90 Aborigines Protection Board, Annual Report, 1946, SAPP, no. 20, 1946; Raynes, 'A Little Flour', pp.52–3

91 See above, pp.140–1

92 This phenomenon has been repeated across Australia and is telling evidence of Aboriginal people's ongoing disenfran-chisement and the subjugation of their interests when these conflict with non-indigenous economic interests. This has been powerfully captured on film, as well as recorded in other ways. See for example, *Exile and the Kingdom*, 1993, which tells the story of the people of Roebourne in Western Australia, repeatedly assaulted by waves of non-indige-nous economic activity, and *State of Shock*, 1989, which is based on the impact of the enforced move of Aboriginal people from Mapoon to Weipa in north Queensland, to make way for a bauxite mine. Re the Mapoon/Weipa story, see also DA Dunstan, SAPD, House of Assembly, 30 August 1962, p.815.

93 For an account of missionary and other non-indigenous involvement at Ooldea, and the enforced move to Yalata and its

was clearly not calculated to encourage their assimilation into the broader community.[93]

The increased movement of Aboriginal people into the general community at this time, either as a result of direct encouragement by the Board, or as a result of economically driven 'drift', had significant repercussions for the government. In 1955 the Board reported on increased business arising from 'certain developmental policies' and the need for 'increased effort in social and welfare activities'. Some of this was relatively easy to deal with, such as providing furniture and domestic equipment to Aboriginal families being settled in houses in the general community, to enable them to avoid the embarrassment of not meeting prevailing standards.[94] Other issues were more problematic. Ensuring that Aboriginal people who moved from segregated settlements into the general community were accepted and offered genuine opportunities to become part of it depended on non-indigenous good will. This was not something that the Aborigines Department could ensure, and the Protection Board recorded evidence of non-indigenous reticence in welcoming indigenous neighbours. For example, in 1954 the local council in the riverland town of Berri objected to homes for 'natives' being built in the town and declared that 'the most suitable sites were the allotments selected at Glossop' – that is, in a nearby area of sparser settlement and lower land values and social prestige. In the following year local government in the Eyre Peninsula town of Kimba rebuffed the Board's suggestion that they establish a reserve for Aboriginal residents 'where reasonable types of dwellings could be erected together with toilet and bathing facilities'. Instead, the council wanted their town to be proclaimed an area in which it would be unlawful for unemployed Aboriginals to remain.[95]

Employment was often as hard to come by as accommodation. The Board noted that 'many aborigines, usually part-aborigines' living in or near country towns were sometimes 'actually destitute' and inclined to return to the reserves because they could not find jobs. It authorised police officers to issue relief to such people, to ensure that they were not in want as a result of sickness or unemployment. The Board said nothing of non-indigenous attitudes and prejudices that may have contributed to indigenous underemployment and therefore to the need for the continuation of rationing at many depots throughout the state. However, it did suggest that the indigenous contributed to their own problems: 'unfortunately the native is not inclined to remain in one position for any lengthy period, and is constantly changing employers'.[96] The Board was nevertheless undeterred, and, in particular, remained convinced of the value of the provision of 'proper' housing. Its assertion that, without it, 'little progress is likely to be made with the aboriginal problem towards their absorption in the white community' was both a straightforward statement about material needs of indigenous people and a coded reference to the non-indigenous prejudices

---

aftermath, see Mattingley and Hampton, *Survival In Our Own Land*, chapter 29. See also, Aborigines Protection Board, Annual Report, 1951, 1952, *SAPP*, no.20, 1951, 1952.

94 Aborigines Protection Board, Minutes, for example, 3 November 1954, p.7, 17 November 1954, p.10, 2 March 1955, p.31, 16 March 1955, p.32, GRG 52/16/2; Annual Report, 1955, *SAPP*, no.20, 1955

95 Aborigines Protection Board, Minutes, 17 November 1954, p.11, 7 December 1955, p.106, GRG/52/16/1

96 Aborigines Protection Board, Annual Report, 1954, *SAPP*, no.20, 1954

97 Aborigines Protection Board, Minutes, 18 May1955, p.47, GRG 52/16/2

and expectations that continued to make such absorption unlikely, or at least difficult.[97]

The Aborigines Protection Board's dream of supplying assimilation packages of Housing Trust homes in country towns, complete with fences, clothes-lines, time-payment furniture and employment for male bread-winners was realised in the case of small numbers of approved Aboriginal families.[98] However, in most cases, under-resourcing, community hostility or indifference and continuing assumptions that Aboriginals did not have the same material needs as the rest of the community, nor the same aptitude for work, meant that this goal was not realised. The records of the Board frequently exposed the distance between the reality and the dream. Some examples from this period, outlined below, illustrate the severity of the problems, especially in relation to the provision of accommodation, and the Aborigines Department's limited capacity to respond to them.

After months of 'almost constant complaint' from many quarters about conditions at Colebrook Home, the Board requested an investigation into its functioning and care. Bartlett's report to the Board in August 1956 was damning. He found that the home was inadequately supervised, had incompetent staff, was poorly furnished, was generally dirty and untidy, had inadequate and malfunctioning sanitary arrangements, and offered an insufficiently varied diet. He recommended that the Colebrook children be removed from the care of the UAM and the home taken over by the government to enable the children to 'be given every opportunity as they are in similar Government Institutions for white children'. The problems were not limited to Colebrook: Bartlett suggested that he 'did not know of any aboriginal children's home in South Australia which could be con-sidered as satisfactory, perhaps with the exception of Tanderra'. These trenchant criticisms and continuing adverse reports about conditions at Colebrook resulted in ministerial action. This eventually led to the appointment of new staff, increases in government expenditure for the maintenance of the children, plans to provide separate accommoda-tion for the older boys at Campbell House, a recently established farm-training institution, and directives to the UAM concerning maintaining the property in decent order. In announcing this action to the parliament, the minister took the opportunity to reiterate the government's commitment to the 'total assimilation of aborigines into the white community' through the mechanisms of compulsory education to fourteen years, followed by vocational training to sixteen, and assistance in finding jobs and rental homes in country towns or in Adelaide.[99]

Around the same time, the Aborigines Department received complaints from the General Secretary of the UAM that its capacity to pursue the 'spiritual work' which was its main objective was hampered by the necessity to perform 'social service' for Aboriginal people in its care. Bartlett was unsympathetic. He was 'surprised' to hear that the UAM

---

98 See Doris May Graham and Cecil Wallace Graham, *As We've Known It: 1911 to the present*, South Australian College of Advanced Education, Adelaide, 1987, p.66, for an example of this working well. By 1962, 105 families had been accom-modated by the Aborigines Department. Joyce Steele, *SAPD*, House of Assembly, 17 October 1962, p.1525

99 Aborigines Protection Board, Minutes, 27 May 1955, p.49, 25 January 1956, p.16, 5 September 1956, pp.208–9, 5 December 1956, p.234, 19 December 1956, p.239, 6 February 1957, p.254, GRG 52/16/2; M McIntosh, *SAPD*, House of Assembly, 5 February 1957, pp.172–3

carried out any 'social service', and judged its institutions as 'far from satisfactory', and housing conditions on its missions as 'deplorable'. He made specific mention of the mission at Gerard, where 'the houses were definitely substandard and unfit for human occupation'. Subsequent requests from the UAM to be relieved of the burden of 'social service' met with a similar response: the Protection Board refused to bolster the UAM's over-stretched institutions, predicting they would soon have to be taken over by the government.[100]

Also at this time, investigations by officers of the Aborigines Department into conditions at Koonibba, Ceduna and Coober Pedy revealed serious departures from standards that the department deemed acceptable. At Koonibba, cottages were overcrowded, and lacked sanitary facilities, lighting and adequate ventilation. In addition, staff shortages meant that neither the hospital nor the children's home was operating. On the outskirts of Ceduna, between 100 and 150 Aboriginals, dissatisfied with the overcrowding and the dearth of health services and work opportunities at Koonibba, were camped on a reserve, living in wurlies 'in highly unsanitary conditions'. At the 'native encampment' at Coober Pedy, where no reserve had been officially created, 'sanitation and hygiene requirements' included such basic amenities as pit latrines, shade houses with rooves to provide water catchment, a camp site located so as not to pollute the water catchment area, and an issue of DDT to fumigate 'native wurlies and native clothing'. The disenchanted Superintendent of the settlement was also concerned about moral hygiene and wanted the Aboriginal population removed from the 'unsavoury atmosphere brought about by the close proximity of so many undesirable white people'. In these cases, deficiencies in amenities could be attributed partly to remoteness and the frontier nature of the settlements. However, this could not be proffered as a reason for the deplorable condition of the accommodation provided for Aboriginal women and girls visiting Adelaide for department-approved reasons and staying at the Aboriginal Women's Home in Sussex Street, North Adelaide. Bartlett believed that the Protection Board 'would be open to severe censure if the public were aware of the nature of the accommodation provided both for the matron and the aborigines'.[101]

This widespread inability to provide decent amenities and services for Aboriginal South Australians reveals a continuing reality of segregation and deprivation greatly removed from the assimilationist objectives of the 1939 act. The Aborigines Department believed that the provision of good housing, along with education and training that would lead to employment, was both a means of encouraging indigenous preparedness to become part of the general community and a reward for demonstrating it. However, neither the department nor the missions and other institutions supporting Aboriginal people was able to provide it. They all struggled against chronic underresourcing, which resulted in an inability to take action, even though they were aware of deficiencies that needed to be addressed. The Protection Board and the Aborigines Department regularly reiterated their policy goal: 'the promotion of the welfare of aborigines to a standard whereat they are considered capable of complete assimilation into the white community'.[102] However, they also regularly reported evidence that the policy was not working

---

100 Aborigines Protection Board, Minutes, 20 June 1956, p.180, 21 November 1956, p.232, GRG 52/16/2

101 Aborigines Protection Board, Minutes, 4 April 1956, p.145, 18 April 1956, pp.149–51, GRG 52/16/2

as intended: the lives of many Aboriginals continued to be characterised by poor health, substandard housing, minimal educational achievements, exploitation or lack of opportunity in employment, ongoing need for rationing, and in some cases, destitution.

While the policy was clearly not working as intended and the 'absorption' of indigenous people into the 'white' community was proving to be an elusive goal, Aboriginals were, inevitably, being assimilated to some extent. Indeed, none could resist some degree of assimilation once they had been brought into contact with the authoritative legal and economic structures of the dominant non-Aboriginal culture. When Aboriginal people 'came in' or were removed from their 'country', when they adopted, even if only for some of the time, a settled life on pastoral stations or reserves or in towns, when they accessed rations, when they sought work within the 'white' economy or places for their children within schools established by non-Aboriginals, when they embraced Christianity, or sought an accommodation between its claims and their traditional beliefs, when they submitted themselves to western medical services, and when they tried to comply with the confusing intricacies of the exemption and welfare systems, they were demonstrating varying degrees of assimilation to non-indigenous culture. Some of them had been doing some of this from the earliest days of colonial settlement, long before their assimilation became a legislatively backed policy goal. But this did not mean that they were achieving the 'standards' that would allow them to be 'absorbed' into the dominant culture, to enable them to disappear and 'become white', as was often predicted by proponents of the assimilation policy in the 1930s, 1940s and 1950s. Nor did it mean that they were accessing all the opportunities, rights and privileges of what at that time was loosely called 'citizenship' and thereby experiencing 'assimilation' as a positive and liberating process.[103]

The Board and the Department were largely unreflective about this complex process. They did not record, except indirectly and then usually in the context of dealing with complaints, how Aboriginals experienced, understood and felt about it, nor speculate on why they chose to accept some aspects of what was on offer and rejected others. Nor did they reveal any awareness of why some Aboriginal people identified themselves as Aboriginal, and as not 'white', and did not accept that 'absorption' into western culture was a reasonable price to pay for access to the material goods it offered.

This lack of awareness is not surprising. The 'Aboriginal question' hardly impinged on the consciousness of the many South Australians who had nothing to do with the administration of Aboriginal affairs and had no contact with Aboriginals in the course of their daily lives. It was a different matter, of course, for others such as staff of the Aborigines

---

102 Aborigines Protection Board, Minutes, 18 May 1956, p.163, GRG 52/16/2

103 This sometimes causes confusion for people who have attached positive meaning to the term 'assimilation', in situations where one 'race' has struggled against suppression by another. For example, in the 1960s, the term 'assimilation' carried strong connotations of liberation because of its association with the struggles of black South Africans and Afro-Americans against suppression and exclusion. For them, to be assimilated was to be freed and to have their rights as human beings and as citizens of a democracy acknowledged. Thus 'assimilation' in these contexts was not about 'absorption' or becoming someone else, as it was in Australia: it was about emerging, and being themselves.

Department, members of the Protection Board, managers of Aboriginal institutions and missions, and pastoralists who employed and supported Aboriginal workers and their families. However, their very closeness to the question, and their uncritical acceptance of the conventional wisdom that the only future for the indigenous population lay in assimilation into the general community diminished their capacity to hear and take seriously indigenous reactions that implied an alternative view. Nor did they register the claims of Aboriginal people that they frequently experienced what 'the general community' offered not as opportunity, but as loss. Admittedly, these reactions were not always articulated clearly, or in places where they would have a wide audience, or in ways that prevented their easy dismissal.

If the Aborigines Protection Board, the Aborigines Department and staff of Aboriginal institutions gave little thought to the impact and meaning of the processes of assimilation, these were issues that still engaged scholarly interest. Anthropological analysis during the period when assimilation was still the dominant policy goal reveals the extent to which even the most sympathetic observers believed that, for most people of Aboriginal descent, genuine 'Aboriginality' had been lost and any hope for the future lay in being afforded opportunities to join 'the general community'. The remaining 'traditional aborigines' or 'full-bloods' continued to be routinely considered as a separate group whose survival depended on the continuation of special protective measures. But 'part-aborigines' were frequently assumed to have lost their culture and to be more akin to the poorer sections of white society. For example, the influential anthropologists Ronald and Catherine Berndt, discussing Aboriginals living in Adelaide in 1950, argued that 'the main trend of their behaviour is towards assimilation into white society'. Most had no real knowledge of Aboriginal life and culture, which they had in any case been taught to regard as inferior, and 'consider that their main hope for the future lies in their identification with the white community'.[104] In the Berndts' view, this future was a limited, historically determined and *non-Aboriginal* (my emphasis) one:

> As they intermarry and their offspring become progressively lighter, it seems likely that they will in time merge into the white community, but particularly into that section now resident in the West End. That is, it is with people of this social grouping, living at present in sub-standard houses, and often in restricted economic circumstances, that these 'aborigines' will finally become identified. And their aboriginal background, with all its valuable as well as dispensable traits, will in time become to them no more than a fantastic echo of the long-ago past.[105]

While the extent to which the Berndts were describing rather than prescribing is not entirely clear, it seems that they had difficulty in envisaging a variety of viable futures for Aboriginals or the possibility that there might be more than one legitimate way of 'being Aboriginal'. In this same discussion of Adelaide Aboriginals they contemplated the disappearance of 'Aboriginal' as a meaningful category, and argued that:

---

104 Ronald and Catherine Berndt, *From Black to White in South Australia*, FW Cheshire, Melbourne, 1951, p.263

105 The 'West End' refers to the residential areas of the western quadrant of the city of Adelaide which were among the poorest and 'roughest' in the city and metropolitan area, with some sections warranting the description of slum. Berndts, *From Black to White*, p.268

in matters affecting their economy and employment, these people should be studied as part of the general urban community and not as a separate group. As they become increasingly similar to their white counterparts in the city, they tend to relax their extended family and relationship ties and obligations, and to become more individualised in their approach. The more thoroughly they are merged into the white community, the less they depend on their near and distant relatives for mutual help and economic assistance in times of difficulty. The stress is rather on immediate members of their own families; and even then, since it is usually as individuals rather than as family groups that they are accepted into white society, there is some selection among those close relatives. A man or woman passing into the general community is apt to discard, for all practical purposes, any but those who will conform to the new pattern of life as opposed to the old, and to ignore the majority of 'aborigines' in Adelaide and elsewhere.[106]

However, they acknowledged that this process of 'merging into the white community' is not a straightforward one, and that Aboriginals who choose to pursue it may well find that it involves painful choices and is simply 'too hard'. Their reaction to these difficulties may include putting up resistance, taking refuge in their own community and asserting their rights – in short, being pushed to claim an identity as Aboriginals by the very processes of assimilation that were aimed at absorbing them. The Berndts concluded:

It seems that they are anxious to cling to [their] association, however slight, with the old ways, rather than to merge themselves completely into the culture, which, however, is steadily absorbing them.[107]

Both the tone and content of their analysis suggests that they believed that the opportunity for things to be different – for the process of assimilation to be experienced more positively – had been lost:

This resistance would probably have been less apparent had some elements of the aboriginal culture been incorporated in the new. If for instance, something of the songs and dramatic ballets had been retained, this could have enhanced the self-respect of these people, and averted the feeling (which many of them have) that they are only the inferior recipients of a 'progressive' culture.[108]

Despite its negative and fatalistic tone, this is prescient: it is an embryonic precursor of what has developed into an important theme in indigenous policy development, perhaps most obviously in the case of health policy. It is now a commonplace understanding that 'Aboriginal culture' – and the term can accommodate varying meaning and content – has not been completely and permanently lost and that its recovery and rehabilitation yield positive health outcomes. These include restored pride and confidence,

---

106 ibid., p.244
107 ibid., pp.274–5
108 ibid., p.275

replacing of negativity and despair with hope, and reclaiming connections that contribute to a sense of identity and belonging. This cultural reclamation involves much more
than the revaluing of certain aspects of 'traditional Aboriginal culture', such as the 'songs
and dramatic ballets' mentioned by the Berndts, although that is a vital part of it. It is also
about acknowledging that even those people of Aboriginal descent who are most thoroughly 'assimilated' within western culture, have not ceased to be 'Aboriginal'. For them,
'being Aboriginal' is not about conforming to a prescribed cultural type, but about
valuing a dynamic 'culture of Aboriginality' that may have less to do with ancient traditions than with more recent experiences of survival and resistance to absorption. Of
course, this raises scepticism and hostility now as it did in earlier times. It is frequently
asserted by non-indigenous people that 'real Aboriginals' are a rare breed, that there are
only a limited number of ways of 'being Aboriginal' and that expansiveness about this is
tantamount to fraud and evidence of trying to 'have it both ways', in order to gain
improper access to public resources. The distinguished anthropologist Elkin, in his
Introduction to the Berndts' 1951 publication, was alert to such restrictive thinking. He
saw it as a 'fundamental error' that Aborigines should be denied the privileges of citizenship if they chose to live on settlements or reserves. He called for a more imaginative
approach, warning that it was 'unwise sociologically, to make the breaking of the
Aborigines' own communal ties, the price of their citizenship'.[109]

Such thinking did not have a major impact on the public imagination in the 1950s.
Much of what is now known about indigenous reactions to 'white' society in the period
when assimilation was official policy is a result of later testimony. The increasing confidence with which this testimony has been offered in more recent times, and the ways in
which it has been received have been mediated by a changed political consciousness, and,
in particular, a more critical assessment of the place of assimilationist ideologies within
Australian society.

This testimony has taken several forms. Firstly, there has been a proliferation of
published individual and family memoirs written by indigenous people. These are often
explicit about 'setting the record straight' and use recollection of the details of domestic
life, schooling, and relationships with the Protection Board, the police and 'the welfare' to
record the hostility and prejudice they encountered as they tried to make their way in the
non-Aboriginal world. They also reveal the authors' pride in their identity as Aboriginals,
an identity that survived attempts to denigrate it or 'exempt' them from it. Such writings,
including South Australian examples already mentioned, often contain errors in relation
to dates and contextual details and misunderstandings of the origins of policies and practice, errors that are characteristic of oral testimony and of the process of remembering.
Despite this, they are authentic subjective accounts of indigenous experiences, of the
meanings that the writers attached to these experiences, and of the ways in which they
shaped their identity and ambitions. Indeed, the value of these writings lies in this very
subjectivity and its capacity to tell the stories that remain untold by government and institutional records. From such accounts we also know that the bitter experience of trying to
survive and gain respect as Aboriginals in a context of hostility and marginalisation led

---

109 ibid., pp.14–16

some to hide their identity and to seek acceptance and opportunity through painful denial of who they were.[110]

A second kind of writing which provides insights into the impact of the policies and practices of the assimilation period on the lives and self-concept of indigenous Australians are non-indigenous histories which have intentionally set out to accomplish this by uncovering indigenous stories from archival sources, locating these within broader social and political contexts and making them the focus of their historical inquiry. These histories, of which Rosalind Kidd's *The Way We Civilise* and Anna Haebich's *For Their Own Good* are acclaimed examples, demonstrate that indigenous people have not been merely the objects of political processes, although often they have been profoundly damaged and disempowered by them. On the contrary, they have frequently exercised agency, and responded in a discriminating fashion to the dominant culture. For example, in an account that mirrors what occurred in South Australia, Haebich tells how in Western Australia 'ultimate absorption' was foiled not just by legal and administrative inconsistencies, low levels of funding and government commitment, racist community attitudes and competing economic priorities, but by the emergence of a distinctive Aboriginal identity in response to the official policy of assimilation.[111]

A third source of insight into how Aboriginal people experienced one of the central strategies of 'assimilation' has emerged from the National Inquiry into the Separation of Aboriginal and Torres Strait Islander Children from their Families. *Bringing them Home*, the official report of this inquiry, chronicles the stories of 535 indigenous people removed from their families and communities as infants or children, in the interest of their assimilation into the general community. These were stories that remained hidden behind the bland official reporting during the assimilation period of the growing numbers of Aboriginal children being cared for in institutions and in foster homes. They revealed a 'less cautious and less progressive approach' to the separation of Aboriginal children from their families than was suggested by the Protection Board's official policy or by its formal relationship with the Children's Welfare and Public Relief Board, as defined by the 1939 *Aborigines Act.*[112] They also revealed that, once removed, many, although not all children's lives lacked the safety, stability, opportunity for 'advancement' and loving care that the system promised.[113] South Australian witnesses before the inquiry, like those from the rest

---

110 Prominent examples of this are Sally Morgan, *My Place*, Fremantle Arts Centre Press, Fremantle, 1987, and Roberta Sykes, *Snake Cradle*, Allen and Unwin, Sydney, 1997. Sykes's writings and political stances as an activist for Aboriginal rights are regarded by some as contentious and inappropriate, since her own ethnic identity – she identifies as a 'black woman' – remains ambiguous. Nevertheless, her nuanced account of growing up in north Queensland, her analysis of her mother's attempts to raise her to 'fit in' via 'respectable' domestic and public behaviour, and her acute awareness of the stratified nature of society and the gains and losses entailed in claiming one identity rather than another, shed considerable light on how assimilationist policies and racist community attitudes can shape the self-concepts of marginalised groups.

111 Anna Haebich, *For Their Own Good: Aborigines and Government in the South West of Western Australia, 1900–1940*, University of Western Australia Press, Nedlands, 1992 [1988], p.356

112 Human Rights and Equal Opportunity Commission, *Bringing Them Home*, pp.126–7

113 *Bringing Them Home* suggests that at Colebrook Home 'the encouragement of close attachment' between the older girls and the younger children 'went some way to overcoming the many other damaging effects of institutionalisation'. It also

of Australia, told how their culture and kin were denigrated and the truth about their origins or their families hidden or denied:

> She [foster mother] would say I was dumb all the time and my mother and father were lazy dirty people who couldn't feed me or the other brothers and sister.

> I grew up sadly not knowing one Aboriginal person and the view that was given to me was fear towards [my] people. I was told not to have anything to do with them as they were dirty, lived in shabby conditions and, of course, drank to excess. Not once was I told that I was of Aboriginal descent.[114]

They told of severe treatment:

> I remember the beatings and hidings . . . I remember if you played up, especially on a Sunday, you got the cane. You play chasing, you had to drop your pants, lie across the bed and get 3–5 whacks. If you pissed the bed, another 3–5.

> They used to lock us up in a little room like a cell and keep us on bread and water for a week if you played up too much.[115]

They told of the failure of the system to take them seriously or protect them from various kinds of abuse:

> They[foster family] started to get very nasty towards me . . . I couldn't even see anybody to tell them what was happening. A lady from the welfare came to see me. I told her how I was feeling. She just took no notice of me and done her reports saying I was very happy with [them].

> I remember when my sister came down and visited me . . . and I couldn't tell her that I'd been raped. And I never told anyone for years and years . . . I've been sexually abused, harassed, and then finally raped, y'know, and I've never had anyone to talk to about it . . . nobody, no father, no mother, no-one. We had no-one to guide us. I felt so isolated, alienated . . . That's why I hit the booze. None of that family bonding, nurturing, nothing.[116]

They told of the long-term effects of their removal on their ability to form personal relationships, their relationship with the law and their sense of identity:

> It's wrecking our relationship and the thing is that I just don't trust anybody half the time in

---

provides examples of fostering that provided 'love, care and comfort, and often a considerable measure of understanding of their indigenous heritage', pp.169–70. See also Barnes, *Munyi's Daughter*, for a positive account of the influence of Colebrook home and of many later experiences that involved a high level of assimilation into non-indigenous culture.

114 ibid., pp.156–7, confidential submission 483; confidential evidence 5
115 ibid., pp.160–1, confidential evidence 251, 358b
116 ibid., pp.168, 184, confidential evidence 253, 248

my life because I don't know whether they're going to be there one minute of gone the next.

If you grow up with no love ... I thought sex was love. That's why I probably had all those kids, cause I was trying to get all this love, y'know. Cause I never got it when I was in the Home.

It did lead to a career in crime ... it was getting back at society. It was kicking them, y'know? ... it was the fact that, well, I'm going to pay back now for twenty odd years. Now, I served something like five years in prisons, not because I wanted to be a criminal, but because I didn't know where I was, I didn't know who I belonged to.

... I felt, growing up, that I wasn't really a blackfella. You hear whitefellas tell you you're a black-fella. But blackfellas tell you you're a whitefella. So you're caught in a half-caste world.[117]

When these things were happening, the ideology of assimilation rendered the practice of child removal as a benefit to the children involved and as a humane response to the 'Aboriginal problem' and blocked contemplation of the experiences of loss, grief and abuse behind it.[118] It did this so effectively that when the revelations contained in *Bringing Them Home* were published in 1997, they came as a genuine shock to many Australians. Indeed, the report was so unsettling that it evoked attempts to deny or min-imise the inquiry's findings and to discredit its methodology. There were also suggestions that instances of 'stolen' children having later done well in life disproved claims that the policy had been misguided.

In the 1950s, however, all this remained hidden or could be rationalised or ignored.[119] In the main, Aboriginal people themselves remained silent about it, at least in public, or expressed their resistance in individual behaviour that cost them dearly and brought them more firmly under 'white' authority. They did not protest about it in an organised way. In fact, the most forthright organised protest the South Australian Aborigines Department had to contend with at this time was not a protest against assimilation, as much as a request that the government provide genuine opportunities for assimilation to occur.

In February 1957, bearing a petition signed by 66 residents, a deputation of four

---

117 ibid., pp.185, 221, 190, 203, confidential evidence 379, 383, 354, 289

118 My own experience attests to the effectiveness of this blocking. I was born in Adelaide in 1945 and grew up there during the assimilation period. My family was deeply involved in a church that supported Aboriginal missions in Western Australia. I knew a good deal about these missions and contributed to their upkeep from my pocket money, but it never occurred to me, at that time, to wonder where the children who lived in the mission homes came from, or where their families were. Nor did I ever wonder about how the one Aboriginal I knew as a teenager came to be a resident at Colebrook Home. I did not ask, and was not aware of anyone else asking, about his family, his pre-Colebrook life, his experiences as a target of the assimilation policy, or his aspirations for the future.

119 It is important to note that the removal and institutionalisation of indigenous children occurred at a time when the removal and institutionalisation of non-indigenous children – for different reasons and at nothing like the same rate, but with many of the same tragic consequences – was also routine and largely unquestioned. See Senate Community Affairs Committee, *Forgotten Australians: a report on Australians who experienced institutional or out-of-home case as children*, Commonwealth of Australia, Canberra, 2004.

Aboriginals from Point Pearce approached the Protection Board with a series of complaints about the management of the station and requesting greater indigenous involvement in its administration and access to farming opportunities on reserve land. They asked for the removal of the station manager and his wife on many grounds: unfair treatment of individuals; high-handedness and lack of civility and respect; poor administration and unnecessary restriction of nursing and medical services; poor maintenance of the water supply, sanitation systems and housing; underpayment of girls working as domestics at the station; lack of encouragement or support for young people seeking employment; and neglect of fences and farm stock. They voiced their sense of injustice that non-Aboriginals continued to be employed as share-farmers on Aboriginal reserve land at Point Pearce, while all but four Aboriginal residents were unable to gain such employment or have access to land. They asked the Board to consider 'a form of self-government by the native people so that they could be given the opportunity of operating Point Pearce as a co-operative settlement', and suggested that if this were granted, and they could retain a primary and secondary school and a welfare officer, they could dispense with special assistance from the Aborigines Department.[120]

This amounted to a significant display of initiative on the petitioners' part, and was surely evidence of a desire to work, contribute to the community and take responsibility for their future – in short to do what government, missionaries and Protectors had been telling them to do since the earliest days of non-Aboriginal settlement. It was certainly evidence of willingness to participate in the project of assimilation, although not expressed in these terms. However, neither the Protection Board nor the Secretary of the Department saw it in this way. They were dismissive of complaints about the behaviour of the manager and his wife towards the residents and found that there were 'no grounds whatsoever' for pursuing the request for their removal. They were defensive about complaints regarding maintenance of the water supply, but promised action in the future, 'when sufficient finance and labour is available'. They dismissed allegations about lack of employment opportunities and poor pay as 'ridiculous' and said they would continue to employ white share-farmers. They judged the plan for a locally run cooperative, based on division of the land into 200 to 300-acre blocks, as 'simply fantastic' and 'quite preposterous'. Finally they decided that the suggestion that the Point Pearce people do without special assistance from the Aborigines Department be 'ignored as not being in the interests of the natives themselves'.[121] Assimilation, apparently, was to be on non-indigenous terms and was not a matter for negotiation.

In reacting as they did to the Point Pearce petition the Protection Board and Aborigines Department were actually subverting the process of assimilation and falling back on the more comfortable strategies of segregation and protection. This episode highlights a number of the complexities that existed by the end of the period under discussion in the relations between the government and the older, more settled Aboriginal communities such as those at Point Pearce, Point McLeay and Koonibba. These complexities constituted significant policy challenges for the future.

---

120 Aborigines Protection Board, Minutes, 27 February 1957, pp.261–4, GRG 52/16/2

121 Aborigines Protection Board, Minutes, 13 March 1957, pp.276–8, GRG 52/16/2

For example, as already discussed, one of the strategies that the government had been pursuing in order to achieve its assimilation goals was moving 'suitable' Aboriginal people out of the segregated missions and government institutions, into which they had been congregated at an earlier time, and into the general community. In the meantime, however – and for some this meant a period spanning several generations – many people had formed genuine attachments to these missions and settlements which had provided protection, sustenance and even survival in earlier times. For people whose links to traditional country and sometimes to kin had been severed, they had become home. In conventional economic terms they were artificial communities, set up and governed under protectionist legislation. Their farms, fishing ventures, stores, butcheries, bakeries, schools, churches and clinics lent them an appearance of self-sufficiency, or at least self-containment, but in reality, they were never able to provide adequately for the needs of their residents and always relied on varying levels of government subsidy. These settlements had been envisaged as temporary, but for administrative reasons, as well as those relating to sentiment and attachment, they exhibited 'a practical tendency to entrenchment'.[122] In the 1950s this was a problem for state and federal governments committed to assimilation, and in 1955 Hasluck warned against perpetuating 'a series of flourishing native settlements in which the majority of the native peoples were living apart from the rest of the community'.[123] This was a situation which resisted change, however, since what may have begun as enforced segregation from the wider community and an unwelcome mixing of different indigenous groups had in some cases grown into something more positive. Indigenous embrace of manufactured, separate communities, clearly discernible from this time and set to strengthen in the following decades, in conjunction with growing demands for the rights and opportunities enjoyed by other Australians, constituted a major challenge to non-indigenous notions of assimilation and prudent use of public resources.

An alternative mission experiment begun on a remote and theoretically 'inviolable' Aboriginal reserve during the time South Australia was adopting assimilation as its official policy provides a further example of the complex intertwining of assimilation, segregation and protection that continued to characterise both ideas and practice, and, in the long term, to shape indigenous relations with the rest of the community. In 1936, at the instigation of influential layman Dr Charles Duguid, the South Australian Assembly of the Presbyterian Church undertook to establish a mission at Ernabella in the North-West Reserve, the country of the Pitjantjatjara.[124] Increasing encroachment by non-Aboriginal hunters and pastoralists in this area had raised concerns about the effects of this on the well-being of the Pitjantjatjara who were still living largely traditional lives.[125] Duguid

---

122 Rowse, *White Flour, White Power*, p.111

123 ibid., p.111

124 *Presbyterian Banner*, September 1936, p.6. See also Duguid's Moderatorial Address, *Presbyterian Banner*, April 1935, pp.6–10. The mission was too large a financial burden for South Australian Presbyterians and became the responsibility of the Australian Presbyterian Church in 1937. Duguid, as already noted, was an inaugural member of the Aborigines Protection Board.

125 The AFA was vigilant in relation to threats to Aboriginal Reserves throughout the 1930s and maintained that well-run missions were the best hope of protecting their 'inviolability' and contributing to the welfare of their indigenous

envisaged the mission as a buffer that would protect them from the degradation that frequently accompanied contact with western culture, while allowing for their gradual assimilation without the obliteration of their culture and identity. This was in line with the view of the Chief Protector, who, in 1936, argued:

> [i]t appears to be impossible to stop the progress of the white race, even if it does upset the life and habits of the indigenous people. It therefore becomes our duty to buffer the contact in some way so that the clash will not only be gradual, but will in the first instance be with persons who have the welfare and love of the aborigines at heart.[126]

During the 1940s and 1950s the Ernabella experiment developed as Duguid had envisaged, while also satisfying various agenda of the Aborigines Protection Board.[127] Growth in population numbers without an increase in mixed-race births and the maintenance of cultural and economic independence were signs of the health and vigour of the community and of the effective protection offered by the mission. In 1954 the Board declared Ernabella to be

> an efficient buffer between the near primitive natives and white civilization. The Presbyterian authorities in control of this mission have adopted the policy of very gradually preparing the aborigines for their eventual contact with civilization. Tribal customs and ceremonies are permitted, in fact encouraged, and every opportunity is taken to encourage the natives to retain their self-respect and natural dignity. As little relief as possible is issued and the menfolk, where not employed, must hunt for their natural food. Although the children are taught to speak some English, they are also instructed in their own dialect, and few of the natives converse in other than their own language.[128]

The Board's 1961 report indicated some capacity by the mission to accommodate the Pitjantjatjara's discriminating responses to the services it offered, and an openness on the part of mission staff to Aboriginal ways of doing things.[129] However, there is no evidence that the Board generalised from the experiences at Ernabella to reflect on a healthy balance between assimilation and protection, or on what was likely to make the inevitable trend towards assimilation less destructive of indigenous identity and well-being than it might otherwise be. These remained as challenges for the future.

---

populations. See for example, AFA Committee minutes, 2 July 1930; AFA Annual Reports, 24 March 1931, 6 March 1935, AFA Minute Books, SRG139/2, vols v and vi.

126 Report of Chief Protector of Aborigines, 1936, *SAPP*, no.29, 1936

127 Aborigines Protection Board, Annual Report, 1947, *SAPP*, no.20, 1947. For further insight into Duguid's views, see Charles Duguid, *No Dying Race*, Rigby, Adelaide, 1963, and *Doctor and the Aborigines*, Rigby, Adelaide, 1972.

128 Aborigines Protection Board, Annual Report, 1954, *SAPP*, no.20, 1954

129 Aborigines Protection Board, Annual Report, 1961, *SAPP*, no.20, 1961. This was particularly in relation to birthing and post-natal care.

At the end of its 23 years of guardianship of the lives of South Australia's indigenous population, the Aborigines Protection Board admitted that attempts to assimilate the Aboriginal
population into the general community had not been successful: 'a great number of our
aborigines simply have no desire to be assimilated, but understandably would rather lead
a life of their own choice'. While believing that 'forced assimilation is simply not practicable nor possible and can only end in tragedy for the aborigine concerned', the Board
nevertheless insisted that 'every effort must be made to create a desire on the part of the
aborigine for his ultimate assimilation'. This could be done through 'such measures as persuading and enticing him to improve his standard of living and education'.[130] Thus 'ultimate assimilation' was constructed as relying entirely on indigenous desire for it rather
than on the non-indigenous structural and attitudinal changes necessary to allow it to
happen. It was all up to the Aboriginals themselves: if they shaped up they would be
accepted, and if they did not, they were simply throwing away their chances for a better
life. That was what the Board had tried to make them understand:

> Aboriginals living in substandard conditions are being continually encouraged to better their
> conditions in the hope that this type of native will eventually desire to live in a home with the
> added responsibility of paying a nominal rental. There is no doubt that he or his family will not
> be accepted in the community until such time as they have the desire to be properly housed and
> are capable of living in a home in the normal manner.[131]

In its frustration, the Board resorted to simplistic victim-blaming. In addition, it ignored
the indigenous consciousness and aspirations that had been generated by previous attempts
to achieve assimilation and failed to consider how these might shape future choices made
by Aboriginal people. The next chapter explores how this emergent indigenous consciousness, supported by a more liberal social and political climate, modified the assimilation project and the relationship of the indigenous population to the public.

---

130 Aborigines Protection Board, Annual Report, 1960, 1961, *SAPP*, no.20, 1960, 1961
131 Aborigines Protection Board, Annual Report, 1961, *SAPP*, no.20, 1961

Chapter 7

1963–1973: A New Age?

Individual aborigines have demonstrated that they can manage their own affairs efficiently, to be rewarded in many cases by the granting of full citizenship rights. Each time this is done, there is an agitation from other aborigines for similar rights and privileges. But they have to be refused if these applicants are unable to shoulder the inescapable responsibilities which accompany them ... A surprising number of aborigines are contributing a full share to the Australian way of life as is shown by a singer, a clergyman, nurses and athletes who are well known. Every effort must be made to aid and encourage others to do likewise.

Norman B Tindale and HA Lindsay 1963[1]

The people of the State have their own part to play by accepting the Aboriginal into their midst as he becomes fitted for life in a predominantly white community.

Advertiser **1 February 1963**

Increasingly, Aborigines all over the State are taking the initiative in bringing about changes in their conditions and are airing the frustrations and dissatisfactions that they have quietly suffered for the past 150 years.

Aboriginal Affairs Board 1969[2]

The *Aboriginal Affairs Act, 1962*, aimed to place 'all Aborigines and persons of Aboriginal blood under the same legal provisions as other South Australians with the same opportunities and the same responsibilities'. Thus it spelled a formal end to protection, and to the binary legal system that had clouded efforts at assimilation during the life of the previous act. Legally, it made all persons of Aboriginal descent part of the public. It provided for new definitions: 'full-blood' descendants of the original inhabitants were defined as 'Aborigines', henceforth to be accorded the dignity of a capital letter, and those who were of Aboriginal descent, but not 'full-blood', defined as 'persons of Aboriginal blood'. The act placed no restrictions on Aborigines or persons of Aboriginal blood, other than

1 Norman B Tindale and HA Lindsay, *Aboriginal Australians*, Jacaranda Press, Brisbane 1963, p.134

2 Aboriginal Affairs Board (AAB), Report 1969, *SAPP*, no.20, 1969, p.19

those applying to all citizens, except in the case of the supply and consumption of alcoholic liquor. This remaining restriction could be lifted, in relation to particular areas, by the proclamation of the Governor. The lack of restriction in the act was complemented by provision for 'assistance ... of a positive nature, calculated to assist development and assimilation', including the provision of housing, fostering and education of children and encouraging engagement in 'primary, mechanical or business pursuits'. The objectives of the Department of Aboriginal Affairs and the Aboriginal Affairs Board (AAB) which had been created by the act were focused

> more on real welfare than perhaps has been the case in the past, concentrating more on help and encouragement to Aborigines and persons of Aboriginal blood to accept their full responsibilities and thus promote their social, economic and political development until their assimilation into the community.

In short, it assumed that 'the stage of development has now been reached where most of the Aborigines and part-Aborigines need guidance rather than protection'.[3]

When he introduced the bill for a new Aboriginal affairs act into the South Australian parliament on 16 August 1962, the responsible minister, the Hon. GG Pearson, reminded his colleagues that 'time marches on and that circumstances and concepts change'. He argued that the bill reflected

> the progress made over the years in development towards normal standards of living by Aborigines and progress, too, towards the enlightened public mind which has come to an awareness of our individual responsibilities towards Aborigines as our fellow citizens. The difficulties to be overcome are ours as much as theirs.[4]

He claimed to be well aware of these difficulties. In exercising his ministerial responsibilities he had travelled around the state and 'developed a considerable respect for Aboriginal people'. At the same time he had

> learnt to be somewhat wary of the starry-eyed idealists and those people who become subject to spasmodic enthusiasms regarding what ought to be done for Aboriginal people, because the question of their assimilation into our community is not one of short duration. It cannot be so. That is impossible, and the scientific world has agreed that assimilation is something that must take place over several generations if we are not to tear apart the fabric and psychology of the people whom we are trying to help.[5]

---

3 *An Act to repeal the Aborigines Act, 1934–1939, and to promote the welfare and advancement of persons of Aboriginal blood in South Australia, and for other purposes*, no, 42, 1962; AAB, Report, 1963, *SAPP*, no.20, 1963, p.6

4 GG Pearson, *SAPD*, House of Assembly, 16 August 1962, pp.564–5

5 ibid., pp.567–8

If assimilation was something that could not be hurried, it was also something which, for Pearson, needed neither precise definition nor defence as a policy goal. Like many others before him, he assumed it to be self-evidently the inevitable and desirable future for the indigenous population. The bill met with a positive response from both sides of the house, and there was general agreement that it was not a party-political measure.

The tone of the debate was set by DA Dunstan, the Labor member for Norwood and chief opposition spokesperson on Aboriginal affairs. He had suggested a new framework for thinking about indigenous issues in the previous year when he argued against the maintenance of protective legislation and ideas. He acknowledged that there was an ongoing need for assistance towards integration but saw this as

> quite different from the business of monitoring protection of aborigines by saying that they are not to have the same rights as other citizens, and that they may have their property or their children disposed of by an administrative decision of the department.[6]

Three weeks later he presented a petition to parliament. Signed by 11,842 South Australian electors, it protested against Aboriginals being 'subject to diverse disabilities in law and restrictions upon their freedom, not because of their individual characteristics but solely because of their race', and sought removal of these disabilities and restrictions by amending the *Aborigines Act* and the *Licensing Act*.[7]

In 1962, Dunstan entered the debate on the new bill well armed, since the Labor Party had already prepared its own 'comprehensive measure' for consideration during the current session of parliament, and had adopted as a 'general principle' that

> legislation on Aborigines should be only welfare legislation, in effect, and that all restrictions on Aborigines should be removed, which were restrictions by virtue of their race rather than the individual characteristics of the persons to whom these restrictions would be applied.

In a long speech that revealed close acquaintance with the outcomes of protection and assimilation policies and practices in South Australia, Dunstan insisted that protective legislation and its underlying assumption that Aboriginals needed to be treated as 'wayward children' and have their lives 'managed for them' was 'completely wrong' and incompatible with 'either assimilation or integration':

> Assimilation and integration will never take place unless these people are simply subject to the same laws as operate for every other member of the community who has freedom from restriction ... it is vital that Aborigines be encouraged to stand on their own feet, but they never will while there is a continuance of protective legislation or a continuance of assistance known fairly accurately as the 'hand-out' system.[8]

---

6 DA Dunstan, *SAPD*, House of Assembly, 3 October 1961, p.1015

7 ibid., 24 October 1961, p.1447

8 ibid., 30 August 1962, p.812

Dunstan's focus on integration is significant. What he meant by integration is indicated not only by his statement of definition in which he distinguished it from assimilation, but by the outlining of policy directions that went well beyond the familiar pious generalisations about training opportunities that would encourage Aboriginals to take their place in the community as responsible citizens. He characterised assimilation as a policy and a process whereby Aboriginals were to become 'indistinguishable from other members of [the] community apart from their different coloured skin'. He argued against that approach, claiming:

> in numbers of cases the Aboriginal, although he is detribalized, still retains a very close feeling of family and of group; he does not want to be separated from family and group and put amongst what is still to him something of an alien community. He wants to be taken into the community as a group and maintain some of the features of his own way of life within the group.

Being able to maintain features of the Aboriginal 'way of life' while being 'taken into' the wider community was what Dunstan meant by 'integration', and he believed that 'in many cases [it] was wise'. This position recognised that Aboriginal people might have other ambitions apart from absorption into the general community, and that being 'detribalized' and assimilated to some aspects of non-Aboriginal culture need not mean the loss of traditional bonds with kin and country or constitute a relinquishing of Aboriginal identity. As a key means to achieve integration he advocated that Aboriginal people living on reserves be guaranteed 'proprietary rights' to the land. In the case of the discovery of minerals on the land, the Aboriginal proprietors would be entitled to royalties, and in the case of resumption of the land by government, to the payment of compensation. Dunstan reminded the parliament that this was in line with the directives under which the province of South Australia had been established and warned them that 'this business of giving no sort of proprietary rights to Aborigines gets them jumping'. He argued also for the development of Point Pearce and Point McLeay as indigenous cooperatives, and for indigenous representation on the AAB that was proposed as the successor to the Aborigines Protection Board.[9] In addition, he developed detailed arguments about particular provisions of the bill that the Labor Party believed needed amendment, specifically, the dismantling of particular restrictions and protective mechanisms. In doing so he displayed familiarity not only with the situation in South Australia, but also with that in the rest of Australia and in other countries with analogous 'problems'.[10]

Another major contributor to the second reading debate was RR Loveday, Labor member for Whyalla. Like Dunstan's, his speech was distinguished by its appeals to history and experiences in other countries, and, in addition, to contemporary research findings. He supported Dunstan's line on indigenous representation in government administrative structures and on recognition of indigenous property rights in land. He reminded the parliament that land had been 'filched' from the original inhabitants in

9 ibid., pp.814–16
10 ibid., pp.816–23

breach of colonial law and that in their attempts to 'Christianise' the Aboriginals the colonists had forgotten 'many of the more important things regarding their material welfare'.[11] To support his case against assimilation as absorption he referred to the research of Adelaide geographer, Fay Gale. In pointing to the diversity of settlement and living patterns within the indigenous population and the varying degrees of their involvement with and accommodation to non-indigenous society, Gale demonstrated that assimilation was not a simple, unified matter. For example, the fact that Aboriginals made up 71 per cent of the population of the far north-west and the pastoral regions, but only 24 per cent of the 'detribalized' areas of Eyre Peninsula, the opal fields and the northern towns and agricultural areas, and a mere 1.3 per cent of Adelaide and its surrounds and the south-east meant that 'the problem of assimilation, so termed, is a different problem in each place'. Loveday was of the opinion that some indigenous people would never be assimilated, but could be integrated into the community as long as non-Aboriginal people recognised that they were not 'the ones who have everything to offer'. He believed that the situation was so complex that 'research [was] badly needed' and hoped the new legislation would provide for it.[12] These were large issues that went beyond the scope of the 1962 bill. They foreshadowed directions that were pursued when Labor achieved office and when Aboriginal people became increasingly involved in shaping their political futures.

LG Riches, Labor member for the northern seat of Stuart, which included the town of Port Augusta and the nearby Umeewarra Mission, welcomed the bill and claimed it had widespread support among organisations working in the interests of Aboriginal people. He also sounded some warning notes and offered some challenges to prevailing views. He noted that many commentators saw the bill as a means to end a culture of 'handouts' which they claimed had characterised and bedevilled indigenous–non-indigenous relations. He rejected the notion, implicit in this, that Aboriginal people had had it easy. On the contrary, he claimed that 'the Aborigines I have been amongst have never had an opportunity to make good and nothing they have received can be regarded as a handout'. Certainly the government had issued 'enough rations to keep body and soul together' when no work was available, but they did this for 'white people' as well, including Riches himself. Thus he saw no reason for saying that

> out of a benevolent and kindly attitude of the State we have been over-generous to Aborigines ... If any criticism is to be made it is that we have been niggardly towards Aborigines and that they have not had a chance.[13]

In other words, he was rejecting the double standard that had operated since the earliest days of the colony. This was the assumption that Aboriginal people did not have the same

---

11 RR Loveday, *SAPD*, House of Assembly, 17 October 1962, pp.1526–27

12 ibid., pp.1529–31. Loveday was up to date, as Gale's research was recent. 'The role of employment in the assimilation of part Aborigines' was published in 1959 in *Proceedings of the Royal Geographical Society of Australasia, South Australian Branch*, vol.60, pp.49–58, and her University of Adelaide PhD thesis, 'A Study of Assimilation: part-Aborigines in South Australia' was completed in 1960.

13 LG Riches, *SAPD*, House of Assembly, 17 October 1962, p.1540

claim on government resources as the rest of the population and that any government provision, however slight, was an act of benevolence and generosity. By contrast, he was constructing the indigenous population as part of the public.

Riches went on to demonstrate insight into some of the difficulties that were frequently glossed over by advocates of assimilation and integration. He pointed out that the 'new deal' expected by some to result from the new legislation depended on 'the co-operation of all our people', and he was aware this was something that could not be guaranteed. He illustrated the difficulties by referring to the situation in Port Augusta, where about 400 'assimilated' Aboriginals lived. Many of these 'attend the picture shows and concerts, walk about the streets, attend our churches and generally are accepted into the community life'. Children from Umeewarra 'who are able to take their place with the white children are brought into the white schools and are treated in every respect in the same way as white children'. But Riches judged that these experiments had

> been successful because of the good behaviour of the Aborigines. If this had not been so, the move for assimilation could have been set back for years. The Aborigines must be careful to see that their actions are above reproach. In Port Augusta we are accustomed to Aborigines being in the streets and we welcome it, but if an Aboriginal should be under the influence of intoxicating liquor no mother would allow her children to go out into the street where he was ... The Aborigines who attend town hall functions are well-behaved and cleanly dressed. It would be easy to build up an objection to them if they were not so well-behaved and dressed.

In short, Riches was acknowledging that, in the ordinary situations of daily life, acceptance of Aboriginals as members of the community depended on non-Aboriginal judgements about their behaviour and demeanour. In parliament and elsewhere where assimilation and integration were discussed as matters of principle there was ready agreement that Aboriginal people had the same rights as all other South Australians and that judgements, restrictions or exclusions based on 'race' were unacceptable. However, on the streets of Port Augusta and other centres with concentrations of Aboriginals, opportunities for 'assimilation' and 'integration' still appeared more as privileges offered to those who shaped up and passed arbitrary tests set by non-Aboriginals. In addition, crude racist prejudices still supported instances of segregation. As Riches admitted, when an orchestral concert or other similar event was held in the Port Augusta Town Hall, tickets for the front seats, normally the most expensive for a concert, 'cannot be given away', since when 'picture shows are held ... Aborigines sit in the front seats'. In this fragile context of limited tolerance, he was surely right to suggest that the success of the proposed legislation depended on 'sympathetic understanding and a strong administration with adequate power to deal with problems as they arise', as well as vigilance by Aboriginals 'to see that their actions are above reproach'.[14]

In committee, Pearson responded with some flexibility to the opposition's case, presented by Dunstan, for a number of amendments to the bill. Key amendments that

---

14 ibid., pp.1541–2

were approved included making the minister rather than the AAB responsible for the administration of the act and limiting the AAB to an advisory role; tightening the clause referring to existing Aboriginal reserves so that no portion of them could be alienated from use by indigenous people; the inclusion of additional paragraphs clarifying the purpose of the act as promoting development leading to integration, and providing for research into the problems of the indigenous population and the collection of data concerning their regional distribution; and, after lengthy debate, provision for the repeal of those sections of the *Licensing Act* that had hitherto prohibited the purchase and consumption of alcoholic liquor by indigenous persons. Henceforth, restrictions would apply 'in such areas of the State as shall be proclaimed', rather than, as in the original bill, to persons of Aboriginal blood but not to Aborigines.[15] The 'drinking rights' question was widely regarded as of crucial importance: 'wrongly handled, this will do more harm to assimilation than anything else we can think of'.[16] Amendments that were not passed included dispensing with the definitional difference between Aborigines and persons of Aboriginal blood and the restrictions placed on the former; requiring that a prescribed number of members of the AAB be of Aboriginal descent; and abolishing the power of the AAB to authorise a medical officer to examine Aborigines and persons of Aboriginal blood believed to be suffering from an infectious disease, and to insist on their treatment. Dunstan argued strongly against this discriminatory treatment in relation to health and believed that the matter could be dealt with under the general *Health Act*. However, Pearson would not budge, insisting that this clause was needed to protect the health of the Aboriginals who were a 'people of a primitive way of life, far removed from medical care and with no knowledge of drugs, antidotes or medical matters of any sort, as we understand them'.[17] Perhaps behind this assertion of the need for blanket protection for an apparently homogeneous primitive population – a position at odds with the rest of the debate – lurked residual fears of contamination of the 'white' population by the 'black'.

An Act to repeal the Aborigines Act, 1934–1939, and to promote the welfare and advancement of Aborigines and persons of Aboriginal blood in South Australia, and for other purposes, no. 45 of 1962 – henceforth referred to as the *Aboriginal Affairs Act, 1962* – was assented to on 15 November 1962 and came into operation on 28 February 1963. The membership of the inaugural AAB, which was established under the act to advise the Minister of Aboriginal Affairs on matters affecting the welfare of Aboriginal people, was gazetted on that day. It had seven members from the university and scientific community, the churches, the Education Department, the pastoral industry and organisations committed to furthering the interests of the indigenous population, and, as the AAB rather coyly reported in its first official report, 'amongst [its] members was for the first time a person

15 *SAPD*, House of Assembly, 17 October 1962, pp.1546–51; 23 October 1962, pp.1629–36

16 GA Bywaters, *SAPD*, House of Assembly, 23 October 1962, p.1631

17 *SAPD*, House of Assembly, 17 October 1962, pp.1546–1551; 18 October 1962, pp.1569–80; 23 October 1962, pp.1629–42; 24 October 1962, pp.1683–4

of Aboriginal blood'.[18] Its first meeting, held on 26 March 1963, was attended by
CJ Millar, Acting Head of the Aborigines Department since Bartlett's retirement in mid-
1962, and subsequently the first Director of the Department of Aboriginal Affairs.[19] The
AAB's first report, for the year ending 30 June 1963, was submitted before it had been able
'to formulate firm recommendations on administration and future policy'. Despite this
prematurity, the report provides an invaluable summary of the state of services, provisions
and existing policies relating to the indigenous population at a time of major transition,
and of the expanded capacity and agenda of the new department. It acts as a useful template against which to consider the work of the AAB and other activities and developments
impinging on Aboriginal affairs over the next decade.[20]

Members of the AAB appeared to be taking their advisory role seriously, and by June
1963 had already visited many reserves and other centre of indigenous population. They
noted that people of Aboriginal descent were living in many different situations and
included 'spear-carrying nomadic people living under tribal conditions' as well as those
living in country towns or the metropolitan area 'under exactly the same working and
living conditions as their non-Aboriginal neighbours'. There were perhaps 6000 in total,
2000 of whom were Aborigines, living mainly in the far north and west of the state, and
4000 persons of Aboriginal blood who were more widely dispersed, with concentrations
on missions and reserves.[21] Because of the 'valuable work' done by the Aborigines
Protection Board, most of these 6000 were now deemed to be more in need of guidance
than protection. The objective of the new AAB and the Department of Aboriginal Affairs
was to promote their 'real welfare' by pursuing the 'social, economic and political development' that would enable them to be assimilated into the general community. The AAB
commended recent initiatives towards this end undertaken by its predecessor, the
Aborigines Protection Board. These included the government's purchase of the Gerard
Reserve from UAM, the establishment of Musgrave Park Station on the North-West
Reserve, the establishment of welfare centres in the opal mining townships of Coober Pedy
and Andamooka, the building of 100 houses for Aboriginal families, and the trend
towards placing 'rescued' Aboriginal children in foster homes rather than in institutions.
To carry out its mandate under the new legislation, the staff of the Department of

---

18 The members of the first Aboriginal Affairs Board were Professor AA Abbie (Chairman, Professor of Anatomy, University
of Adelaide), Professor JB Cleland (Deputy Chairman, Emeritus Professor of Pathology, University of Adelaide),
Mr J Whitburn (Superintendent of Primary Schools, Education Department), the Rev. GW Pope (Congregational
minister, formerly in the Riverland and at the time of his appointment, in suburban Hindmarsh), Mr RJ Barnes (senior
electrical fitter and mechanic, Post Master General's Department), Mr IR McTaggart, (pastoralist and company director,
Nonning Station, via Port Augusta) and Mrs FM Hunt-Cooke. The person of Aboriginal blood was Barnes, a Second
World War veteran, and a protege of Duguid who was active within the Aborigines Advancement League. *SAGG*, 28
February 1963, p.507; AAB, Minutes, 26 March 1963, p.1, GRS 4343/1/P

19 ibid.

20 AAB, Report, 1963, *SAPP*, no.20, 1963

21 The terms 'Aborigines' and 'persons of Aboriginal blood', as defined under the *Aboriginal Affairs Act, 1962*, were not always
used with precision. I will use these terms as they are used in the legislation when it is important to distinguish between
the two groups, but otherwise will continue to use 'Aboriginals' or 'indigenous people/population'.

Aboriginal Affairs had been expanded to 17, and included new senior positions – a Senior Administrative Officer, who acted as secretary to the AAB, a Supervisor of Reserves and a Senior Welfare Officer – as well as an Employment Officer and additional welfare staff. There were many 'serious problems connected with the Aboriginal in employment', since some of those seeking work had 'no idea of the responsibility entailed when they enter it'. Thus the Employment Officer's role was not only to assist Aboriginals to find work, but also to 'ensure its continuance'. The main role of the Welfare Officers was to provide training in domestic management and child-rearing for women on the reserves. It was difficult to find suitable applicants for this job, and three positions for resident female Welfare Officers on reserves remained unfilled.[22]

The AAB's comments on specific aspects of the department's responsibilities – employment, provision of relief, care of children, secondary education, health, housing and community education for assimilation – are superficial and incomplete. However, they reveal that achieving the desired balance between guidance and protection, while bringing Aboriginals under the same legal provisions as other South Australians, was a complex challenge. Something of this challenge is indicated by the following examples.

The Department of Aboriginal Affairs had assisted 166 males and 36 females to enter employment, the nature, location or conditions of which were unspecified. An unknown number of others were already in employment or had recently secured jobs without recourse to the department. The AAB was aware that, late in 1962, 158 Aboriginals were working for the Commonwealth or South Australian Railways and in other state and local government positions. It claimed, without reference to any comparative substantiating data, that the fact that about 21 per cent of these had completed at least five years of service indicated that 'there was no real reason to suppose that persons of Aboriginal blood are any more unstable in employment than any other class of person'. However, the report suggests that not all those employed were paid like 'any other class of person': in 'a number of cases' the department was having to subsidise the costs of board for 'younger boys and girls' whose wages did not cover the cost of their basic needs or enable them to be self-supporting.[23]

Meanwhile, the historic practice of rationing had not disappeared. While the provision of 'relief' to 'necessitous Aborigines' was being brought in line with the provision of social service benefits to other Australians, actual access to benefits, especially in the case of 'nomadic Aborigines' and those living outside the metropolitan area, was still subject to paternalistic departmental control. The department also continued to exercise another historic role: it still regarded 'the proper care' of 'neglected' or 'orphan' Aboriginal children as one of its most important responsibilities and was no more forthcoming about definitions of terms than had been the case in the past. This care was now administered by the Children's Welfare and Public Relief Department under the terms of the *Maintenance Act, 1926*. As at 30 June 1963, 155 Aboriginal children were in private foster homes, 164 in institutions, and 11 had been legally adopted by non-Aboriginals in the last year. The provision of education for Aboriginal children, once left largely to missions, was now the

---

22 AAB, Report, 1963, *SAPP*, no.20, 1963, pp.6–7

23 ibid., p.7

responsibility of the Education Department, which had taken over reserve and mission primary schools. In addition, the Department of Aboriginal Affairs was meeting the costs of secondary schooling for those who showed 'the necessary ability'. The report did not indicate how many indigenous children were deemed to have such ability or give any idea of the extent to which indigenous children were engaged with the 'mainstream' education system or of their levels of achievement or acceptance within it.

Housing was still seen as a major aid to integration into the wider community. The department believed it needed to provide housing of different standards, depending on 'the various standards of development achieved by Aborigines in various parts of the State'. It owned 105 houses on minor reserves and in towns and a few on major reserves, and rented these to Aboriginal tenants. In addition, about 50 Aboriginal families were living in South Australian Housing Trust homes in the metropolitan and country areas. The report was silent about whether supply matched demand, whether indigenous tenants were welcomed and integrated into the areas in which they took up housing, and whether this part of the department's policy undermined or confirmed existing racial prejudice and discriminatory behaviour.[24]

Under the heading of health, the AAB reported on surveys and treatment for tuberculosis, trachoma and venereal diseases, and on high levels of immunisation against poliomyelitis, influenza, whooping cough, tetanus and diphtheria, in remote areas and on reserves. Those employed and living in the general community had, under the previous regime, been enrolled by the Aborigines Department in medical and hospital benefits funds in the hope that this would encourage them to seek medical attention when necessary. The AAB offered no comment on whether this had worked or not, but gave notice that 'in view of the changed tenor of the Act' indigenous people would be 'encouraged to accept more responsibility in this respect'. The report noted that diseases associated with low standards of hygiene, especially gastroenteritis, were not well controlled among the indigenous population, particularly in remote areas. It made no link between this and any other factors, such as income, employment or housing. Nor did it provide any insight into patterns of morbidity and mortality across the age groups within the Aboriginal population, or comparative rates of morbidity and mortality in the Aboriginal and non-Aboriginal populations. It merely suggested that the answer to the problem of poorly controlled disease was 'elementary education in hygiene', to be provided by women welfare officers.[25]

The AAB reported that, at the minister's direction, it had embarked on a program of community education. This was designed to acquaint the indigenous population with the provisions of the act, to 'promote an informed general public' and to stress that the new law would be ineffective unless all Australians were prepared 'to accept the Aboriginal as a person and to acknowledge ... that, with suitable encouragement, he is able to take his place in society'. To this end, 28 public meetings had been held in Adelaide, in country towns and on Aboriginal reserves. This 'Education for Assimilation' was being undertaken in conjunction with the United Churches Social Reform Board, and the report suggests

24 ibid., pp.7–8
25 ibid., p.8

that, despite its broad remit, a major focus was preparation for the day when Aboriginals would have unrestricted access to alcohol. Although the AAB claimed that 'the Aboriginal people have very much appreciated this work on their behalf', their own Senior Welfare Officer, AA Glastonbury, had in fact warned them, in a report discussed at their April meeting, that the United Churches Social Reform Board's total abstinence stance

> would not only be resented by the residents [of reserves], who had not the right to exercise free choice yet, but would also be ineffective as far as a significant percentage of adult male residents was concerned, many of whom already have a serious problem with alcohol.[26]

The report then provided a summary of the population, conditions, activities, achievements and problems at all the reserves, missions, welfare centres and other institutions administered by the Department of Aboriginal Affairs in 1963. This is telling in its optimism, its lack of detail about what lay behind bland generalisations about 'good health' and smoothly functioning schools, and its failure to comment on levels of deprivation and dependence and the continuation of protective practices that were difficult to reconcile with progress towards assimilation or integration.

At Point Pearce Reserve, where many of the 291 residents were 'in the final stage towards assimilation', farming, grazing and pig husbandry continued under the supervision of a farm overseer. After almost a century of activity at Point Pearce, the farm work was still seen as training, and 'the whole subject of training' was 'currently undergoing review'. Buildings were in need of repair, but one successful attempt at building using only Aboriginal labour 'could have much significance in the future'. The reserve was 'very fortunate' to share Yorke Peninsula's reticulated water and electricity supplies. Point Pearce children were able to attend kindergarten and primary school up to grade four on the reserve and were taught by trained teachers provided by the Education Department. Schooling beyond grade four was available at Maitland Area School but the report indicated that the children's progress was retarded by 'lack of parental interest'. Health care was provided by a resident nurse orderly, a 'well-equipped dispensary', a visiting medical officer and dentist, access to an ambulance, and transport to Adelaide for specialist care.[27]

At Point McLeay Reserve 247 people lived on what the AAB described as 'a final training ground from which families are eventually settled outside'. During the past year, eight families had been established in homes away from the reserve. Health care arrangements were similar to those at Point Pearce, and the children were transferred from the Point McLeay School to Meningie Area School after grade five to encourage them to 'mix freely with other children from the surrounding districts'. Farm work, of which the most successful was dairying, was referred to as training, and training opportunities were also provided by building and maintenance work on the reserve. This work involved bringing the dairy up to required health standards, providing sewerage for bathrooms and laundries and 'engender[ing] pride in the occupants'. The settlement was yet to be connected to the state electricity supply. Efforts were being made to 'brighten up the village' in an attempt

26 ibid., pp.8–9; AAB, Minutes, 29 April 1963, pp.10–11, GRS 4343/1/P

27 AAB, Report, 1963, *SAPP*, no.20, 1963, pp.9–10

to 'preserve morale', but much remained to be done. The AAB concluded its assessment of these two long-established Aboriginal institutions with a throwaway line that revealed an ongoing lack of clarity about whether they were staging posts on the way to integration into the wider community or segregated communities seeking self-sufficiency: 'in the interest of the training of Aborigines the Board anticipates that it may proceed further to improve the efficiency of these Reserves'.[28]

At Gerard Reserve, which the government had taken over from the UAM at the end of 1961, about 130 Aboriginals were living. The department had provided them with 25 houses and commented favorably on the 'improved outlook' of many of the residents and on their willingness to 'settle down to do a job of work'. Again work was described as 'training'. On the reserve itself this consisted of fruit-growing, building and maintenance for the men, and, for the women, 'domestic labour in the homes of the staff'. Beyond the reserve, the men could also find building work and seasonal employment in the fruit industry. There was a preschool kindergarten on site, and older children attended the nearby Winkie Primary School. Health care, as elsewhere, was provided by a resident nurse who ran a dispensary and small clinic and who could call on a medical officer from a nearby town when necessary. A 'vigorous education campaign' had significantly reduced the reserve's drinking problem.[29]

The government was responsible also for other Aboriginal reserves with no history as missions and no claims to being final training grounds for people on the verge of integration into the broader community. The largest and most remote of these was the North-West Reserve, 'virgin country in which Aborigines reside in accordance with their age old customs, but under the supervision of the Superintendent and staff of the Reserve'. Here men were employed in fencing, road-making, and construction of an air strip. Supplementary daily feeding maintained the nutritional requirements of young children, and weekly rations alleviated the hardship experienced by women and children as a result of 'the tribal social structure and the nomadic habits, together with tribal rituals and ceremonies'. A reserve store provided 'essential food stuffs and clothing' as well as training in use of money. Medical treatment was provided by a resident nurse, and regular clinics were conducted by the Northern Territory Aerial Medical Service. The report gave no indications of the numbers living on this large reserve.[30]

Another remote reserve was the one recently established at the Coober Pedy opal fields, where there were 400 indigenous people among a total population of 1100. The AAB claimed that there had been 'outstanding' change in the two years since a superintendent had been appointed by the department: 'the Aboriginal population who were formerly developing into a state of dependency have been converted into an almost independent community'. In this 'almost independent community', increases in health and prosperity had been achieved through a 'positive approach to welfare'. The men were being encouraged to mine, the women and children were served nutritious supplementary meals in a communal dining room, and this, together with the services of a nurse had 'dispelled malnutrition'. Six two-roomed houses, built with outside voluntary labour

---

28 ibid., p.10

29 ibid., pp.10–11

30 ibid., pp.11–12

were now owned by Aboriginals – 'a major step forward as these former nomadic people have now become 'house proud". However, there were 'no scholastic achievements to laud' so far at the school, and communal ablution and laundry facilities were needed to counteract the effects of the poor hygiene standards of some families. Alcohol was a problem at Coober Pedy as on other reserves, since 'unscrupulous persons charge exorbitant prices for cheap wines and almost any fight or argument springs from the consumption of liquor'.[31]

At Port Augusta about 300 Aboriginals lived on the reserve, with another 150 in the town. In 1964 Dunstan called it a 'central staging camp' which linked Aboriginals from the north of the state with the settled areas further south and with various government services. The Department of Aboriginal Affairs stationed a Welfare Officer there, with additional responsibility for the welfare of other Aboriginals in northern areas where there were no departmental officers. This officer had been successful in gaining employment for Aboriginals on pastoral properties or with the Commonwealth Railways, and in the previous year, ten families had moved to Whyalla, where they worked with Broken Hill Proprietary Limited and were accommodated by the South Australian Housing Trust. Aboriginal people from this reserve, as we have already seen, received a tentative welcome into the town life of Port Augusta, as long as they met non-indigenous expectations regarding dress and deportment.[32]

This period was one of significant transition for South Australia's remaining Christian missions. Umeewarra, the Open Brethren mission situated on the Port Augusta Reserve and in 1963 renamed Davenport Reserve, retained its status as a mission for a few more years, while its services were gradually superceded by those provided by the government. In 1963 the AAB reported that the mission ran a children's home where 70 boys and girls lived in dormitories and were provided with sporting and recreational facilities. In familiar mission style, the boys were trained in woodwork and in the 'minor phases of engineering work', and the girls in needlework and homecraft. A 'babies' dormitory' had recently been opened. The AAB made no mention of where these children and babies came from or where their parents were, nor offered any assessment of the UAM's work or indicated where it might be leading. A later assessment saw the Umeewarra Mission as an attempt to meet, 'at their own level in their own environment', the needs of 'fringe-dwellers', who were attracted to Port Augusta because of employment and other opportunities. However, it was also claimed that, from its earliest days, non-indigenous support for the mission was related not to any contribution the mission made to assimilation or integration, but to its contribution to cleaning up the environment of the reserve and providing a rationale for keeping black children out of white schools.[33]

The Lutherans were in the process of relinquishing control of their missions at Koonibba and Yalata. Two thousand acres of the 20 000 acquired at Koonibba, along with the mission's plant and stock, were to be purchased by the government on 1 July 1963 and

---

31 ibid., p.12

32 ibid., p.15; DA Dunstan, *SAPD*, House of Assembly, 29 July 1964, pp.1084–5, cited in Raynes. '*A Little Flour*', p.59

33 AAB, Report, 1963, *SAPP*, no.20, 1963, p.14; Arthur Maxwell Hart, 'A History of the Education of Full-Blood Aborigines in South Australia', MEd. thesis, University of Adelaide, 1970, pp.110–12

the land gazetted as an Aboriginal reserve. The rest of the land, except for a small section around the church and manse, was to be leased under renewable ten-year leases to neighbouring farmers, with a right to purchase. The AAB noted the mission's historic inability to provide sufficient work for its residents, who in 1963 numbered about 300. The nearby port of Thevenard had once provided significant numbers of Koonibba men with seasonal work on its wharves, but bulk handling had changed this. Similarly, mechanisation on surrounding farms had diminished work opportunities and now only 'spasmodic' employment could be found outside the mission. On the mission itself, building and renovating continued to provide 'good training' but only for a small number.[34] The Lutherans' more recently established mission at Yalata was being run under a ten-year agreement with the government, scheduled to expire on 30 June 1964.[35] The church had been expected to run the mission as a pastoral enterprise to promote the welfare of the 350 indigenous people associated with it, but the AAB's 1963 report indicated a high level of dependence on government, which was providing

> all clothing, blankets, rations, medicines ... the salary of the nursing sister and expenses of any medical practitioner in connection with medical treatment ... the cost of transport and payment of rates and taxes ... [and] financial grants-in-aid for capital improvements effected on the property.

Finding sufficient work for the Yalata population was an ongoing problem, and the sale of 'curios' was providing the main source of income for many. The health of the Aboriginals was 'good' and the Education Department school was 'working smoothly'.[36]

Government takeover of missions was something for which there was bipartisan parliamentary support. In October 1961 Dunstan had expressed the Opposition's approval of government plans to assume responsibility for Gerard and indicated that 'for some years' he had been discussing a similar arrangement with the Lutherans, at their request, in relation to Koonibba. He said the Lutherans were 'desperately anxious for the future' since they did not have 'sufficient capacity to do the kind of vocational training and development work that they see is necessary for the development of this aboriginal group'. He believed that previous governments had left to missions a job that they were insufficiently resourced to perform, and, while missions should have the opportunity of providing for spiritual development, they 'should not have on their shoulders the responsibility for the whole development and integration' of Aboriginal people. That was a responsibility that he thought was 'far more properly the duty of government'.[37]

However, although financially stretched, relying on government subsidies to survive and ill-equipped to fulfil an assimilation or integration agenda, some missions hung on a little longer. In 1963 the UAM mission at Nepabunna was still providing for the spiritual welfare of about 110 Adnyamathanha people. Their health needs were being met through

---

34 AAB, Report, 1963, *SAPP*, no.20, 1963, p.14

35 This arrangement was subsequently extended until 30 June 1970. AAB, Report, 1968, *SAPP*, no.20, 1968, p.20

36 AAB, Report, 1963, *SAPP*, no.20, 1963, p.13

37 DA Dunstan, *SAPD*, House of Assembly, 3 October 1961, p.1015

'the usual facilities' of a nurse, a dispensary, and access to the Royal Flying Doctor Service. The Education Department had taken over the school. But the mission still had no adequate water supply or sanitary arrangements and could neither provide employment nor decently house the residents. The government took control in 1973, after protracted discussion and in response to repeated requests from the Adnyamathanha.[38]

The Presbyterian mission at Ernabella, with its outstation at Fregon,[39] was distinctive among South Australian missions and was never taken over by government. On a pastoral lease in the remote country of the Pitjantjatjara, in the North-West Reserve, the mission had a population of about 400, whom the AAB described as 'still basically nomads'. It had been established to protect these people by providing a buffer against the encroachment of non-indigenous population and interests and did not discourage the 'nomadic habits or adherence to custom' of the Pitjantjatjara. It provided Christian teaching, education for the children, initially in their own language, and employment for some of the adults, in pastoral pursuits, bore sinking, fencing, construction of windmills and stockyards, and the making of handcrafts and artifacts for sale. As on the North-West Reserve, a hospital and dispensary were run by a nurse, medical help was provided by the Northern Territory Aerial Medical Service, and a communal kitchen provided supplementary feeding for school children and others deemed to be at nutritional disadvantage. A site and plan for a future village had been prepared and one prototype house built.[40]

The AAB made no mention in 1963, or subsequently, of the impact on the well-being of the indigenous people involved, of the timing, nature and conditions of government takeover or church relinquishment of the missions. However, these factors could be highly significant. For example, the relinquishing of Koonibba was initiated by the Lutheran church at a time when assimilation was still official policy and when the notion of self-determination had exerted almost no impact on government or community thinking. The Koonibba Aboriginals, like the Poonindie people before them, finished up with no stake in their land. Ten years later, in a changed political climate in which self-determination was the new policy goal, the Adnyamathanha did much better. They initiated the government takeover of the mission from the UAM and eventually gained freehold title to the Nepabunna land. At Ernabella, remoteness, the comparative lateness of sustained contact with settler culture and the distinctive philosophy of the mission put the Pitjantjatjara in a stronger position than other missionised Aboriginals in South Australia. Together these factors ensured that the Pitjantjatjara never lost their country, their language and many other aspects of their culture. Similarly, in other parts of Australia, the transition from mission to post-mission era has had differing impacts on the indigenous people in whose presumed interests – temporal and eternal – the missions had originally been established, depending on how and when the transition has occurred. In some instances, mission

---

38 AAB, Report, 1963, *SAPP*, no.20, 1963, p.14. See also, Brock, *Outback Ghettos*, pp.141, 153, and AAB, Minutes, e.g. 4 July 1966, p.233; 3 October 1966, p.244; 12 December 1966, p.254; 7 August 1967, p.288; 2 February 1970, p.131; 5 April 1971, p.178 etc., GRS 4343/1/P

39 Established in 1961, Fregon was the first of several outstations which allowed decentralisation of the population and relieved pressure on resources and employment opportunities at Ernabella.

40 AAB, Report, 1963, *SAPP*, no.20, 1963, p.13

authorities negotiated the transition to ensure that the indigenous people were able to assume control of former mission functions and assets, to deal on favourable terms with government, and to maintain a stake in their land. In others, missions simply retreated and left the indigenous people without resources, with the mission societies maintaining control of mission land and other assets, or selling them to non-indigenous interests.

The final section of the AAB's 1963 report detailed the services and oversight provided by the Department of Aboriginal Affairs in areas other than the reserves and missions. For example, the report noted 120–180 Aboriginal people living in Port Lincoln, a town it identified as, 'like Port Augusta ... a focal point at which Aborigines come into contact with the industrial and commercial world'. They found seasonal employment in fishing, pastoral and agricultural industries and permanent employment in the Highways, Railways and Engineering and Water Supply departments. For this population, one house, designed to 'conform to the style of other houses in the town', had been built for the department by the Housing Trust and one more was under construction.[41] At Berri, where the seasonal nature of work in the fruit-growing industry meant there was a fluctuating population of indigenous people, the department had established a welfare centre staffed by one Welfare Officer. By January 1963 he had provided assistance to 30 families and some single men. Substandard houses were being cleared from Berri Flat and the occupants rehoused in departmental houses at Glossop, Barmera, and Gerard, where employment was available. Aboriginal children were reported to be doing well at local schools.[42] Another Welfare Officer had been appointed to Andamooka where the economic opportunities on the opal fields allowed the indigenous population of 170 'to live and work in the same conditions as the rest of the community'. This opportunity appeared to be more potential than realised, however, since, the report went on to say that the Welfare Officer had a 'continual battle' against 'the tendency to live in substandard houses' and that much of his work was 'protecting the Aboriginal from exploitation by the unscrupulous'.[43]

Finally, the Aboriginal Affairs Department supported a handful of institutions which provided various services designed to promote assimilation and integration among people of Aboriginal descent: the UAM's Colebrook and Oodnadatta Children's Homes, which in 1963 had 17 and four residents respectively; the Aborigines Advancement League Hostel in suburban Millswood, which accommodated 15 country girls and women undertaking secondary schooling or receiving medical treatment in Adelaide; the UAM's Tanderra Home, by then in suburban Torrensville, where three Aboriginal girls were living; the department's Campbell House Farm School, designed to provide farming and pastoral training but being used to house orphans and neglected boys; and the Aboriginal Women's Home, North Adelaide, which provided accommodation for small numbers of women and children from the country accessing medical treatment, and for babies awaiting adoption.

As this report indicates, the Department of Aboriginal Affairs was involved in a wide variety of ways and with widely varying degrees of directness and immediacy in the lives of many of the people whom it identified as Aborigines and people of Aboriginal blood. But

---

41 ibid., p.15
42 ibid., p.16
43 ibid., p.16

the numbers of indigenous people referred to in this report amounted to only about 3300, plus an unspecified number living on the North-West Reserve. What of the rest of the total indigenous population of 6000? While the 1963 report had nothing to say about these people, subsequent reports shed some light on this silence and recorded a growing recognition of their existence, their problems and their emerging assertiveness and sense of identity.

In 1964 the AAB reported that the 'general problem' confronting the Department of Aboriginal Affairs was persuading Aboriginals to enter into what it called 'citizenship'. 'Citizenship' was, apparently, demonstrated by being independent of the department. According to this view, those Aboriginals already independent of its support were not its concern: they were assumed to be assimilated or integrated, and therefore no longer regarded as Aboriginals. The 'general problem' among those who were still dependent on the department was 'minor' in the case of the 'sophisticated' and 'nearly white' people of Point Pearce and Point McLeay: 'intensive work on these two reserves could eliminate any problem they present within a comparatively short period'. The problem was 'major' in the north and west of the state among the nomadic 'full-bloods'. Even so, there were some 'bright spots': there were some 'moderately well-educated and quite sophisticated' Aboriginals at Oodnadatta, Maree, Copley and Nepabunna, who would soon be independent of the department, and others such as self-employed opal miners, who were 'making progress towards independence quite on their own initiative'.[44]

This division of the indigenous population into those whom the department regarded as its responsibility – and as either a major or minor problem – and those whom it did not regard as its responsibility, is underlined by its policy and practice in relation to the provision of government relief. Needy metropolitan and non-metropolitan Aboriginals could access relief from the state government which matched Commonwealth Department of Social Security scales until payments from the latter became available. However, while metropolitan Aboriginals had to apply through mainstream channels, that is, the Children's Welfare and Public Relief Department, their remote counterparts dealt with the Department of Aboriginal Affairs. In the case of the latter, practices more akin to protection persisted, with the Department of Aboriginal Affairs providing *ad hoc* payments and rations in cases of unemployment, food shortages and destitution. In adopting this approach, it seems that the department and the AAB, when first established, subscribed to an historic underestimation of the complex social and economic marginalisation of Aboriginal people. They applied simplistic and pauperising solutions to the problems of non-metropolitan Aboriginals and revealed little awareness of ongoing need, as well as the growth of a distinctive identity and assertiveness, among the metropolitan group whom they deemed to be already assimilated and not their responsibility.[45] However, this view did not

---

44 AAB, Report, 1964, *SAPP*, no.20, 1964, p.5

45 There were some technical difficulties in relation to this question that seem not to have been anticipated. People of Aboriginal descent who had been exempted from their status as Aboriginals under previous legislation were, formally, not the responsibility of the Department of Aboriginal Affairs. While some members of the AAB argued that such distinctions should no longer carry weight, they also regretted 'a tendency to bring back under Aboriginal Affairs Department influence families which have prior to the passing of the new Act been independent', AAB, Minutes, 16 December 1963, p.71; 20 April 1964, p.100, GRS 4343/1/P.

go unchallenged for long, and the annual reports soon became less bland and began to acknowledge problems and adopt a more analytical approach to responding to them.

An important early AAB insight into the well-being of the indigenous population concerned the complex issue of employment, an issue clearly of fundamental importance to any program of integration. The AAB recognised that efforts to get Aboriginal people into employment had thus far been hampered not only by insufficient vocational training but also by the powerful legacy of inappropriate past emphases and assumptions which had focused on farm-work and pastoral activity. In a bold departure it declared: 'The land, formerly the accepted destiny of the Aborigines, can absorb relatively few; the majority must seek other fields, and particularly in secondary industry'.[46] This position was supported by a consistent advocacy of greater involvement of Aboriginal children in general education, beginning with pre-school kindergarten in order to counteract the disadvantage associated with late starts, and extending beyond the customary few years of primary schooling into secondary education, in order to provide greater occupational choice. Numerical data on the department's support for education were provided regularly, along with assessments of the negative impact of the children's home circumstances on their scholastic progress.[47]

The Department of Aboriginal Affairs demonstrated the possibility of occupational destinies for indigenous people other than the land and secondary industry by itself becoming an employer of suitably educated indigenous people. In its 1967 report the AAB enumerated the Aboriginal staff of the department. There were 11 employed at head office: six clerks, two typists and one escort officer, all of whom were females, and two males, one in accounts and one working as a messenger. In addition, there were 11 youths in the housing maintenance section, one welfare officer and two welfare assistants at Davenport Reserve, three reserve staff, employed as foremen or building overseers, at Koonibba, Point McLeay and Point Pearce reserves, and 'most of the staff', including the Matron and Deputy Matron, at the North Adelaide Women's Home, all of whom were indigenous. The AAB 'proposed that the practice of bringing Aboriginals into responsible permanent public service positions will be continued'. In line with this goal, the Board was supporting increasing numbers of Aboriginal young people to remain at secondary school and reported that eight were enrolled at technical colleges, four at adult education centres, one at the School of Art, two at Teachers College and two at Flinders University.[48]

There were other complicated aspects to the issue of employment of Aboriginal people. The government's commitment to ending protection and moving towards integration called into question the employment practices that had been pursued on reserves, whereby all able-bodied residents had been required to work, some being 'employed for

---

46 AAB, Report, 1964, *SAPP*, no.20, 1964, p.6

47 See, for example, AAB, Report, 1964, *SAPP*, no.20, 1964, pp.6, 10; *SAPP*, no.20A, 1965, p.8; *SAPP*, no. 20, 1967, pp.10–11

48 AAB, Report, 1967, *SAPP*, no.20,1967, pp.10–11

welfare reasons' and others engaged in 'training employment'.[49] If Aboriginals were to be integrated into the state's economy on a non-discriminatory basis and be paid at the same rates as non-Aboriginals, they had to meet normal work expectations, which included facing dismissal if they did not measure up, and living in places where there were genuine jobs available. The government agreed to raise pay on the reserves by £1 per week from 1 July 1965, and in July 1967, the AAB reported that all Aboriginals working on reserves, except on the North-West Reserve, were being paid the basic wage. It noted, however, that most of those working on pastoral properties were not. Even when the Federal Pastoral Industry Award was broadened to include indigenous workers from December 1968 and the payment of award wages to Aboriginals working on pastoral properties was made mandatory, many were still not receiving them.[50]

Maintaining wage justice meant maintaining vigilance. In February 1970 the AAB was made aware that, although male Aboriginal workers on reserves were being paid 'the State living wage' of $36.70 per week, they were the only government employees to receive this rate: for all other male government workers the 'absolute minimum wage' included a margin that bought it up to $41.90. The AAB recommended that this 'untenable position' be rectified by the payment of the minimum wage of $41.90 to all adult male employees on reserves, except those at Amata and Indulkana.[51]

These changes to the protective 'jobs for all' economy meant that some reserve residents had to look elsewhere for employment. This highlighted problems with qualifications and housing and revealed an interim need for study grants and hostel accommodation, especially for people moving to Adelaide. In addition, community prejudice against Aboriginal workers, who could no longer be employed at a discounted rate compared with non-Aboriginals, closed avenues that had once been open. This was probably most apparent in the pastoral industry. These problems, and the challenge of solving them without recourse to old models of protection, were sufficiently serious for the South Australian office of the Commonwealth Department of Labour and National Service to establish a program targeting indigenous people as part of its employment services.[52]

The ending of the 'experiment of full employment on reserves' and the introduction of award wages was associated with a raft of other changes: rent for government housing was charged from 1964, and by 1969 was at normal South Australian Housing Trust levels; medical and pharmaceutical benefits fees were no longer paid by government; free transport from reserves to towns to access health or other services was scrapped, as were the issue of free milk and the sale of reserve farm produce at minimal prices. Furthermore, parents were expected to be responsible for ensuring that their children were

---

49 The practice was a long-standing one. This terminology, however, is from 1970. AAB, Minutes, 2 February 1970, p.126, GRS 4343/1/P.

50 AAB, Minutes, 7 June 1965, p.178; 3 July 1967, p.285, GRS 4343/1/P; AAB, Report, 1967, *SAPP*, no.20, 1967, p.9. On the Coober Pedy Reserve in 1967 as many as 90 per cent of Aboriginal workers were not being paid the basic wage, AAB, Report, 1969, *SAPP*, no.20, 1969, p.13.

51 AAB, Minutes, 2 February 1970, pp.126–8, GRS 4343/1/P. At the relatively new remote centres of Amata and Indulkana work was still considered to be training, and wages were being raised incrementally.

52 AAB, Report, 1969, *SAPP*, no.20, 1969, pp.13–14

participating in schooling. These changes were a practical demonstration of what integration entailed, and were implemented in the face of the challenging 'attitudinal legacy' of the protection era.[53] The minutes of the AAB from time to time reveal how perplexed its members were by the task of providing sympathetic and flexible support to the indigenous population as they responded to the new demands on them, while at the same time avoiding any appearance of resorting to protectionist or discriminatory practices.[54]

Nevertheless, the AAB was prepared to insist on discriminatory treatment when this was necessary to safeguard indigenous welfare. This was clearly demonstrated in its defence of its policy at Indulkana. In the face of complaints from the pastoralist holding the lease over the area, that the presence of the Aboriginals 'imped[ed] development' and a request from the Chairman of the Pastoral Board for the removal of the Indulkana people to Oodnadatta, the AAB took the side of the Aboriginals. Indulkana had been established as an Aboriginal reserve for 'welfare reasons at a site long occupied by Aborigines for camping and ritual', and was serving as 'a refuge for age and invalid pensioners ... [and as] a camping site for men and women when work is not available on the adjacent cattle stations'. A pre-school centre and primary school were soon to be provided and a nursing sister was already providing health care. The AAB rejected the implication that 'developments' for these people were less important than the economic development of the pastoral industry and considered that the suggestion that the Indulkana people be moved to Oodnadatta was 'offered in complete disregard or ignorance of the Aboriginal situation':

> Indulkana is an ancient tribal and sacred site which the Aborigines would certainly leave with the utmost reluctance and a mass transfer to Oodnadatta would be a serious violation of their rights; also, it would not succeed because the people would almost certainly drift back to the north. Moreover, it would be little short of criminal to take these unsophisticated people from a protective environment where they have some chance of developing at their own pace to a region where they would be exposed to western drink and vice and where they would lose all incentive to progress any further. Amata (Musgrave Park) has already been rejected by this group of Aborigines and to divide them between Amata and Oodnadatta would be both inhuman and unsuccessful.[55]

This forthright defence of the Indulkana people, while it was clearly a form of protection, revealed a number of new attitudes: a preparedness to listen to rather than impose on indigenous people; respect for their attachment to particular land; and the valuing of Aboriginal rights over others', or at least the insistence, in a stance that foreshadowed future events, that the two could 'coexist'.

---

53 AAB, Report, 1970, *SAPP*, no.20, 1970, p.11

54 See, for example, AAB, Minutes, 7 February 1966, p.209; 7 March 1966, pp.215–16; 1 April 1968, pp.33–4; November 1970, p.164, GRS 4343/1/P

55 AAB, Minutes, 2 February 1970, pp.133–5, GRS 4343/1/P

Other events during the 1960s led the integration project in new directions. Two developments of practical and symbolic significance occurred at the federal level and reflected changes in public opinion about what was appropriate in a modern and progressive nation. In 1962, the Commonwealth Government legislated to give all Aboriginal and Torres Strait Islanders the right to vote in Commonwealth elections.[56] Secondly, in a referendum in 1967 the electors of Australia voted overwhelming for constitutional change to allow for Aboriginals and Torres Strait Islanders to be counted in the census and for the Commonwealth Government to make special laws in relation to them. The campaign to push for this referendum and to promote a 'yes' vote, initiated by New South Wales political activist Jessie Street in 1956, was heir to an older movement seeking additional powers for the Commonwealth on the assumption that this would advance indigenous interests. From the beginning Dunstan and Duguid were involved, as individuals and through their leadership of the Federal Council for the Advancement of Aborigines[57], which was a key player in the referendum campaign.[58]

Other developments which furthered the cause of indigenous 'advancement' in this period were encouraged by the election of a Labor Government in South Australia in March 1965. This ended 32 years of Liberal administration, which, in the account of the long-serving Liberal Premier, Thomas Playford, had been so taken up with establishing secondary industry and basic economic infrastructure that it had not been able to attend to public health or social welfare issues 'on a generous scale'.[59] The Labor victory brought Dunstan to prominence, firstly as Minister for Aboriginal Affairs from March 1965, and subsequently as Premier from June 1967 to April 1968, and Premier again from June 1970 to February 1979. Developments in Aboriginal affairs during this period were certainly not entirely of his making and were generally supported by successive state administrations.[60] However, Dunstan's reformist social vision and energetic commitment to the welfare of the indigenous population provided considerable momentum for change.

---

56 Scott Bennett, *Aborigines and Political Power*, Allen and Unwin, Sydney, 1992, chapter 6, 'Elections and Representation', and especially p.114. See also, Pat Stretton and Christine Finnimore, 'Black Fellow Citizens: Aborigines and the Commonwealth franchise', *Australian Historical Studies*, vol.25, no.101, October 1993, pp.521–35.

57 See below, p.247

58 The constitutional changes secured by the 1967 Referendum have been widely misunderstood to be about voting and citizenship. For a lucid analysis of the background to the referendum and of the circumstances in which it has acquired symbolic meanings that go far beyond the constitutional change it brought about, see Bain Attwood and Andrew Markus, in collaboration with Dale Edwards and Kath Schilling, *The 1967 Referendum, or when Aborigines didn't get the vote*, Australian Institute for Aboriginal and Torres Strait Islander Studies, Canberra, 1997.

59 Stewart Cockburn, assisted by John Playford, *Playford: benevolent despot*, Axiom Publishing, Adelaide, 1991, p.205. See also essays on many aspects of South Australia's political, social and economic development in the period 1933 to 1968 in Bernard O'Neil, Judith Raftery and Kerrie Round (eds), *Playford's South Australia: essays on the history of South Australia, 1933–1968*, Association of Professional Historians Inc, Adelaide, 1996.

60 The Dunstan Labor Government of June 1967 to April 1968 with RR Loveday as Minister for Aboriginal Affairs was succeeded by a Liberal Country League (LCL) administration with Steele Hall as Premier and RR Millhouse and Joyce Steele as Ministers for Aboriginal Affairs. In June 1970, Labor again achieved office, with Dunstan as Premier and LJ King as Minister for Aboriginal Affairs.

In 1966 the context in which the government attempted to further the welfare of indigenous people was altered, formally at least, by the passage of the *Prohibition of Discrimination Act*.[61] This legislation, the first of its kind in Australia, made it an offence to discriminate against any person on the basis of race, country of origin or skin colour in relation to employment and access to services, accommodation and public places. In introducing the bill, Premier Dunstan claimed that, while there was no 'racial or colour problem in Australia ... certain minor but known discriminatory practices exist in South Australia'. It was his government's intention to ensure that these did not continue. Opposition members, although not opposed in principle, doubted the need for the legislation and worried that its implementation might actually represent discrimination against those found to be in breach of it.[62] The members of the AAB also were initially wary. Before the bill was introduced into parliament, they had expressed their disapproval on the grounds, albeit illogical, that it reintroduced the concept of special Aboriginal legislation, which the government had made a commitment to avoid. Furthermore, they believed it to be unnecessary, since public opinion was becoming more 'tolerant', and potentially counter-productive, since 'the threat of coercion could arouse an antagonistic reaction that cannot but delay the course of Aboriginal acceptance and assimilation'.[63] However, as more indigenous people tested the levels of 'tolerance' in the general community, the need for anti-discrimination legislation or, perhaps more properly, for the community opinion of which such legislation was an expression or a driver, became obvious.[64]

The AAB welcomed the increase in services for Aboriginals that followed Labor's assumption of office in South Australia. It wasted no time in aligning itself with Dunstan's integration stance and his emphasis on indigenous self-reliance:

> Those wishing to merge into the social, economic and political life of the community will be assisted to do so with practical assistance and advice in making the necessary adjustments. Policy objectives are centred on positive welfare and the assistance granted will be of a nature calculated to promote self-help, self-reliance and self-determination so that Aborigines may assume more and more responsibility for the management of their own affairs. Thus

---

61 *Prohibition of Discrimination Act, 1966*, no.82 of 1966, assented to on 1 December 1966.

62 DA Dunstan, *SAPD*, House of Assembly, 14 July 1966, p.492. For opposition views see ibid., 25 October, 1966, pp.2522–6; 26 October 1966, pp.2554–90.

63 AAB, Minutes, 22 January 1966, p.206, GRS 4343/1/P

64 Dunstan and the AAB were coy about the extent of the problem. Memoirs and life stories of indigenous people indicate that they experienced racial discrimination regularly during this period. The AAB was aware of instances of discrimination, sometimes disguised as concerns about 'hygiene' in schools and hospitals, and of a more generally discriminatory climate in country areas. See, for example, AAB, Minutes, 2 August 1965, p.185, 8 November 1965, p.188, 4 March 1968, p.26, GRS 4343/1/P; AAB, Report, 1969, *SAPP*, no.20, 1969, p.7. Occasionally allegations of discrimination made headlines in the press. See, for example, *News*, 21 April 1969, p.7; 22 April 1969, p.22; 1 May 1969, p.7.

Departmental services will be designed to help the Aboriginal to act for himself rather than for the Department to act for him.[65]

From the period before the passage of the *Aboriginal Affairs Act* of 1962, Dunstan had been a consistent advocate of indigenous representation on government bodies, and growth of such representation was a feature of his period of office. The nature of this indigenous involvement invites scrutiny. Aboriginal people had never been considered to have the required expertise for membership of the Aborigines Protection Board, which, as an executive board, had direct influence on government policy. The AAB onto which they were welcomed had advisory powers only, thus making their presence easier to achieve and less contentious.[66] Furthermore, it is not clear whom Aboriginal members on the AAB were representing. Their presence appeared to reflect how well they were known to the minister, to other members of the AAB or to senior officers in the Department of Aboriginal Affairs. They did not in any real sense 'represent' other Aboriginal people and were not answerable to any Aboriginal constituency.[67] While these circumstances constrained their influence, their appointment was nevertheless of symbolic and material importance and represented a shift in government attitudes.

The first indigenous member of the AAB was Reginald Jeffery Barnes, originally from the far north of South Australia. He had been brought up by non-Aboriginal foster parents, was the first person of Aboriginal descent to join the RAAF in South Australia, a Second World War veteran and an electrician employed by the South Australian Government. He had come to public notice in Adelaide in the 1950s through his association with the Aborigines Advancement League and Dr Charles Duguid, and was one of the speakers at a much-publicised Adelaide Town Hall meeting arranged by Duguid in 1953 to draw attention to injustices suffered by indigenous people.[68] Barnes remained on the AAB until March 1970. Other persons of Aboriginal descent to serve as members of the AAB were Nancy Brumbie (May 1965–February 1967), Gladys Elphick (December 1966–March 1972), Bert Clark (April 1967–March 1972), and Faith Thomas (March 1970–March 1972).

It is difficult to gauge the impact of these indigenous members on the AAB's thinking and activity. Brumbie was a 'Colebrook girl' and a trained and experienced preschool kindergarten director. Like Barnes, whom she later married, she was a protégée of Duguid, and well known in Adelaide among 'assimilated' people of Aboriginal descent. When she joined the Board, expectations were high: 'her knowledge of her people and her special training in the field of pre-school activities should afford valuable assistance'. Prior to her appointment she had been part of a group from the Kindergarten Union and the Department of Aboriginal Affairs which had visited remote Aboriginal reserves

---

65 AAB, Report, 1965, *SAPP*, no.20, 1965, p.6

66 Margaret Macilwain, 'South Australian Aborigines Protection Board (1939–1962): tensions between expertise and the idea of representative government', paper presented at Australian Political Science Association Conference, September 2004.

67 Of course the same could be said of non-Aboriginals on the AAB. Though chosen from different sectors of the community, they were not representative of or answerable to those sectors.

68 See below, p.248. See also Barnes, *Munyi's Daughter*, pp.83–8, 91–3.

with a view to establishing pre-school services. Of her membership of the AAB, she wrote:

> Being on the Board was, for me, one of many firsts, but it was probably the one most critical in my goal of helping Aboriginal people and creating bridges. This appointment gave me the opportunity to discuss, at high decision-making levels in the Government, the needs of Aboriginal children and families and the way these needs could be met.[69]

However, she had nothing more to say either about the AAB's work or her contribution to it, and there is no discernible evidence of her impact in its minutes or reports. The same could not be said of Gladys Elphick. Originally from Point Pearce, Elphick had been living in Adelaide since 1939. By the time she joined the AAB she had developed considerable political and strategic awareness and was well known in government circles as an advocate for her people. She used her membership of the AAB to encourage government support for the Council of Aboriginal Women in South Australia, of which she was a founder and driving force, and to draw attention not only to the problems faced by indigenous people but to indigenous initiatives in response to these problems.[70]

At the same time as a few hand-picked Aboriginals were being invited to serve on the AAB, a different and potentially more influential form of indigenous involvement and leadership was being encouraged by the government through the formation of Aboriginal Reserve Councils. The councils were initially introduced on an informal basis pending the passage of legislation to provide for their formal establishment. It was envisaged that these organisations would cooperate with the Superintendents in the running of the reserves. The expectation was that given time, encouragement and training, they would provide effective administration of the reserves, independent of protective departmental supervision.

In 1964 the AAB reported that the first two Aboriginal Reserve Councils had been formed – at Gerard and Koonibba. The Gerard council was concerned mostly with welfare and social activities, and although not all members had 'sustained their interest . . . in the main most [had] shouldered their responsibilities well'. At Koonibba the council was advising the Superintendent on residents' complaints and suggestions and helping to adjudicate in cases of infringement of regulations. In addition, the council had 'taken a further step towards assimilation' by advocating the payment of standard wages on the reserve, thus gaining 'the satisfaction of knowing that so far as wage-earning and spending goes they are on a par with white men'. By 1965 Aboriginal Reserve Councils had been formed on most reserves and were 'gaining in efficiency as people get a better grasp of their functions and learn to use them more freely'. In 1967 the AAB reported that the Point Pearce council had 'functioned conscientiously', but the Point McLeay council had not been 'as active as hoped' and needed 'to be alerted to its responsibilities'. These responsibilities were clarified by the passage of the *Aboriginal Affairs Act Amendment Act 1966–67*, no 11 of 1967, which provided the Aboriginal Reserve Councils with a legal framework

---

69 Barnes, *Munyi's Daughter*, p.123

70 See for example, AAB, Minutes, 6 February 1967, pp.261–2; 6 March 1967, p.263, GRS 4343/1/P See also, Forte, *Flight of an Eagle*, pp.69, 83–106.

and also allowed for the establishment, incorporation and registration of organisations for the pursuit of economic activities on reserves. In the following year, the AAB reported that 'the Councils of the five southern Aboriginal Reserves continue[d] to mature', and were handling permit systems for visits to the reserves, undertaking village improvements and planning celebrations. By 1970, this growing 'maturity' of the councils was reflected in the willingness of the Department of Aboriginal Affairs and the AAB to entrust them with some financial responsibility: they agreed that grants be made to them, 'subject to appropriate budgeting and accounting procedures being instituted', and for additional funds to be paid as subsidies for council earnings. However, in a summary statement issued that year, the AAB's assessment of the councils was equivocal: while they had 'grow[n] in authority' and 'modified the authority of the Superintendents ... problems remain[ed] in maintaining stable functioning'.[71]

There were other views about this situation. The Select Committee Inquiry into the Welfare of Aboriginal Children in South Australia, reporting in July 1969, criticised the situation on the reserves: there were too many non-Aboriginal staff, not enough training to equip Aboriginals to take over from them, and the Reserve Councils needed to be invested with more authority. Witnesses before the select committee had 'complained bitterly at the failure to give worthwhile responsibilities to the councils'.[72] Given the long history of protection and its 'attitudinal legacy' in both Aboriginal reserve residents and departmental staff, it is hardly surprising that the significant culture change required for the stable and effective functioning of the Aboriginal Reserve Councils was not easily achieved.

In retrospect, AAB member Geoff Pope considered that one of the problems was that some reserve staff were poorly equipped to implement Department of Aboriginal Affairs policy and more 'old school' in their attitudes than was needed to facilitate the transition to indigenous control.[73] The testimony of Rex Orr, clerk at Point Pearce from 1966 to 1970 and Superintendent at Koonibba from 1970 to 1975, lends weight to this claim and sheds further light on Pope's assessment. Orr recalled the 'enormously pressured situation' at Point Pearce and the inability of many staff to cope with it, 'presumably because they didn't come from a community-based, social training, educational background. They came in to manage the reserve'. While he understood his role as implementing 'policies which were designed in the longer term to hand responsibility over to Aboriginal people', his staff often saw things differently. Faced with drunkenness, violence and 'horrendous social interaction', he found it a 'very difficult social task ... to pass over that responsibility', but nevertheless 'couldn't see that it was better to maintain a European salvaging of the situation'.[74]

Another government scheme that involved the acceptance of leadership and respon-

71 AAB, Report, 1964, 1965, 1967, 1969, 1970, *SAPP*, no. 20, 1964, pp.8, 14, 16; ibid., no. 20A, 1965, p.5; ibid., no.20, 1967, pp.9, 17; ibid., no. 20, 1969, p.11; ibid., no.20, 1970, p.11; AAB, Minutes, 6 April 1970, p.139, GRS 4343/1/P

72 Report of the Select Committee of the Legislative Council into the Welfare of Aboriginal Children, July 1969, p.13, cited in Raynes, *A Little Flour*, p.62

73 Rev. Geoffrey Pope, Interview, Adelaide, 11 March 1999; tape and transcript in possession of author.

74 Rex Orr, Interview, Adelaide, 26 February 1999; tape and transcript in possession of author.

sibility by some Aboriginal people was the development and operation of the Aboriginal Lands Trust. *The Aboriginal Lands Trust Act, 1966*, no.87 of 1966, was assented to on 8 December 1966. It provided for the transfer of crown and reserve lands to the trust, which had the authority, with ministerial consent, to sell, lease, mortgage or develop land vested in it, as long as such activity preserved the benefits and values of the land for the Aboriginal people concerned. It also provided for the payment of royalties to the trust in relation to minerals found on or under its lands. The trust was to be administered by an all-Aboriginal board of up to 12 members, the initial three being appointed by the Governor on ministerial recommendation, the remainder to be nominated by the Reserve Councils of communities which chose to vest their lands in the trust.[75]

This was a scheme close to Dunstan's heart and reflected his belief that indigenous welfare and integration would be enhanced by granting Aboriginal reserve populations what he called 'proprietary rights' to reserve land.[76] For him, this was a matter of justice. In proposing the legislation to establish the Lands Trust, Dunstan claimed that the indigenous people of Australia were alone among comparable people in not having rights in their own land and argued that they were, not surprisingly, 'bitter that they have had their country taken from them, and been given no compensatory rights to land in any area'. While not suggesting that there was a 'short and simple solution' to the problems associated with the integration of Aboriginal people into the broader community, he believed that the Lands Trust would cope with

> one real facet of the Aboriginal problem ... [and would] provide areas of land for Aborigines, titles for Aborigines, and a feeling on the part of Aborigines that at least they [were] getting their just dues which were so unjustly taken from them over a century ago.[77]

The debate on the bill was vigorous, with the opposition exhibiting considerable scepticism about not only the indigenous population's ability to use land productively, to act independently, or, except in a few cases, to 'make good', but also about the injustices from which the government claimed that they suffered. The member for Alexandra, the Hon. DN Brookman, led the opposition's case against the bill and concluded that: 'We are too loose in our descriptions of the wrongs done to Aborigines'. He was 'satisfied that injustices spoken about over the years do not exist at the present, and that Aborigines do not require the land in the form that is proposed'.[78] Much of the opposition comment displayed unease with the essence of the proposed legislation which, as well as recognising Aboriginal rights to land, gave considerable authority to Aboriginal Reserve Councils in relation to how that land should be used. Some of the views expressed were frankly racist, many betrayed an inability to conceive of the value of Aboriginal people having land unless they farmed it, and in one case, there was resentment about the 'unfair advantage' the Aboriginal population would gain from the legislation, especially if there were signi-

---

75 AAB, Report, 1967, *SAPP*, no.20, 1967, p.8

76 See above, pp.222

77 DA Dunstan, *SAPD*, House of Assembly, 1 December 1965, p.3452; 13 July 1966, pp.478–9

78 DN Brookman, *SAPD*, House of Assembly, 13 July 1966, pp.549, 554

ficant mineral royalties paid.[79] Dunstan was adamant that the key issue was respect for the indigenous population's right to choice:

> The only people who have a right to [decide about use of their land] are the representatives of the Aborigines themselves. They can make up their minds; it is not for us to tell them what they are to do; it is for the representatives of the Aborigines to make up their minds.[80]

Well before the legislation had been passed, or even debated in detail, Minister Dunstan was trying to sell the idea to reserve residents and canvassing for possible inaugural Lands Trust board members. This was the focus of a special meeting between him and members of the AAB in December 1965. Dunstan expected that the work of the trust would begin slowly. While the transfer of unoccupied reserve lands would take place with relative ease, the transfer of the lands of the occupied reserves would be complicated and dependent on 'numbers of things yet to be done'. Getting Reserve Councils established and operating effectively was, in both the minister's and the AAB's view, a key factor in preparing the ground for the Lands Trust. This was not an easy task. Dunstan told the AAB of his recent visit to Point McLeay when the residents had made clear their wish to remain a closed and supervised reserve and not to become an 'open village' with responsibility for their own affairs, or their own land, 'this side of five years hence'. He had discussed the further development of Reserve Councils with the Gerard, Davenport and Point Pearce people as well, but did not 'seem to be getting any rush on their part to take the responsibility'.[81] This was hardly a fair comment. None of the legislation or regulations relating either to Reserve Councils or to the Lands Trust had been passed, and the Aboriginal people were being asked to embrace far-reaching change, whose details and implications were yet to be spelled out and for which they had been ill-prepared.

Undeterred by these difficulties, Dunstan was keen to recruit Aboriginal people to be the inaugural members of the proposed Lands Trust board and suggested names to the AAB based on his 'personal knowledge of the people concerned' and discussions with 'some officers in the Department'.[82] He was looking for people who were:

> experienced on the land, who knew something about rural economy and who had their heads screwed on the right way, who were not the kind of people who would come up with the sort of suggestion that Point McLeay be divided into irrigation fruit blocks.

Despite his later vigorous defence of indigenous choice and self-determination as he piloted the Lands Trust Bill through parliament, there was no hint of it here. What he wanted were people who would be sympathetic to the government's agenda and capable

---

79 See for example, *SAPD*, House of Assembly, 19 July1966, pp.548–54; 21 July 1966, pp.626–8; 28 July 1966, pp.656–73

80 DA Dunstan, *SAPD*, House of Assembly, 2 August 1966, p.801

81 AAB, Minutes, 16 December 1965, pp.197–8, GRS 4343/1/P; AAB, Report, 1965, *SAPP*, no.20A, 1965, p.5

82 Barnes and Brumbie, the indigenous members of the AAB at this time were present at the meeting, but took no part in the discussion and had no suggestions to make, even when directly asked.

of bringing others along with them. The chairman of the AAB agreed: 'If you are going to appoint this Trust, you don't want it to fail'. It seems that the bottom line was not, after all, respect for self-determination, but political pragmatism.

Dunstan had two front runners. The first was Gladys Elphick's son, Tim Hughes, who had a 'soldier's settlement' block at Lucindale, knew 'what the land is capable of and can see what is possible and what is simply out of the question', and was 'a very good type'. The second was Garnet Wilson, formerly of Point McLeay, a young man who had 'really pulled himself up by his boot straps' and had 'made his way excellently'. He was a quali-fied wool classer who worked all over South Australia and was 'much in demand'. A revealing discussion followed about who else should be on the board. Several other men were suggested, but it was clear that AAB members had doubts about them. Dunstan wondered if there should be a woman, and Millar, Director of the Department of Aboriginal Affairs and Secretary to the AAB, endorsed Geoff Pope's suggestion of Natascha MacNamara, 'a very able girl', apparently with skills, although no formal qualifications, in accounting. There was no dispute about her suitability but Hunt-Cooke thought that it might be more important to have someone 'from the north', than to have a woman. However, no one seemed to know anyone 'from the north' who would be suitable. Pope's suggestion of elections for the Lands Trust Board, based on nominations from Aboriginal groups, was met with some concern about 'an unpredictable result' and the need to 'have people you can rely on at the beginning'.[83]

This conversation foreshadowed concerns that have become both commonplace and problematic in subsequent years, as non-indigenous people of good will have struggled to act consultatively and to balance a desire to ensure opportunities for indigenous self-determination with a fear of its unpredictable consequences. Within that struggle, notions of representation and delegation continue to be difficult and divisive issues. AAB member Frances Hunt-Cooke was alert to this. She commented in 1965 that the problem of running elections for the Lands Trust 'boil[ed] down to whether any community would ever [accept] a nominee from another community'. In the event, there were no elections and no consultation with Aboriginal groups or communities. The initial members of the Aboriginal Lands Trust were the two men whom Dunstan had endorsed at his December 1965 meeting with the AAB and the one woman mentioned at that same meeting: Tim Hughes, Garnet Wilson and Natascha MacNamara.[84]

As expected, once established, the Aboriginal Lands Trust was not overwhelmed with business. In its 1968 report the AAB noted that eight unoccupied reserves totalling 5774 acres had been transferred to the trust by the Department of Aboriginal Affairs.[85] However, the communities on most occupied reserves continued to be cautious about the implications of handing over control of their lands to the trust. In 1969 the Point Pearce community asked for their land to be transferred, but the Point McLeay people, who, as

---

83 AAB, Minutes, 16 December 1965, pp.199–202, GRS 4343/1/P

84 MacNamara later gained formal qualifications in business administration. She was prominent within the Aboriginal Women's Council, whose incorporation, constitution and formal administrative procedures were her doing, and in the Aboriginal Legal Rights Movement. See Forte, *Flight of an Eagle*, pp.9, 84.

85 AAB, Report, 1968, *SAPP*, no.20, 1968, p.12

noted already, had reacted strongly against the Lands Trust and Reserve Councils proposals, were, as late as 1971, expressing such significant anxiety and disgruntlement about the future of the reserve that the AAB decided:

> whilst the long term goal for this reserve might still be the creation of an open village the degree of threat and community breakdown is such as to make it impossible for this to be considered or proceeded toward by the people at this stage.[86]

As well as seeking ways of involving selected indigenous people in government activities and encouraging residents of reserves to accept increasing responsibility for running their own communities, the government also began to acknowledge and respond to voluntary organisations established to further indigenous causes in the general community. The growth of such organisations reflected the post-Second World War movement of indigenous people into Adelaide and country towns and into mainstream employment, a movement encouraged by the government's assimilation policies. Similar developments were occurring in other states, and the presence of greater concentrations of Aboriginal people, especially in the capital cities, increased their capacity for organisation and political influence and exposed them to greater media attention. While, 'by the late 1960s European control of most Aboriginal organisations had melted away as Aboriginal people of ability stepped forward to take their destiny in their own hands', initially such organisations relied on non-indigenous initiative, leadership and advocacy.[87] The most prominent national example of this is found in the history of the Federal Council for the Advancement of Aborigines, later the Federal Council for the Advancement of Aborigines and Torres Strait Islanders, formed in 1958 with a largely non-indigenous membership. Its first three presidents were non-indigenous and two of these were South Australians. Both were deeply involved in supporting the 'Aboriginal cause' in the community and in parliament: Dr Charles Duguid and Donald Dunstan. However, by 1961, an Aboriginal, Joe McGinnes, was president, and indigenous membership and control of the council's agenda grew from that time.[88]

The Aborigines Advancement League was formed in South Australia in 1946. The league had a mostly non-indigenous membership and was associated particularly with Charles and Phyllis Duguid. Indigenous people who benefited directly from its efforts were mostly Adelaide-based 'part-Aboriginals' who were making their way in the general community, such as Nancy Brumbie and Jeff Barnes, or children from distant settlements or from Colebrook home whom the Duguids 'adopted'. The standing of the Duguids and their capacity to provide their protégés with material and experiential advantages that helped them to 'assimilate' conferred considerable benefits on a few individuals.

---

86 AAB, Minutes,16 December 1965, pp.198, 202–3; 8 December 1969, p.122; 4 November 1971, p.202, GRS 4343/1/P

87 Broome, *Aboriginal Australians*, pp.173–5

88 ibid., p.175. See above, p.239, and Susan Taffe. *Black and White Together FCAATSI: the Federal Council for the Advancement of Aborigines and Torres Strait Islanders, 1958–1973*, University of Queensland Press, St Lucia, Queensland, 2005.

However, the Aborigines Advancement League also acted to further the Aboriginal cause in more general ways. The best known example of its public advocacy was the Adelaide Town Hall meeting which it sponsored in August 1953. At this meeting, 'without any resentment and in excellent English', five young Aboriginals, including Jeff Barnes, told the large audience 'of the difficulties under which their people lived'. Duguid used this occasion to highlight one particular difficulty which had recently incensed him and had led him to organise the meeting: the refusal of the matron at the Royal Adelaide Hospital to accept three appropriately qualified young 'part-Aboriginal' women for training as nurses. The publicity resulting from Duguid's exposé of this blatant racism ensured that the hospital's decision was quickly modified. The other 'difficulties' mentioned by the indigenous speakers on behalf of their people were less politically volatile and easier to ignore.[89] However, one practical outcome of the meeting was an increase in the Aborigines Advancement League's membership, which facilitated the establishment, in 1956, of a hostel for young indigenous women pursuing secondary education in Adelaide. A survey carried out earlier by Jeff Barnes and two others had identified this as a pressing need among Aboriginals in Adelaide and some other areas, including Point McLeay and Point Pearce.[90]

Another instance in the 1950s of Aboriginal protests making it into the public arena was initiated by the Aborigines Protection Board and the Aborigines Department's Consultant Medical Officer at the Royal Adelaide Hospital, Dr Dudley Packer. They actively encouraged Aboriginal participation in the 1958 congress of the Australian and New Zealand Association for the Advancement of Science (ANZAAS), held in Adelaide. Two Aboriginal men – Percy Rigney from Point McLeay and Robert Wanganeen from Point Pearce – took up the challenge. The Adelaide *News* of 22 August 1958 pictured Rigney and Wanganeen at the congress with Paul Hasluck, the Commonwealth minister responsible for Aboriginal affairs and a forthright advocate of assimilation. The newspaper summarised Rigney's address on 'the future of the Australian aboriginal':

> What can the future hold for my race when we are denied equal rights, recognition, and full rights as to citizenship? Liquor bars us from full citizenship and we feel it is a drastic restriction. If a man is good enough to fight for a country in a world war, he is good enough to enjoy its citizenship rights. We have been asked what kind of work we would like to do. Our answer is: the work we are capable of doing. Men on the mission [sic] can do various kinds of work efficiently, such as carpentry, plumbing, farm work, and shoeing. It is well known that we are among the State's best shearers.

Rigney was concerned that his people's work be justly recompensed. Pointing out that the average weekly wage at Point McLeay was about £7, he continued: 'Granted we are rent-free, given free milk (two pints a day), and granted medical expenses, but that still

---

89 For Duguid's own account of the Adelaide Town Hall meeting, cited in Barnes, *Munyi's Daughter*, pp.91–3, see Charles Duguid, *No Dying Race*, Rigby, Adelaide, 1963, pp.100–1. For the trainee nurses affair, see above, footnote 83, p.200, and also Forte, *Flight of an Eagle*, pp.76–8.

90 The hostel was in suburban Millswood. Barnes, *Munyi's Daughter*, p.85

does not bring us to the basic wage'.[91] It is not known what Hasluck thought of Rigney's address, but he could not have failed to hear its plain message that, if assimilation was to be the future for Aboriginal Australians – and significantly Rigney raised no other possibilities – then it had to be on the basis of a just and proper recognition of their contribution to the public good.

Publicised events such as Rigney's and Wanganeen's ANZAAS appearance probably had symbolic value only. Of greater significance to the Aboriginal cause was the burgeoning of indigenous organisations that built on the foundations laid by the Aborigines Advancement League. In 1954 Laurie Bryan, a non-indigenous man who wanted to 'do something practical' for Aboriginal people after becoming acquainted with their living conditions in Port Augusta joined the Aborigines Advancement League but soon broke with it to form the Aboriginal Progress Association, an organisation whose membership was almost entirely indigenous, although leadership was exercised by Bryan and another non-indigenous man, Eugene Lumbers. While the Progress Association attracted and maintained the support of well-educated and assertive Aboriginals, established the Aboriginal Education Foundation to encourage indigenous engagement in secondary and tertiary education, and later involved itself in broad political issues such as police harassment and land rights, it did not suit all indigenous activists.[92] Gladys Elphick found its membership too male and its leadership too white, and left it to work with a group of indigenous women who, in 1966, formed the Council of Aboriginal Women in South Australia.

Elphick's concerns, which set the agenda of the Women's Council, were of two kinds. She wanted to provide support, including knowledge about 'where to turn' for help, to the many Aboriginal families in Adelaide who were living in poverty. She also wanted to encourage Aboriginal people to '[act] more decisively in their own affairs', and to 'project a better and more positive Aboriginal image', to ensure an increased focus on the 'many Aboriginal people living lives of achievement and social success' and less on 'those who were failing'. She claimed:

> There was a real need for us. We wanted to show people, and to show the government, that we could do things for ourselves. They couldn't seem to accept us as intelligent adults. Even Dr Duguid who was such a true friend, saw us as 'his children'.[93]

The Council of Aboriginal Women did indeed 'show the government' what they were capable of. This occurred partly through Elphick's advocacy on the AAB, but also through the initiative, energy and vision of their community work and direct contact with Dunstan, and later with Ian Cox, Director-General of the Department of Social Welfare

---

91 *News*, 22 August 1958, p.12; for background to Rigney and Wanganeen's involvement at the ANZAAS Congress see GRG 52/1/1958/123. It appears that no written version of Rigney's presentation survives and it is likely that he spoke 'off the cuff'.

92 Forte, *Flight of an Eagle*, pp.70–1, 99

93 ibid., pp.70–2, 78–9, 83. Other founders of the Council of Aboriginal Women were Ruby Hammond, Margaret Lawrie, Natascha MacNamara, Faith Thomas and Maude Tongerie.

and Aboriginal Affairs.[94] The council succeeded in attracting financial support from the government which enabled it to employ trained staff and expand its services. Strengthened by strategic alliances with like-minded Aboriginal groups, the council was instrumental in the development of other indigenous organisations which were to have a significant and ongoing role from the early 1970s: the Aboriginal Legal Rights Movement; the Aboriginal Community Centre, which through various changes in focus and scope became an Aboriginal Community Controlled Health Centre, most recently known as Nunkuwarrin Yunti; and the Aboriginal Community College, now known as Tauondi College.[95]

These developments reflected the changing political climate, the greater openness to diversity and the extension of rights of various kinds that characterised Australian society in the post-Second World War period, and especially in the 1960s and 1970s. Some of the radical actions taken by indigenous groups and their supporters in other parts of Australia at this time to protect reserve and traditional land, expose racial discrimination and protest against unjust work conditions have since achieved iconic status in the history of the struggle for indigenous rights.[96] The Aboriginal people who participated in these activities, as well as the South Australian women who, with less public exposure, established the Women's Council, were not merely beneficiaries of that changing climate: their assertiveness and their insistence on being the agents of their own political destiny were part of what changed it.

This gathering momentum for change and an increasing willingness to consider what Aboriginals themselves were indicating as their concerns and priorities are evident in the records of the AAB. Early in 1965 the modest proposal of AAB member Geoff Pope that the Department of Aboriginal Affairs sponsor a conference of organisations interested in Aboriginal welfare, in relation to the establishment of an Aboriginal welfare council, drew a sharply negative response from minister Pearson:

> Whilst he welcomed imaginative and stimulative [sic] constructive criticism and expression of ideas, he did not find it necessary to provide support to organized collective public criticism when there is obviously not sufficient interest to form a council without Departmental assistance.[97]

However, by 1967 the AAB was freely acknowledging the contribution of voluntary organisations, including indigenous ones, to Aboriginal welfare, and the Department of Aboriginal Affairs was directing support to the Council of Aboriginal Women. In 1969 the organisations were mentioned again, and the AAB acknowledged the contribution of

---

94 See below, p.258

95 Forte, *Flight of an Eagle*, chapter four. See also David Hollinsworth, 'Aboriginal Protest and Politics', in Wilfrid Prest, Kerrie Round and Carol Fort (eds), *The Wakefield Companion to South Australian History*, Wakefield Press, Adelaide, 2001, pp.16–17; Mattingley and Hampton, *Survival in Our Own Land*, pp.153–4.

96 Broome, *Aboriginal Australians*, pp.175–7

97 AAB, Minutes, 7 December 1964, p.151; 8 February 1965, p.154, GRS 4343/1/P

Aboriginal people to the community education program that the department was running in response to the 'ceaseless' demand from the public for information about its work. Aboriginals who offered themselves as public speakers were 'hoping to create an environment for their children which is more tolerant than the one they have had to conquer'. Far from echoing Pearson's 1965 defensiveness about indigenous criticism – implicit or explicit – of past and present government policies, the AAB seemed by then to welcome it. It noted indigenous initiatives which went beyond those 'imposed ... by their non-Aboriginal neighbours or by legislation': the Whyalla Aborigines Group, whose purpose was to help families new to the town to settle in; the Port Lincoln Aboriginal Helpers Association set up to deal with local problems; the establishment by the Council of Aboriginal Women of an Adelaide social welfare agency employing indigenous staff; and further development of the work of Reserve Councils at Gerard, Koonibba, Davenport and Yalata. The AAB saw these developments as positive signs:

> Increasingly, Aborigines all over the State are taking the initiative in bringing about changes in their conditions and are airing the frustrations and dissatisfactions that they have quietly suffered for the past 150 years.[98]

The 1968 AAB report went even further by acknowledging an issue over which a great silence normally prevailed in non-indigenous society: the persistence among Aboriginals with a significant level of involvement with non-indigenous society of a distinctive indigenous identity connected to traditional values. As the AAB noted, this could, in some cases, be strong enough to determine where and how such people wanted to live. Thus the AAB noted:

> While Aboriginal culture and ceremonies play very little part in the overt lives of the Aboriginal community at Coober Pedy, they still have some influence on the adults. Many of the older people whose lives are still very largely dominated by Aboriginal rites and customs are now moving either north to Indulkana or south-west to Yalata; those who stay on at Coober Pedy complain of their loss of authority. Although it seems that the Aboriginals at Coober Pedy are disillusioned by the failure of their own concepts and values to explain their present circumstances, they have not, except on a superficial level, accepted European culture to any significant extent.

The same report noted that people who had moved from Ooldea in 1945–46 and were now living on the Gerard Reserve had also retained their local identity. Some still spoke their native Pitjantjatjara, exercised traditional skills and retained links with their kin from the north of the state. One man had been initiated and others were said to be considering this. They did not themselves observe traditional ceremonies, but had a 'deep respect' for those practised elsewhere. This retention of traditional culture, links and identity among people who were living and making their way – in the government-approved fashion – in the non-indigenous world had not been reported before. It was done so here without

---

98 AAB, Report, 1967, 1969, *SAPP*, no.20, 1967, pp.12–13; ibid., no. 20, 1969, p.19

judgement and not perceived as a 'problem'. Not surprisingly, such traditional ties persisted in the more remote areas as well: the AAB noted that, in the North-West Reserve, although the seductions of the 'market economy' were becoming more significant among the younger generation, 'European contact has done little to erode the culture of the older generation who still exert a powerful influence'.[99]

However, it would be naïve to make too much of this new-found 'sensitivity' on the part of the non-indigenous commentators or of their apparent acceptance of indigenous choice, including the choice to be different. Such acceptance was easy enough to claim in a report or to summon in relation to traditional people or those living in relatively remote situations. It was less likely to be forthcoming in relation to more substantially 'assimilated' urban Aboriginals exercising their political muscle in Adelaide. In any case it needs to be considered alongside indigenous assessments of how far things had actually moved. Elphick, for example, claimed at a conference in 1969 that, when Aboriginal people moved from the reserves or other country areas to the city in order to 'better themselves', their problems were often exacerbated. Jobs were hard to find, accommodation was expensive, leading to overcrowding, health suffered, the benefits of improved education could not be realised and Aboriginal people ended up feeling insecure in an environment that was 'not home'.[100] In seeking to address these problems, government and non-indigenous institutions seemed incapable of little real consultation with indigenous people, or accommodation to their wishes:

> It is so often the way. They ask you for your suggestions, but then it is their own ideas that they want to put into practice . . . we are trying to help ourselves, but we get knocked back on it all the time. They don't want our ideas. They want to do things their way, not ours, and that's most of the trouble'.[101]

What is significant about this statement from an 'assimilated' woman whom many would have judged as no longer a real Aboriginal, because of admixtures of 'white' blood and a mission upbringing, is her insistence that there are two ways of thinking, and two ways of doing things – 'theirs' and 'ours'. A distinctive 'Aboriginality' had not been extinguished, even amongst the most 'assimilated'. Failure on the part of the general community to realise this, and an ongoing privileging of non-indigenous views over indigenous was a fundamental source of the problems and injustices experienced by Aboriginal people.

All the developments discussed so far in this chapter – all of the legislative, regulatory, constitutional and organisational changes that dismantled the old system of protection, encouraged integration, and extended basic 'citizenship' rights and opportunities to the

---

99 AAB, Report, 1968, *SAPP*, no.20, 1968, pp.12, 14, 15

100 Gladys Elphick, 'The Council of Aboriginal Women', in Department of Adult Education, University of Adelaide, *The Aborigines of South Australia: their background and future prospects, proceedings of a conference held at the University of Adelaide, 13–16 June 1969*, pp.93–5.

101 Forte, *Flight of an Eagle*, p.106

indigenous population – were developments which influenced the health of the indigenous population in the broad sense in which health is understood in this book. In theory these changes had the potential to promote health by extending rights and freedoms, for example, voting rights, access to 'normal' wage scales and government benefits, educational opportunity, protection from racial discrimination, choice about domicile, and limited title to land. All of these contributed significantly towards the indigenous population being recognised as part of the public, as citizens who were 'taking their place' in society, and contributing to it. Such recognition and social inclusion, as the argument presented in chapter two suggests, is crucial to the health of all sections of the population, and especially the most marginalised. In practice, however, in Australia in the 1960s it was difficult for the indigenous population to realise these theoretical gains. Many of them were negated or severely compromised by the challenges involved in making the necessary transitions in a social context characterised by personal and institutional racism, major economic inequalities, and various disabling legacies of the past.

These legacies included the learnt helplessness displayed by many Aboriginal people who had been 'protected' and treated as mendicants, and the corresponding paternalism and cultural arrogance of many non-Aboriginal people, practices and structures. In addition, there was what Koonibba missionary Eckermann had earlier called the 'self-respect wound', a wound carried by Aboriginal people whose old world had gone and whose experience of the new world left them 'baffled, frustrated, and often devoid of hope', with a 'smouldering resentment' born of a 'sense that they had been sold short'.[102] Such legacies clearly undermined both physical and mental health and stood in the way of improving it. The growth of indigenous organisations during this period symbolised the complexity of these legacies, while demonstrating both the health and the absence of health within the indigenous population. On the one hand, the assertiveness, cultural pride, self-esteem, insight and energy that established and sustained these organisations were evidence of individual and community health. On the other, the reasons for the advent of these organisations – the poverty, lack of education, insecurity, abusive behaviour, crime, violence and individual and family dysfunction they sought to address – were potent signs of lack of health.

Within this complex context, the Department of Aboriginal Affairs continued to focus on specific issues identified as health issues, but there is evidence that it reflected on these with somewhat greater sophistication and insight than had been the case in earlier times. For example, the extension of 'drinking rights' to people of Aboriginal descent – in 1963 to those in the Adelaide metropolitan area, and by 1965 to all except those living on missions and reserves – led to concerns about the levels of consumption, drunkenness, violence and other alcohol-related problems within the Aboriginal population.[103] It also led to non-Aboriginal exaggeration of the problems and a marked tendency to construct

---

102 CV Eckermann, 'Aboriginal Missions: the church's problem child', *Australian Lutheran*, 27 August 1958, pp.281–2; 10 September 1958, pp.295–6

103 'Drinking rights', as they were popularly known, were extended by amending the discriminatory sections, 172 and 173, of the *Licensing Act 1932–60*. See AAB, Report, 1964, 1965, *SAPP*, no.20, 1964, p.8; *SAPP*, no.20A, 1965, p.5. See also, Raynes, *'A Little Flour'*, pp.59, 152–3.

them as problems of race. The AAB, while not minimising the 'drink' problem, was also concerned about community perceptions and reactions. In 1967 it reported:

> It is disturbing to discover how frequently behaviour which is readily tolerated in the general community ... becomes a matter of condemnation when committed by an Aboriginal. It is also disturbing to note how often behaviour which is individually censured when committed by a non-Aboriginal is regarded as a racial characteristic when committed by an Aboriginal.[104]

Distancing itself from such a view and also from the moralism of many earlier responses to alcohol-related problems among indigenous people, the AAB supported research to understand the issues more fully.[105]

The AAB was also aware of other health problems, especially malnutrition among infants and children in the stock camps and northern reserves. It acknowledged the inadequacy of the remedial medical service that the government provided and listed discussions with the Department of Public Health about a more preventive approach as part of its future plans. The AAB also indicated an awareness that health problems were often complex in their aetiology and could not be rectified by health services, no matter how 'preventive'. For example, commenting on reports from Department of Aboriginal Affairs Welfare Officers about children starving at Maree, it noted:

> lack of income was not a factor in these children being inadequately cared for or fed. Boredom, the depressing environment and climate encourages the mothers to the hotel where they soon lose any sense of responsibility.[106]

By 1970 the AAB had abandoned the old bland, superficial and often optimistic style that had been a feature of earlier government reporting on indigenous health and was frankly acknowledging problems. It was also recognising the need for better health data in response to a recent focus on this issue at joint Commonwealth–states Native Welfare Conferences. At the 1961 conference there had been a call for 'all native welfare authorities [to] maintain accurate vital statistics' in order to provide information particularly on needs in the area of infant welfare.[107] At the 1963 conference, statistical comparisons between a number of Aboriginal and non-Aboriginal population groups were presented, revealing, among other things, stark differences in infant mortality. In the Northern Territory, for example, mortality of Aboriginal infants in the period 1957–61 was somewhat higher than it had been among non-Aboriginal infants in Australia in 1903, and more than five times as high as among non-Aboriginal infants in Australia in 1959.[108]

---

104 AAB, Report, 1967, *SAPP*, no.20, 1967, p.7

105 See below, p.255

106 AAB, Report, 1968, *SAPP*, no. 20, 1968, pp.12, 14, 17, 21; AAB, Minutes, 27 November 1967, p.11, GRS 4343/1/P

107 Proceedings and Decisions of Native Welfare Conference, Commonwealth and State Authorities, Canberra, 26–27 January 1961, p.35, GRG 52/18/6

108 Proceedings and Decisions of Native Welfare Conference, Commonwealth and State Authorities, Darwin, 11–12 July 1963, agenda paper: 'Northern Territory, Aboriginal population as at 31/12/1961', table 2, infant mortality, GRG 52/22/13

These were incomplete data, but they were nevertheless a clear indication that the social, economic and medical advances that had underwritten substantial saving of non-indigenous infant lives during the first half of the twentieth century had not been extended to the indigenous population. In 1967 the NHMRC reported that, despite an increase in research activity on various aspects of indigenous life and culture, 'there is very little factual information available on the incidence and prevalence of ill health in Aborigines, or indeed in the Australian population as a whole'. It hoped that since the indigenous population would henceforth be included in the Commonwealth census, comparative mortality data would become available and predicted that these would 'certainly pinpoint a number of fatal conditions requiring special investigation and measures for their prevention'.[109]

In South Australia, in response to the prompting of the Native Welfare Conferences and the NHMRC, and to the need for the research identified in the 1962 *Aboriginal Affairs Act*, the Department of Aboriginal Affairs initiated a number of research activities in the late 1960s. The AAB's 1969 report listed three projects: the first, in collaboration with the Commonwealth Government, the Alcohol and Drug Addiction Board of South Australia and the Psychology Department at the University of Adelaide was a study of Aboriginal alcohol consumption; the second was the development of a training program for Aboriginal Reserve Councillors; the third was a trial of a 'community method of working' with people of Aboriginal blood in Port Lincoln, which aimed

> to restore the self-confidence and pride of Aboriginal people in themselves and their heritage
> and to develop skills in leadership and working together in order to identify their own partic-
> ular needs and to overcome them by their own efforts.[110]

This modest research agenda reflected what was to become – and remain – an increasingly complex tension between various approaches to health improvement: the need to respond to specific and entrenched health problems, while at the same time supporting broadly developmental projects which, in ways not always easy to predict or measure, have the potential to prevent illness and perhaps even produce health.

The Department of Aboriginal Affairs and the AAB kept their feet firmly on the ground, despite increased sophistication in their activities and insights. In 1970 they cautioned against complacency: 'significant advances have been made towards documenting the problems, but solutions are little nearer, particularly in the far north of the State'. Malnutrition was again singled out as an issue and, for the first time, diabetes was mentioned: there was an 'alarmingly high percentage of Aboriginals with diabetes in one urbanized Aboriginal community'. The AAB enumerated specific services and strategies to help combat these problems: skilled health personnel and Aboriginal people to work with them; better housing; adequate and safe water supplies; more hygienic sanitary arrangements; and pre- and post-natal services. Although the Board did not make a specific connection to poor health, in the same report it noted that severe unemployment

---

109 Aboriginal Welfare Conference of Commonwealth and State Officers, Perth, 18–19 July 1967, Report on NHMRC
       actions and recommendations and work in progress relating to Aboriginal health, GRG 52/18/11

110 AAB, Report, 1969, *SAPP*, no.20, 1969, p.11

persisted among indigenous people, not only those without western education and living in remote areas, but also among school leavers in the settled areas. There were 'urgent needs' for housing as well, and the AAB believed that generally the department had 'not begun to cope with the relocation needs' of Aboriginal people who were 'drifting' to the metropolitan area in search of employment and access to services and education.

In 1971, the final report filed by the AAB celebrated the achievements of John Moriarty, former president of the Aboriginal Progress Association, part-time employee of the Department of Aboriginal Affairs, outspoken critic of government policy, and the first Aboriginal to graduate from a South Australian university. However, the AAB also issued a warning. Moriarty's case was exceptional. For many Aboriginal people the experience of education and of seeking inclusion in the 'white' community had less healthy and fulfilling outcomes:

> It is not in the interests of Aborigines either to be educated for a place in a world they will never see, or to be forced to leave the surroundings which provide them with their social and spiritual security in order to drift from place to place on the fringes of an alien and rejecting culture.

Since, despite these difficulties, 'many will find a future only in the towns and cities', the message was clear: the means had to be found to make integration a reality. There would be no security, achievement or health for indigenous people unless the community could actually deliver the opportunities for inclusion and participation that were promised by laws and policies.[111]

On 1 July 1970, as a result of a decision of Steele Hall's Liberal Country League government, which was in office from April 1968 until June 1969, the Departments of Aboriginal Affairs and Social Welfare were formally amalgamated to become the Department of Social Welfare and Aboriginal Affairs. The AAB had been opposed to this from when it was first mooted, believing that it would be 'inimical to the interests of the Aborigines'. In 1970, in what they imagined would be their last report, AAB members expressed their hope 'that the interests of this special minority will not be swamped out of sight by the combined reports that are likely to be issued in the future'. As a precaution, they provided an immediate agenda for the new department: it would need to make more funds available for the development of services in the north of the state; it would need to ensure that Aboriginals in the south did not feel that their special status and needs were no longer recognised; its staffing arrangements must not reduce the likelihood of staff gaining experience with the specialised problems of Aboriginal people; and it needed to take care that Aboriginal needs were not overlooked in policies which responded to the needs of a predominantly 'white' community. The AAB's alarmed and protective response to the new regime was understandable. Given the niggardly response of governments to the needs and aspirations of the indigenous population during most of the period since European

---

111   AAB, Report, 1970, 1971, *SAPP*, no.20, 1970, pp.13, 17, 22, 26; *SAPP*, no.20, 1971, pp.5–6

settlement, the AAB was anxious to preserve the positive moves towards recognition and inclusion with which it had been associated during the last decade. And given the small size of the Department of Aboriginal Affairs compared with the Department of Social Welfare, AAB members may well have wondered whether amalgamation would in fact be a takeover. As it turned out, the AAB's 1970 report was not its last: it submitted one more in 1971, and used it to draw attention to the 'increasingly focused and vocal desires of the Aboriginal people' whose fulfillment must be taken into account in future policies.[112]

The establishment of the Department of Social Welfare and Aboriginal Affairs was an ironic outcome of a period in which there had been much talk of furthering the welfare of indigenous South Australians. As already indicated, both before and after he achieved office, Dunstan had suggested that 'legislation on Aborigines should only be welfare legislation'; that is, legislation designed to promote the welfare, or wellbeing, of Aboriginals. This had translated into abolition of restrictions and discriminatory practices, the establishment of rights to land, the extension of services and material goods, and the provision of opportunities for a public voice and for being involved in decision-making about their future. For Dunstan, promoting the welfare of indigenous people had been predominantly concerned with their integration into the general community and their inclusion in the changes occurring in the broader society as citizens, admittedly citizens with special needs, including the need for 'guidance'. However, the linking of Aboriginal affairs administratively with 'social welfare' implied a different stance. It constructed Aboriginal affairs as a 'welfare' issue; that is, a problem requiring a particular kind of response from governments, a response usually associated with an unequal power relationship characterised by paternalism on the part of government and passivity and dependence on the part of the client. In such a construction, the literal meaning of welfare as wellbeing, which was the way Dunstan used it, is frequently lost, and its realisation rendered problematic. It can be argued that, despite the rhetoric of community development in vogue in the new department, the 1970 amalgamation, by moving Aboriginal affairs squarely into the 'welfare' area, confirmed a long historical trend. This trend was obvious as early as 1838 at the Government House garden party described in chapter three, and reinforced, as subsequent chapters have shown, in myriad ways since. Viewing the indigenous population as cases in need of 'welfare', has, demonstrably, usually been at odds with their actual welfare, that is, their well-being and their inclusion as members of the public.

The significant administrative changes following the establishment of the Department of Social Welfare and Aboriginal Affairs did not of course undo all the advances of the 1960s. The Aboriginal Lands Trust, the Reserve Councils, the voluntary indigenous organisations and services, and the moves away from the removal and institutionalisation of children all continued. In 1972, new legislation, the *Community Welfare Act, 1972*, specified 'Special Provisions Relating to Aboriginal Affairs' and charged the minister with the following duties:

---

112 AAB, Report, 1969, 1970, 1971, *SAPP*, no.20, 1969, p.7; *SAPP*, no.20, 1970, pp.7, 29; *SAPP*, no.20, 1971, p.7

to promote, in consultation and collaboration with the Aboriginal people, [their] cultural, social, economic and political welfare and development;

to encourage and assist the Aboriginal people to preserve and develop their own languages, traditions and arts;

to formulate and implement programs of research into matters relating to the Aboriginal people;

to establish, and foster the development of, Aboriginal councils and associations;

to foster and promote the establishment or conduct of any business, trade or industry by the Aboriginal people;

to provide grants of money or other assistance to advance the development of the Aboriginal people;

to provide technical and other assistance to advance the development of the Aboriginal people.[113]

The department was renamed the Department for Community Welfare, and within it the Division of Aboriginal Resources was created to provide 'consultative, planning, and advisory services in relation to the general economic, social, and cultural development of the Aboriginal people'.[114] The new Director-General, Ian Cox, who had a background in social welfare administration in Victoria and who enjoyed bi-partisan political support, was critical of the 'inappropriate' ethos, values, procedures and, in some cases, staff that his department had inherited. He was determined to promote a community development approach to Aboriginal affairs that would foster 'self-management' and he claims to have relied directly on the knowledge and insights of the leaders of the Council of Aboriginal Women.[115]

Within months of the establishment of the Department for Community Welfare, more far-reaching changes were afoot. Developments at the federal level signalled the beginning of a new era in which the Commonwealth Government would become the main driver of policy in relation to the indigenous population. In December 1972, a Labor government under the leadership of Gough Whitlam was elected on a platform which included a new deal for Aboriginals. By the end of 1973, the Whitlam Government had formally taken over responsibility for Aboriginal affairs. This led to legislative and administrative changes whereby the state governments were divested of their specific duties and responsibilities towards the indigenous population. In South Australia, the Aboriginal Resources Division within the Department for Community Welfare was abolished and its personnel formed the South Australian Regional Office of the Commonwealth Department of Aboriginal Affairs.

These changes were much more than merely organisational. They were part of a broad program of reform which reflected Whitlam's commitment to social justice, a

---

113 *Community Welfare Act, 1972*, no. 51 of 1972, assented to 27 April 1972, part V, section 83

114 Report, Director-General of Community Welfare, 1972, *SAPP*, no.23, 1972, p.5

115 Ian Cox, Interview, Goolwa, South Australia, 9 December 2002. Notes in possession of author.

program characterised by enhanced community participation in social planning and the extension of a voice and opportunity to populations who had hitherto been silenced or sidelined.[116] Soon after assuming power, his government embarked on 'a massive spending programme' on the Aboriginal population, announced the establishment of an Aboriginal-elected policy advisory committee and programs to 'revitalise Aboriginal social welfare'. Most significantly it initiated an inquiry, under the direction of Justice AE Woodward, to determine 'the appropriate means to recognise and establish the traditional rights and interests of the Aborigines in and in relation to land'. This was all part of Labor's basic policy commitment, articulated in the Commonwealth Parliament on 6 April 1973, 'to restore to the Aboriginal people of Australia their lost power of self-determination in economic, social and political affairs'.[117] In terms of financial commitment, recognition of rights and expansion of opportunities, this represented a clear break with the past. It has been argued that the Whitlam Government was able to make this break because of a shift in public opinion, encouraged and demonstrated by the 1967 referendum 'event':

> The referendum of 27 May 1967 ... was vitally necessary to the progress of change, not so much because it amended section 51 (xxvi) of the Australian constitution but more because the referendum, as an event, helped create a climate of opinion which provided an activist federal government with a mandate: it bestowed upon the Whitlam and subsequent governments the moral authority required to expand the Commonwealth's role in Aboriginal affairs and implement a major program of reform.[118]

Such moral authority notwithstanding, these changes, as significant and potentially transformative as they were, did not guarantee the structural and attitudinal changes in the broader community that were necessary if indigenous people were to have their lost powers of self-determination restored.[119] Nor did they immediately alter the realities of life for many Aboriginal people or suggest solutions to the historically determined problems they faced. Complex challenges to lofty policy goals such as integration and self-determination, and even to such commonplace desires such as securing a job, a decent house, and a future for one's children, remained. And they remained largely because of tensions between allowing Aboriginal people to be who they were, and especially to live

---

116 This reform program was not restricted to indigenous affairs of course and it affected many areas of government concern, including health. For an analysis of the impact of the Whitlam period on health policy and practice in South Australia see Raftery, 'The Social and Historical Context', in Baum (ed.), *Health For All*, pp.19–37.

117 Broome, *Aboriginal Australians*, pp.181, 185.

118 Attwood, Markus et al, *The 1967 Referendum*, p.63

119 Since the Whitlam period a considerable literature has emerged from indigenous and non-indigenous commentators which critiques both the intention and achievement of the policy of self-determination, records its transformation into a policy of self-management, and claims that it was never seriously committed to indigenous autonomy, since it required indigenous people to be self-determining while effectively withholding from them the means to be so. See for example, Tim Rowse, *Indigenous Futures: choice and development for Aboriginal and Islander Australia*, University of New South Wales Press, Sydney, 2002; Tonkinson and Howard (eds), *Going It Alone?*

where they wanted to live, and the apparently immutable insistence of non-Aboriginal society that access to its benefits was guaranteed only by compliance with its social and economic norms. This dilemma, with its origins in both indigenous tradition and colonial and post-colonial history, was unresolved in 1973 and remains unresolved today. At the heart of it is the difficulty experienced by non-indigenous Australia of finding a way to enable the indigenous population to be both 'Aboriginal', and part of the public.

Chapter 8

Aboriginal – and Part of the Public?

As an Australian nation we aim for one people in one continent and we cannot contemplate the idea of having any group of people permanently submerged and permanently underprivileged in our community. We regard the Aborigines as Australians and we do not wish them to live as a group apart from other Australians.   **Paul Hasluck 1963**[1]

This trend toward Aboriginality is gaining ground. In a way, it is a kind of social movement where, for certain purposes, common identity in contrast to other Australians can mark them off from those others as being unique and somehow different – a status-seeking device, as a reaction against the injustices and discrimination of the immediate past.   **Ronald Berndt 1969**[2]

However much they hate the word that caused so much pain in the past, Aboriginals can't escape, and most of them desire, a high degree of assimilation into today's world of technology, mass culture, education, and Western living standards. Only they can work out how, at the same time, they retain an Aboriginal identity. Some may have to face tough decisions about leaving traditional lands for places of greater opportunity. It is unrealistic to think that the white majority could definitely support settlements with no economic base of their own. It is not unrealistic to think that at the minimum the majority should accept an obligation to help Aborigines to a more equal place without requiring them to sacrifice their identity.   **Hal Wooton 1991**[3]

The Commonwealth Government's assumption of responsibility for indigenous affairs in 1973 brought to a close an era which, in South Australia, had lasted for 137 years, from the beginnings of colonial settlement in 1836. During that time, South Australian governments

---

1 Paul Hasluck, in *'Proceedings and Decisions of Aboriginal Welfare Conference of Commonwealth and State Authorities, Darwin, 11–12 July 1963'*, p.3, GRG 52/18/7

2 Ronald M Berndt, 'The concept of protest within an Australian Aboriginal context', in Ronald Berndt, ed., *A Question of Choice: an Australian Aboriginal dilemma. A collection of papers presented at the Australian and New Zealand Association for the Advancement of Science Congress, Adelaide 1969*, University of Western Australia Press, 1971, pp.25–43

3 Hal Wooton, 'Imprisoned by the Old Ways', *Australian*, 19 April 2001, p.15. Wooton was one of the Royal Commissioners into Aboriginal Deaths in Custody.

attempted to deal with the indigenous population through policies committed to various forms of protection, assimilation and integration. They repeatedly claimed to be interested in affording Aboriginal South Australians the protections and benefits associated with the rule of British law and the extension of Christian 'civilisation', and in equipping them to 'take their place' as 'members of the community'. In this enterprise, governments had at some times and in some places relied on administrative partnerships with Christian missions and with pastoralists. At all times governments had to balance the claims of the indigenous population against those of the much more numerous and economically more powerful settlers.

By any reasonable account this enterprise must be judged a failure. Although some aspects of the protection policy no doubt did protect some Aboriginals from a worse fate, it still rendered them a highly vulnerable group. This is clear from population data alone. Numbering perhaps as many as 15,000 at the time the colony was established, the Aboriginal population declined to a low point of fewer than 3000 by the late 1920s or early 1930s before slowly rebuilding to reach 7299 in 1971, the year of the first Commonwealth census in which Aboriginals were officially included.[4] From then, the indigenous population grew markedly, to 9825 in 1981, 16,223 in 1991 and 23,425 in 2001. Some of this was real growth, related to youthfulness and higher fertility compared with the rest of the population; much of it was artefactual, related to increasingly sophisticated census methodology and to a greater willingness, encouraged by shifts in public opinion and more liberal government policy, for people of indigenous descent to identify as such.[5]

By the 1970s, other kinds of data, underlining the vulnerability of the Aboriginal people, their lack of protection from various kinds of threats to their well-being, and the limited extent to which they had been assimilated or integrated into the main currents of South Australian life, were beginning to accumulate. After the constitutional change achieved as a result of the 1967 referendum, the Commonwealth census provided regular analyses of indigenous birth and death rates, involvement in education and the labour force, and housing and income. These indicated major and persistent inequalities between indigenous and non-indigenous South Australians that amounted to significant disadvantage for the indigenous. The emergence of this information stimulated further interest and investigation in various quarters. In the mid-1970s, the Australian Government Commission of Inquiry into Poverty (the 'Henderson Inquiry') and associated commissioned research, argued that the high levels of poverty and poor health of indigenous people reflected their powerlessness and comprehensive disadvantage within the political and economic structures of Australian society.[6] The 1981 investigation by the World Council of Churches of 'the situation of

---

4 Arriving at accurate indigenous population estimates or counts before 1971 is notoriously difficult. See above, pp.112–13. The numbers quoted here, taken from government year books which rely mostly on census data, are somewhat lower than those obtained from other sources, for example, the counts done by the South Australian Department of Aboriginal Affairs. For a comprehensive anlaysis of the issues involved see Smith, *The Aboriginal Population of Australia*; Gordon Briscoe and Len Smith, 'The Aboriginal Population in South Australia 1921–1944', in Gordon Briscoe and Len Smith (eds), *The Aboriginal Population Revisited: 70, 000 years to the present*, Aboriginal History Monograph 10, Aboriginal History Inc., Canberra, 2002, pp.16–40.

5 Australian Bureau of Statistics, *2004 Year Book Australia*, pp.84, 89, 123

6 Commission of Inquiry into Poverty, *Poverty Among Aboriginal Families in Adelaide*, research report by Fay Gale and Joan Binnion, AGPS, Canberra, 1975

Australian Aborigines' demonstrated that awareness of their 'plight' was not confined to Australia. The investigation proposed solutions that included land rights, the funding of Aboriginal-controlled organisations, such as health and legal services and housing co-operatives, and job creation.[7] The most significant addition to information about Aboriginal health in this period was provided by the 1979 report of an inquiry by the House of Representatives Standing Committee on Aboriginal Affairs.[8]

Based on wide-ranging consultation, this inquiry reported a state of health among the Aboriginal population that 'would not be tolerated if it existed in the Australian community as a whole'. It concluded that this poor health was linked to three main factors: the unsatisfactory environmental conditions in which Aboriginals lived; their low socioeconomic status in the Australian community; and the failure of health authorities to pay attention to their specific health needs or take proper account of their distinctive social and cultural beliefs and practices. However, in discussing the bases for improvements to the health of the Aboriginal population, the report ignored socioeconomic status and its major determinants and focused on environmental conditions, health services and indigenous involvement in planning and decision-making.[9] In summarising mortality and morbidity, the report presented a picture that has subsequently become all too familiar: life expectancy 20 or more years less than that of the rest of the population; infant mortality rates three or four times higher; environment-related conditions such as intestinal infections and parasitic infestations, and infectious diseases, including tuberculosis and leprosy, that were very much less common among the rest of the population; diabetes rates among 20 to 39-year-olds that were 20 times, and among 40 to 50-year-olds, 10 times the rates among the non-indigneous; rates of obesity double those of non-Aboriginals and rates of cardiovascular disease two to five times as high; alcoholism at levels causing 'widespread devastation in some traditional communities'; and 'major psychiatric morbidity' about as high as among non-Aboriginals.[10]

Despite avoiding consideration of the impact of low socioeconomic status on health – the report had almost nothing to say about schooling, family or community income, or employment, for instance – it did go some way to understanding Aboriginal health issues as a function of broader political and social factors. For example, it argued that poor mental health in non-urban communities was related to 'extreme stress' stemming from

the breakdown of traditional and social authority structures, the loss of purpose and self-esteem, a perception that social and personal crises are beyond one's ability to change or control, suppressed fear and anger and discrimination. Further causes of stress include lack of assets, refusal to grant authority to Aboriginals which will enable them to develop viable

---

7 Elizabeth Adler, Anwar Barkat, Bena-Silu, Quince Duncan, Pauline Webb, *Justice for Aboriginal Australians: report of the World Council of Churches team visit to the Aborigines, 15 June to 3 July 1981*, Australian Council of Churches, Sydney, 1981

8 House of Representatives Standing Committee on Aboriginal Affairs, 'Aboriginal Health', *Commonwealth of Australia Parliamentary Papers*, no.60, 1979

9 ibid., pp.iii–iv, xv–xxvi

10 ibid., pp.11–25. The data that the report quoted about diabetes came from the 1969–74 research initiated by the Department of Aboriginal Affairs in South Australia. See above, p.255

communities, and lack of recognition by non-Aboriginals of the right of Aboriginals to retain with pride an Aboriginal identity and culture.[11]

The report focused mostly on remote, segregated communities, largely neglecting the health of urban Aboriginals. The inquiry had not included those living in the capital cities, but the committee 'believed' that 'the physical environment of Aboriginals living in these cities, is unsatisfactory, mainly as a result of frequent overcrowding', which was in turn related to poverty and to 'the kinship ethic'. It suggested that 'fringe dwellers' who wanted to make the transition to urban living needed special assistance to allow them 'the chance to become community members having status and opportunities equal to those of non-Aboriginal community members'. However, the only recommendation for such help was the provision of 'homemaker services', and the report sounded rather nervous about the acceptability of these.[12]

The report recognised that the loss by the indigenous population of its traditional economic basis and its lack of access to 'the economic sector' of non-indigenous society trapped it in an unhealthy and 'self-perpetuating cycle of poverty'. It argued that, 'although Aboriginal health cannot improve dramatically without coordinated action on several fronts', it was 'most practicable to promote a program of community development which is spear-headed by a health service and associated public health program'. It put its faith in such an approach because 'health' was the

> logical cornerstone for the progressive realisation of effective community self-determination . . . and control of a health service [was] likely to heighten the awareness of Aboriginals of the precursors of community problems and to provide a collective momentum which will facilitate action on other issues.

This was a classic community development analysis that reflected the thinking influential within the Department for Community Welfare in South Australia at that time[13] as well as within the World Health Organization, to whose recent pronouncements the report referred. This approach saw 'health' as a fruitful site of intervention to reduce disadvantage, since 'the effects of ill-health resonate throughout all other areas of life'. Its focus was on 'empowering' the indigenous communities in relation to one 'domain of life'; that is, 'health', believing that this would produce the requisite self-confidence and self-respect to enable changes in other domains. Its focus was thus on the indigenous communities themselves. Unfortunately, it underestimated the need for radical change within the political and economic priorities of the 'mainstream' to provide the heightened awareness, collective commitment and structural reform necessary to bring about and sustain real change.[14]

---

11 ibid., p.26

12 ibid., pp.37, 48–9

13 Ian Cox, interview, Goolwa, South Australia, 9 December 2002. Notes in possession of author.

14 House of Representatives Standing Committee, 'Aboriginal Health', pp.112–13, 120 121. This naivety about the extent to which change needed to be made within the non-indigenous sector and to extend much further than changes within 'health' is apparent in the 'health' sections of early reports of the departments that succeeded the Department of Aboriginal Affairs in South Australia. See, for example, report on the work of the Department of Social Welfare and of

The House of Representatives' 'Aboriginal Health' report was the most substantial compilation of data and associated commentary pertaining to the health of the indigenous population that was available at the end of the 1970s. It is therefore worth noting the areas it neglected. It largely disregarded the general relationship between health and socio-economic status; moreover, it ignored two specific examples of that relationship for which data were available: unemployment and incarceration. Unemployment levels among Aboriginals were much higher than among non-Aboriginals. In South Australia this was linked to the fact that about two-thirds of the Aboriginal population lived outside the Adelaide metropolitan area, some of them in country towns, but many still on reserves and missions, some of which were extremely remote.[15] Some indigenous people were economically integrated through employment, although overwhelmingly at the lower end of the wage scale. In many centres of Aboriginal settlement, however, unemployment rates not seen in the non-indigenous community were the norm, economic survival being achieved through comprehensive dependence on government benefits.[16] High unemployment levels were associated with poor educational attainment as well as with remoteness. While numbers of Aboriginals attending school and other educational institutions were provided regularly in government reports, the low level of Aboriginal involvement was camouflaged by the use of raw numbers instead of rates, and there was virtually no reporting on achievement. However, the newly amalgamated Department of Social Welfare and Aboriginal Affairs reported in 1971 that 'very few Aborigines have reached sufficient educational standards to be able to compete with the wider community and gain apprenticeships'. Reflecting on the situation many years later, former AAB member Geoff Pope was certain that lack of educational attainment among indigenous young people had been the norm: among those who attended school – and that was certainly not all – most 'unsuccessfully finished' primary school. This would go some way to explain why unemployment among indigenous school leavers in the southern, settled districts of the state was 60 per cent in 1969.[17]

High rates of Aboriginal arrest and imprisonment were another sign – ignored by the 1979 House of Representatives inquiry – of lack of integration into the 'mainstream', and the lack of opportunity and achievement that this implied. In South Australia, rates increased steeply from the 1950s, that is, when assimilation and, later, integration were the official policy goals. Brock has noted that while 'black and coloured' people accounted for 2.4 per cent of those admitted to South Australian prisons between 1905 and 1930, by 1956 the figure was 13 per cent and by 1968, approximately 25 per cent.[18] This trend, not noted by the Department of Aboriginal Affairs or the AAB at the time, was an unintended and unforeseen consequence of the disruption caused by the dismantling of protection and the

Aboriginal Affairs, 1971, *SAPP*, no.23, 1971, p.15: Director-General of Community Welfare, Report, 1972, *SAPP*, no.23, 1972, p.30.

15 See below, Appendix 6A, 6B

16 Report of Director-General of Community Welfare, 1972, *SAPP*, no.23, 1972, pp.32–4

17 Report on the work of the Department of Social Welfare and Aboriginal Affairs, 1971, *SAPP*, no.23, 1971, p.16; Rev. Geoffrey Pope, Interview, Adelaide, 11 March 1999. Tape and transcript in possession of author.

18 Peggy Brock, 'South Australia', in McGrath, *Contested Ground*, p.232

implementation of assimilation policies. It indicates the extent to which both indigenous people and the wider community were ill-prepared to deal with the changes.

———————

If 137 years of protection, assimilation and integration had yielded, for Aboriginal South Australians, comprehensive vulnerability, exclusion from civic goods and opportunities, and inclusion only at the margins or in the lowest ranks of South Australian society, what did the brave new world of self-determination and federal responsibility offer? Significantly, it allowed an 'indigenous sector' to flourish.

From the 1970s there could be no mistaking the presence of indigenous organisations, indigenous voices, indigenous views and indigenous ways of doing things in many areas of Australian life: in health, legal services, education, housing, sporting associations, the arts, the administration of former missions and reserves, and issues related to land. These voices, views and ways of doing things were by no means unified but they were persistent, and they gathered strength over time. Tim Rowse has called this feature of the political landscape 'the Indigenous Sector' and sees its rise as 'the most important product of the policy era known as "self-determination"'.[19] Its emergence was evidence that Aboriginal Australians had neither died out nor chosen to exercise their citizenship in a way that allowed them to disappear or be absorbed into the general community. On the contrary, it was testament to an assertion of difference, of distinctiveness, of separateness. This assertion, accompanied by an insistence on sharing all the opportunities and choices implied by Australian citizenship and exercised within a social and political context also characterised by many kinds of integration, was far removed from what commentators and analysts of an earlier period had expected.

Government commentary as well as anthropological and historical analysis in the 1940s, 1950s and 1960s is marked by an assumption that the maintenance of 'Aboriginality' and acceptance of a greater role in the general community were incompatible, and that the latter could be achieved only at the expense of the former. It was frequently assumed that this process of 'mergence' was already well advanced and would continue inexorably. The distinction was still made between 'real Aborigines', that is, those retaining significant contact with traditional culture and living far from centres of non-indigenous influence, and the many 'half-caste' or 'mixed race' people who were living in much closer relationship with non-indigenous society and were assumed to retain nothing, or nothing 'real', of their own culture. The assumption that 'real Aboriginality' was increasingly rare was linked to the persistent, although, with time, less crudely expressed notion that 'Aboriginality' was determined by genetic inheritance expressed as proportions of 'Aboriginal blood'. It was also linked to the belief, not borne out by available evidence, that it was being progressively diluted by neat mathematical steps through out-marriage. As the quotient of Aboriginal blood decreased, so 'real Aboriginality', according to this view, disappeared. This biological process could be reinforced by separation from traditional culture and exposure to the influence of non-Aboriginal values and lifestyles. As we

———————

19 Tim Rowse, *Indigenous Futures: choice and development for Aboriginal and Islander Australia*, University of New South Wales Press, Sydney, 2002, p.1

have seen in the preceding chapters, this understanding undergirded the two elements – 'breeding out' and 'socialising in' – of assimilation policies pursued in South Australia, as in the rest of the country.

By the 1970s, these expectations were in tatters. The contention, unanticipated by assimilationists, that maintenance of 'Aboriginality' was not incompatible with inclusion in the general community, and indeed might be valued and pursued, posed perplexing questions. What did the maintenance of Aboriginality mean for those who were largely integrated? What were they asserting or arguing for by insisting on this? Indigenous answers to these questions and non-indigenous reactions to these answers have a signifi-cant effect on the extent to which social inclusion is realised and 'Aboriginality' simulta-neously respected and allowed to flourish. In turn, and in complex ways, this affects health and well-being.

Near the end of the period examined in this book, the anthropologist Ronald Berndt recognised the dilemmas and tensions involved in maintaining 'Aboriginality' and what he called 'simply being Australians'. In an introduction to a volume of papers delivered at the ANZAAS congress held in Adelaide in 1969, he suggested that the choice open to people of Aboriginal descent was a dichotomous one: they could choose 'Aboriginality' as 'a device to express uniqueness' or they could choose anonymity within the wider Australian society'.[20] Although he avoided crude judgements about what constituted 'real Aboriginality', he argued that, for many, their only experience of 'Aboriginality' was

> knowledge about and experience in situations of contact – epitomized by the struggle for sur-vival within the context of prejudice and ignorance ... their Aboriginality is that of a sub-culture, hemmed in by barriers which have only recently begun to break down ... In their emergence they have sought two things: a place within the wider system, and a place outside that system.[21]

He seemed uncomfortable about this. He insisted that there was much 'mythmaking' going on, about 'an imagined Aboriginal past', by people whose 'European side ... far out-weighs anything of an Aboriginal nature', and who cannot reasonably be considered as 'separated or separate from the mainstream of Australian life'.[22] He then noted that people of Aboriginal descent, no matter how attenuated the connection, could, of course, regard themselves as separate, and that this would have implications – unspecified, but the tone suggests challenging ones – 'for themselves and for other Australians'.[23] In this he was prescient: his difficulty in seeing that it might be possible, or reasonable, to 'be Aboriginal' and 'be Australian' at the same time, and that such an identity might be more than a strategic device, is still problematic and a source of discomfort for many people today. It is construed as 'undemocratic', and raises fears of 'unfairness' and potential social and

---

20 Ronald M Berndt, Introduction, in Berndt, ed., *A Question of Choice*, p.xix

21 ibid., p.xvii

22 ibid., p.xviii

23 ibid., p.xviii–xix

political division. Rowse sheds light on these objections and fears by identifying two different perspectives on the indigenous sector and on the project of self-determination.

The first of these perspectives understands the difference between the indigenous and non-indigenous populations negatively in terms of historically and culturally determined disadvantage that needs to be remedied, by government-devised 'catch-up' programs aimed at achieving social and economic equality between indigenous and other Australians. This view implies that, once equality has been achieved, the rationale for government support of special indigenous institutions and programs will have disappeared. It would then 'simply be a matter of private choice, not a responsibility of government, were Indigenous Australians to maintain their many associations, councils and corporations'. The second perspective portrays the difference between indigenous and other Australians more positively as an essential distinctiveness, an ongoing 'indigeneity'. Within this perspective, self-determination involves 'conceding to [indigenous Australians] the right to look after their own affairs'. This will, of course, include 'devis[ing] Indigenous solutions to the problems of 'disadvantage' ', but, more than that, it will involve 'entrenching' the indigenous sector 'in the machinery of Australian Government'. This means that there will not come a time when the indigenous sector, having overcome 'disadvantage' and delivered 'equality', will have served its purpose and therefore cease to be. On the contrary, 'Indigenous people will always maintain their own institutions, for these are the apparatuses of their self-determination, expressing their destiny as a people emancipated from a colonial condition'. Their ability to do this, will depend, of course, on 'security of access to public funds'.[24]

This analysis bears directly on the theme of this book. The first perspective that sees indigenous difference as merely disadvantage and deficit that needs to be made good is clearly linked with past perspectives and the policies emerging from them. These, whether labelled protection or assimilation, did not value indigenous culture highly and saw the merging of the Aboriginal people with the rest of the community as their best hope for future well-being. Although usually denied any effective means of 'taking their place' within the structures and value systems of the non-indigenous world, it was somehow achieving that 'mergence', rather than perversely clinging to their separateness, which was viewed as their salvation. This was the clear message of governments from the beginning of colonisation in South Australia. It was explicit in Governor Gawler's 1838 admonition to the 'natives' assembled outside Government House: '. . . you cannot be happy unless you imitate white men. Build huts, wear clothes and be useful'.[25] It was implicit in Sub-Protector Hamilton's 1875 assessment that 'the difficulties attending first attempts to bring savages under new conditions of life, and accustom them to civilized usages, seem in a fair way to be overcome'.[26] It underpinned the practice of child 'rescue' that Chief Protector South justified precisely in terms of its capacity to obliterate difference: 'rescued' children 'promise[d] to develop into good citizens, as they do not come into contact with the aboriginals. Being nearly white they will have a good chance in

---

24 Rowse, *Indigenous Futures*, pp.2–4

25 See above, p.49

26 See above, p.101

life'.[27] It was most famously and categorically enshrined in the assimilation policy adopted by the 1951 Native Welfare Conference, reinforced at subsequent conferences and associated especially with the Federal Minister for Territories, Paul Hasluck.[28] In 1963 Hasluck, in a fulsome statement, linked the Aboriginal population's separateness with their underprivileged status and declared it to be not what he or anyone wanted for Australia:

> I myself believe, and the last Native Welfare Conference affirmed, that the policy of assimilation is the only goal. As an Australian nation we aim for one people in one continent and we cannot contemplate the idea of having any group of people permanently submerged and permanently underprivileged in our community. We regard the Aborigines as Australians and we do not wish them to live as a group apart from other Australians. On the other hand, I believe too that historical change has gone so far that the time is long since past when it was practically possible for the Aborigines to find any other future than one in close association with all other Australians, except a future of their exclusion and their degradation. Neither they nor we want that sort of future for them. We are bound to live together for the good of each other.[29]

This way of understanding and attempting to deal with the differences between indigenous and non-indigenous Australians has suited many members of the non-indigenous population. As well as promising an eventual end to the need for special funding,[30] it involves no rejection of the dominant culture. In fact, as Rowse argues, it implies that the disadvantages from which the indigenous population has suffered are the 'inherent 'disadvantages' of life shaped by Aboriginal or Torres Strait Islander custom'. 'The process of being uplifted' would involve 'leaving behind inhibiting and self-destructive ways', and allowing 'indigeneity' to become nothing more than 'a fond memory of ancestry'.[31] However, as has been argued throughout this book, this 'process of being uplifted' has not been thoroughly pursued: on the contrary, Aboriginal people have been denied any real opportunity to be become part of the public while simultaneously being urged to do so.

The second perspective on the difference between indigenous and other Australians values indigenous culture and distinctiveness more highly. Far from viewing it as something to be obliterated, it sees it as something to be maintained and protected, and assumes that indigenous people 'already ... have the basic capacities for self-government, whether these ... are of ancient origin ... or have recently been acquired through adaptation to colonial pressures'.[32] This second perspective, then, reflects a genuine embrace of the principle of self-determination. It flourishes within the indigenous sector, although

---

27 See above, p.125

28 See Broome, *Aboriginal Australians*, pp.171–3, and see above, p.183

29 Paul Hasluck, in *'Proceedings and Decisions of Aboriginal Welfare Conference of Commonwealth and State Authorities, Darwin, 11–12 July 1963'*, p.3, GRG 52/18/7

30 As already noted, in South Australia in 1954 the Aborigines Protection Board had remarked on the eventual financial advantage to the state of an assimilated indigenous population. See above, p.175.

31 Rowse, *Indigenous Futures*, p.4

32 ibid., p.4

it is not confined to it. It involves a radical departure from the assimilationist views that persist in the first perspective and which characterised past policies and practices. For Australian governments, and for many Australians, it is an uncomfortable perspective: it is critical of the dominant culture; it suggests that Aboriginal people might never 'merge' into the rest of the population, but continue to claim access to public goods, thus constituting an ongoing drain on funds; and, in any case, its capacity to relieve disadvantage is still to be demonstrated.

These differing perspectives on indigenous difference and the relationship between the indigenous sector and self-determination also involve differing views about the issue of indigenous choice. As has been demonstrated in the history dealt with in this book, Aboriginal people have frequently been assumed not to exercise agency or to do so only within narrow constraints imposed by the settler culture. However from the 1970s, within the indigenous sector, Aboriginal people have emerged as vigorous and distinctive 'choosing subjects', their agency being exercised not just, as in the 'mainstream', by individuals and households, but also by larger collectivities – ' "communities", councils, associations, regions, even "nations"'. This is a further source of difficulty and discomfort for those who are wary of a distinctive 'Aboriginality', have a low view of indigenous culture or are distrustful of where self-determination might lead. They tend to see collective decision-making as a brake on indigenous capacity to overcome disadvantage, and suspect that allowing it to flourish will involve significant costs and inefficiencies assumed to be divisive and unfair to the rest of us.[33]

All of this unease, at government and community levels, has significantly undermined the self-determination policy. In fact, the reluctance of governments of whichever political stripe to leave too much to indigenous choice, or to adequately support distinctive Aboriginal values and ways of doing things has meant that not only has 'self-determination' been narrowed to 'self-management', but the means by which Aboriginal people could become genuinely 'self-managing' have frequently been denied them.[34] Some of this reluctance to take self-management, let alone self-determination, seriously, reflects an ongoing commitment to assimilation which, however politely disguised in conciliatory language, is based on scant regard for indigenous values or for cultural diversity. This failure of government nerve has been matched by community nervousness about what self-determination might unleash in a context of indigenous assertion of distinctiveness. Ironically, this has led to the situation whereby Aboriginals are now told to be part of the public by other Australians who believe that the public cannot safely be plural and heterogeneous. It was acceptable, as the narrative of this book has shown, for Aboriginals not to be part of the public when this meant being seen and provided for as *less than the public*, and being subjected to high levels of control. But there is fear now in some quarters that indigenous freedom to choose to be distinctive might amount to preferential treatment, in effect to being *more than the public*. Such fear and the political stances it spawns are significant obstacles to indigenous well-being.[35]

---

33 ibid., p.5

34 See above, pp.19–20, 259–60

35 This fear of plurality and heterogeneity and its imagined connection with preferential treatment for minorities at the

It needs to be acknowledged, however, that some of the difficulties of governments and citizenry with self-determination stem from a genuine inability to imagine how self-determination can break the historic nexus between 'being Aboriginal' and being 'disadvantaged' and 'unequal'. The continuing poor health, escalating violence and social dysfunction that, since the 1970s, have blighted the lives of many Aboriginal people, especially in remote communities, do not readily encourage faith in self-determination's transformative capacity. This in turn contributes to a view that respect for choice and for difference can be taken too far. Those persuaded by this view will agree with the argument advanced by anthropologist Peter Sutton in the inaugural Berndt Foundation Lecture. Like Sutton, they will not be comfortable with the notion that Aboriginals are 'free to go to hell their own way' or 'have the right to make their own mistakes'. Invoking the duty of care which is owed by the democratic state to its citizens, and especially to the most vulnerable, they will tend instead to the view that 'the state cannot justify its persistent concession of choice to Indigenous Australians when the apparent effects of their choices are so disabling and self-harming'.[36] This position, which attempts to balance choice with other goods, especially equity, undergirds much health literature and many health programs. These, with good reason, given the growing evidence about what produces and maintains health, have a strong focus on reducing inequalities. Getting the balance right, however, is notoriously difficult. The history discussed in this book, and indeed the history of public health generally, make abundantly clear the dangers that lurk in the apparently humane assumption by the state of the 'responsibility to protect the vulnerable from their incapacity to manage their own lives'. As Rowse warns:

> it is not enough simply to assert this principle [the duty of care] and hope that everyone will agree about who is vulnerable and what is the best way to protect them from their own unwise choices with the least infringement of their autonomy.[37]

The threats to autonomy are great enough when the differences between the vulnerable and the protecting agency are those associated with class or socioeconomic status, as the history of infant welfare, or tuberculosis, or the health of 'the poor', or much recent and current 'health promotion' demonstrates. Here the behaviour of individual others or the 'culture' of the socioeconomic group to which they belong are seen to be the sources of illness. Better health can thus be achieved through conformity to the cultural and behavioural norms of the sections of society offering protection and advice. The threats to autonomy are likely to be much greater when the difference between the two groups is more complicated, as is the case with indigenous and non-indigenous Australians. This difference has three elements. The first is the marked difference between the indigenous

---

expense of the majority has found expression in recent times in the politics of resentment, most clearly expressed in the phenomenon of Pauline Hanson's 'One Nation' Party. In my experience, this fear is very common, is encountered informally, and on a regular basis, in conversation, and is associated with historically uninformed and often frankly racist views.

36 Peter Sutton, 'The Politics of Suffering: Indigenous policy in Australia since the 1970s', *Anthropological Forum*, vol.11, no.2, 2001, pp.125–73, cited in Rowse, *Indigenous Futures*, p.15

37 Rowse, *Indigenous Futures*, p.16

South Australians and the Europeans who settled in their country from 1836. They were culturally distinct populations. The presumption by the settlers and their governments that the original population was 'uncivilised', 'backward' and in many ways inferior led to the second element of the differing experience of the two groups, that is, the dismantling of the indigenous population's way of life and their profound marginalisation within the new order established by the settlers. The third element of difference is, for Aboriginal people, a positive one, stemming from their deliberate choice to retain and celebrate some aspects of their distinctiveness. Sorting out how much disadvantage and inequality is linked to this genuine choice to exercise distinctive values and priorities, and how much is the product of a negative history of political decisions taken by others to serve other ends, is central to the challenge facing those interested in the well-being and autonomy of the Aboriginal population.

But the challenge does not end there. It is possible that respect for choice, elevated to an absolute value, can be distorted by romanticism and a failure to be realistic. While defending indigenous right to choice, including the choice to maintain distinctive-ness, we need also to ask, as Sutton does, whether 'the culture of indigenous people . . . is entirely a blessing to them in their efforts to deal with the modern world'.[38] He insists that some distinctive behaviour, values and attitudes, arising from tradition and in some cases distorted by the impact of history, including the history of the self-determination era, need to be rethought. While careful to dissociate his position from the 'oppressive, chauvinistic and racist' policies of the past, 'under which even the most private aspects of life were in many places subject to whitefella scrutiny and control', Sutton argues against turning a blind eye to 'the partially cultural underpinnings of disadvantage'.[39] Instead, he argues for state action, including 'significant economic change' to support indigenous 'cultural self-reassessment'. This will involve not, as in the past, 'the direct co-option of indigenous powers of choice', but rather 'the promotion of new contexts of indigenous choice'.[40]

Promoting 'new contexts of indigenous choice' was a challenge which Charles Rowley wrote about in his influential histories published just before the beginning of the self-determination era. Analysing the situation that existed in 1967, he declared 'Aboriginal politics' to be 'the politics of the asylum, hospital, camp, or other authoritarian institution: of inmates against the management'.[41] That is, he recognised that Aboriginal people were not merely, as in the terms of the Black Report, the lowest socioeconomic group and the most disadvantaged, but a group apart, deprived of an autonomous place within the public, or of normal relations with other members of the public. He also alluded, subtly, to damage and dysfunction within the indigenous population, which undermined its

---

38 ibid., p.16

39 Sutton, 'The Politics of Suffering', pp.149, 151

40 Sutton, 'The Politics of Suffering', *passim* and cited in Rowse, *Indigenous Futures*, pp.16–17. Elsewhere, Rowse makes a similar argument about the need for cultural renovation and the naivety of assuming that the 'restoration of older pro-prieties and authorities' will necessarily yield effective responses to modern health problems. Tim Rowse, *Traditions for Health: studies in Aboriginal reconstruction*, North Australia Research Unit, Australian National University, Casuarina, Northern Territory, 1996

41 Rowley, *Outcasts in White Australia*, p.190

chances of 'decid[ing] what it wanted' and 'operat[ing] within the law to get it'. Aspects of this damage and dysfunction were clearly revealed in the 1979 House of Representatives report on Aboriginal health. Tragically, many of these problems remain unsolved and in some cases have worsened since then. In addition, other kinds of damage and dysfunction have been revealed, for example, through the reports of the Royal Commission into Aboriginal Deaths in Custody and the National Inquiry into the Separation of Aboriginal and Torres Strait Islander Children from their Families.[42] What Rowley understood, earlier than many others, was that simple efforts at redressing disadvantage, or indeed construing the issues as being merely about disadvantage, would not work. He recognised the situation as a complex political problem:

> [a solution] will not be approached through education and training, housing schemes, health measures, the end of all discriminatory legislation, outlawing of discrimination and the like, unless a creative effort can be made to produce leadership and the chance is offered for the leadership to operate. Most of the creative decision-making can only come from the Aborigines. How to enable a poor and depressed group to decide what it wants, and to operate within the law to get it, is the main challenge which faces this nation ... The core of the Aboriginal problem is political in the wider sense. Basically the Aboriginal needs, by his own effort within an administrative framework which makes this possible, freedom to decide with other Aborigines what he wants, and taxpayers' assistance to get it. Above all he requires the kind of organisation which will give him hitting power to advance his interests in legal-liberal society.[43]

In short, Rowley argued for self-determination as the context from which constructive responses to historically and culturally determined damage and dysfunction would have the best chance of emerging. Before the burgeoning of the indigenous sector and its insistence on the right to be self-determining, he recognised that Aboriginals were a group to be negotiated with. More than thirty years later non-Aboriginal Australia remains frightened of Aboriginal 'hitting power'. It prefers to control, to direct, to provide, to administer, rather than to risk the relinquishing of power that is involved in negotiation and in promoting 'new contexts of indigenous choice'.

———

The tension between respect for choice and the maintenance of distinctiveness, on the one hand, and providing for the social and economic inclusion associated with good health, on the other, may be highlighted by specific examples. The desire of some Aboriginal people to continue to live on their traditional land, or on land which the process of colonisation has rendered 'home', is frequently seen as a 'problem' and highlights this tension, perhaps

---

42 This is not to say that there have been no gains in Aboriginal health in the period since the 1970s. Many indigenous people would claim the following as health gains: recognition of their title to land; growth of self-esteem mediated, for example, by the renovation of culture and language; exercise of indigenous leadership in many areas; growth in the scope and sophistication of community-controlled services, including health services; and enhanced respect among some sections of the non-indigenous community for Aboriginal values and ways of doing things.

43 Rowley, *Outcasts in White Australia*, pp.333–4

more vividly than any other issue. The 'problem', according to conventional thinking, is that such land cannot support its occupants economically. In addition, because of remoteness and the small size of the communities, it is difficult, perhaps even impossible, to provide them with the basic infrastructure and services that other Australians take for granted or regard as 'rights'. In this context, many non-indigenous people, including people of good will, are impatient with what seems like an overvaluing of choice at the expense of presumed opportunities to diminish disadvantage and suffering. They stress equity over choice as the paramount good to be pursued. And they may well resent as wasteful and inefficient giving primacy to choice.

This is not just a current question. In the 1940s Ronald and Catherine Berndt predicted that this would become an issue for the people of Ooldea, among whom they were conducting field work. In time, they argued, the mission would become unable to meet the 'more varied and more numerous' needs of the Ooldea people and they would 'come to have increasingly less control and association with their tribal lands' and eventually 'be unable, even if they are willing, to find a living there for themselves and their families'.[44] There was an unspoken assumption here that a living could be found elsewhere and that this was part of the process of moving 'from black to white'. It was something that the Ooldea people would have to choose, although such a 'choice' would be akin to lack of choice. In 1959 the Lutheran missionary CV Eckermann, discussing his church's work at Koonibba, reflected on a similar situation. He noted that the mission, like other missions, had concentrated the population in places where there were few employment opportunities. His solution, plausible in terms of conventional economic wisdom, was no more respectful of possible indigenous preferences than was the Berndts':

> In this district to cultivate intensively is to court disaster. Holdings as large as the mission's are being run by a single family, with the help of a little seasonal labour ... to try to make employment available where the resources do not exist is trying to make the mountain come to Mahommet. The sensible thing would be to take surplus population to districts where employment is available.[45]

This 'surplus' and supposedly transportable population were people whose families had perhaps sixty years association with the mission itself, and perhaps much more with the area, since the mission had been established in country where large numbers of Kokatha, Wirangu and Mining people were already living. Even if such people had been willing to move, where would they find employment? Would a 'choice' to leave their country guarantee elimination of economic disadvantage?

Ten years later, in 1969, in an address to a conference held at the University of Adelaide, the South Australian Director of Aboriginal Affairs, CJ Millar, indicated that Eckermann's confidence might have been misplaced. He acknowledged that there were still significant issues of 'transition' that stood in the way of indigenous people accessing 'mainstream' opportunities. Employment seemed to be the biggest hurdle, and for those

---

44 Berndts, *From Black to White in South Australia*, p.125

45 CV Eckermann, *Australian Lutheran*, 18 February 1959, pp.53–4

in remote areas, 'full employment cannot be anticipated ... in the near future'. The best hope was that the next generation might be induced, by horizon-widening education, to leave their country and move to where the jobs were.[46] Many years later, Rex Orr, the last non-Aboriginal Superintendent at Koonibba, expounded movingly on the same theme. Reflecting on problems during his time on the reserve, and subsequently, and on the continuing restriction of social and economic opportunity for indigenous people within the Australian community, he said:

> One of the great dilemmas is, what is [Koonibba] there for? To me, one of the greatest dilemmas was there is no economic purpose for this particular community. Now if you've got no economic purpose for a community, no matter where it is, you've got a problem, and a major problem because there is no valid economic reason for that community to exist. It's non-productive, and is never going to be in a position where the people can see themselves as gainfully rewarded for activity. And so if you want to make a serious statement it would be best not to have a place like that. And the sooner it breaks down the better chance the people will have to move into an environment which is more, quote, 'normal' ... where the pressures of employment and unemployment are more normalised. You know, you take any community where there's no employment and you've got serious social problems. And that's what it's like – to me that's what it was really about. I mean you could put maybe five families there – maybe three or four families – who'd be able to farm properly, because it was a pretty extensive property, and be employed, but after that what was everybody there for?[47]

Orr's question remains a challenging one: *what is everybody there for?* At one time Aboriginals had been on missions and reserves in order to be protected and to be 'Christianised' and 'civilised'. That agenda included no expectation of individual or communal independence and placed no value on indigenous choice or on providing opportunities beyond a narrow range believed appropriate to inmates of closed mission or reserve settlements. But now Aboriginal people are choosing to live in such places, claiming the right to live in them, despite the persistent disadvantages and inequalities which, to date, have been associated with such choices. Non-indigenous people who are concerned about the effects of inequalities on well-being wonder whether this is giving undue priority to choice. According to Rowse, many indigenous Australians, by contrast, are wary of 'the politics of equity', because of 'its strong implication that 'difference' is a 'deficit' to be remedied, rather than a choice to be respected'. While I would argue that a concern for equity does not necessarily see difference as deficit, and that choice and equity are not essentially at odds, Rowse is surely right, given the post-European settlement history of Australia and the enduring pull of assimilationist ideas, to sound a warning:

---

46 CJ Millar, 'Aboriginal Affairs in South Australia', in Department of Adult Education, University of Adelaide, *The Aborigines of South Australia: their background and future prospects, proceedings of a conference held at the University of Adelaide, 13–16 June 1969*, pp.13–18

47 Rex Orr, Interview, Adelaide, 26 February 1999, Tape and transcript in possession of author.

If choice is not to be terminally buried beneath 'deficit' in current policy debates about what Indigenous Australians are entitled to, there must be a persistent and organised articulation of the Indigenous right to choose.[48]

The need for a shift in emphasis to support 'the Indigenous right to choose' is clearly borne out by the history, analysed in this book, of non-indigenous policies and practices in relation to indigenous South Australians. This history has demonstrated long-term and comprehensive limitation of choice for Aboriginal South Australians which has been linked to the production and maintenance of inequality. Lack of choice accompanied by structured social, economic and political inequality have acted together in a cyclical and self-reinforcing fashion to maintain health inequalities. It was this process that produced the poor health of the indigenous population which, by the 1970s, was deeply entrenched and statistically incontrovertible.

It is clear that opportunity for indigenous choice – about pursuing traditional patterns of living and about involvement in the non-indigenous world – was significantly limited from the beginning of colonial settlement in 1836. This limitation of choice occurred through the alienation of the Aboriginals' land and the consequent disruption or destruction of their livelihood and through the pursuit by the settler community of political, social and economic goals that paid little attention to indigenous needs. Within the colonial society built by the settlers, the original inhabitants were ignored if they were sufficiently remote, or were offered a limited and marginal place, in a context of niggardly support for their welfare and high expectations of compliance with government control.

By 1860, a select committee inquiry recommended and legitimised an ongoing agenda of dispossession and inequality. It dismissed the traditional culture of the Aboriginal people as barbaric, declared them to be in need of 'civilising' and 'Christianising', and without the same claim on basic social and economic goods as other South Australians. Despite talk of 'amelioration' and 'advancement', it proposed levels of government support that allowed merely for survival, at best.[49] By 1911, as a result of the passage of the *Aborigines Act*, Aboriginal people were legally confirmed as not part of the public, a people whose needs were not those of the rest of the population and whose lives could be determined – unless they were still protected by geographic remoteness – by others, in fine and intrusive detail. This legislation and the regulations associated with it demonstrated that it was easier, or more consistent with non-indigenous priorities, to extend control over Aboriginal people than to provide for their 'advancement' or to respect their autonomy. It also constructed the indigenous population as an undifferentiated underclass with no diversity of capacity or expectation. By that time Christian missions were well established as partners in pursuing the government agenda of 'Christianising' and 'civilising', and in confirming, among Aboriginal people, a view of themselves consistent with the limited view adopted by many non-Aboriginals.[50]

---

48 Rowse, *Indigenous Futures*, p.236

49 See above, p.89

50 See above, pp.148–9. See also pp.92–4, where I warn against assuming that the impact of missions, or their relationship with government, was straightforward or uniform.

In 1939, changes in academic, government and public opinion about the capacities of the Aboriginals, and about the future that a society claiming to be humane and demo-cratic should offer them, were reflected in new legislation and new policy directions. Through the processes of 'breeding out' and 'socialising in', Aboriginal people were now to be 'assimilated', to 'take their place' within the general community, and to disappear as a separate group. This was assumed to be an unqualified boon to the indigenous population – indeed to be its salvation – and the policy contemplated no choice or alter-native futures. However, the persistent failure of the non-indigenous community to provide the means by which assimilation could occur ensured that the project foundered. It contributed to the production of the disadvantage and inequality that are associated with poor health by allowing for inclusion of only a few Aboriginal people, and only at the margins of the 'mainstream', while simultaneously disrupting some of the older structures, albeit limited and limiting, of stability and 'protection'.[51] The assimilation policy foundered also because some Aboriginals chose not to be 'assimilated'. In fact, the policy and the system of exemptions whereby some Aboriginals were declared to be no longer Aboriginal in the eyes of the law fuelled resistance. Refusing to disappear, some rejected the chance to 'become white' and claimed instead a distinctive and continuing indigenous identity.[52]

Over time, and especially from the 1970s, these claims to the right to choose to be members of the Australian community as well as to maintain a distinctive indigeneity have become increasingly confident and politicised. They have aroused concerns and fears among other Australians about special dealing and social division and have fuelled calls for a single, unified nation.[53] Government reactions to the failure of assimilation, to the tragic harvest of a history of exclusion and inequality, and to the emergence of an assertive indigenous sector have generally returned to older patterns of segregation and protection. They have lacked the imagination to see that maintenance of identity, cultural renovation and choice, *per se*, might be productive of health and even be a means to social and economic integration.

Where, then, is the place of indigenous people within the Australian public? In chapter four I suggested that, in the late nineteenth century, missionaries and protectors saw it as somewhere between the wurley and western civilisation.[54] It was a place of arrested development: it represented progress from the presumed darkness and barbarism of tra-dition, but not so far as to reach the enlightenment of modernity. Whether the failure to arrive at that goal was the result of innate lack of capacity or of historical circumstance, including the most recent historical circumstance of colonisation, was still a matter for debate. The finding and maintaining of that half-way place between the wurley and western civilisation involved compulsion, mission- or government-run segregated

---

51 See above, pp.204–7

52 See above, pp.182–3

53 See above, pp.184, 268–70

54 See above, p.104

settlements and restricted opportunities and choices, all of which resulted in marginalisation and profound inequality.

Later, during the period of assimilation, Australian governments attempted to find a
new place for indigenous Australians. They would leave behind both the wurley and the
controlled staging-post of mission or reserve and become part of the 'mainstream', indistinguishable from other Australians, living as 'members of a single Australian community'.
When Aboriginal people, perversely in the view of many non-indigenous Australians,
rejected this opportunity, preferring to 'lead a life of their own choice'[55], the question
about their place in Australian society emerged as more complicated and problematic than
previously supposed. Other Australians have been fearful of what it might mean for the
whole population if indigenous people, rejecting the offer of assimilation and taking
self-determination seriously, insist on their ongoing 'indigeneity' and their right to choose
a distinctive place for themselves, while also being part of the Australian public. This was
not a choice that non-indigenous Australians or their governments had expected, and as
discussion in this chapter has indicated, it has revealed deep uneasiness. But even when
such fear and uneasiness is outweighed by a genuine respect for indigenous choice, it still
presents all Australians with the fundamental challenge raised by self-determination.
This challenge is to find ways to support indigenous choice that are not associated with the
continuation of historically entrenched inequality, dependence and diminished life
chances.

This is ultimately a challenge about health in the broad sense in which health has been
understood in this book. There is little chance of Aboriginal Australians experiencing
better health until their autonomy and distinctiveness are recognised, respected and
accepted as reconcilable with their membership of the Australian public. And there is little
chance of this happening until the colonial and post-colonial history that constructed
them as not part of the public is understood, and until, as a nation, we respond to that
history by building the more equal, heterogeneous, inclusive and 'civic' society that
research now tells us is the basis of good health for all.

---

55 See above, pp.104, 183, 217

Summary of Australian Indigenous Health, February 2005

Australian Indigenous HealthInfoNet Summary of Australian Indigenous Health, February 2005.

INTRODUCTION

This summary includes facts about common health problems and risk factors among Australian Indigenous people. More detailed information about the health of Indigenous people, associated social and economic circumstances, and health risk factors, is available from the HealthInfoNet's website www.healthinfonet.ecu.edu.au

INDIGENOUS POPULATION

There were around 483,990 Indigenous people living in Australia in 2004 (around 432,560 Aboriginal people, 30,740 Torres Strait Islanders, and 20,690 people of both Aboriginal and Torres Strait Islander descent)[1, 2]. Indigenous people comprise around 2.4 per cent of the total Australian population. Most Indigenous people live in New South Wales, followed by Queensland, Western Australia, and the Northern Territory. The Northern Territory has the highest percentage of Indigenous people among its population and Victoria the lowest. Most Torres Strait Islander people live in Queensland, with New South Wales the only other state with a large number of Torres Strait Islanders.

The Indigenous population is much younger overall than the non-Indigenous population[2]. According to the 2001 Australian census, about 40 out of 100 Indigenous people were aged less than 15 years, compared with 20 out of 100 non-Indigenous people. About 3 out of 100 Indigenous people were aged 65 years or over, compared with 10 out of 100 non-Indigenous people.

BIRTHS

In 2003, there were 11,740 births registered in Australia where one or both parents were

---

1 Australian Bureau of Statistics (2003) *Australian demographic statistics quarterly.* March quarter 2003. (Cat. no. 3101.0), Canberra: Australian Bureau of Statistics.

2 Australian Bureau of Statistics (2004) *Experimental estimates and projections, Aboriginal and Torres Strait Islander Australians.* (Cat. no. 3238.0), Canberra: Australian Bureau of Statistics.

Indigenous (five out of every 100 births)[3]. Overall, Indigenous women had more children and had them at younger ages than did non-Indigenous women.

Based on the pattern of births in recent years, Indigenous women would have, on average, around 2.15 births in their lifetime, compared with less than 1.8 births for non-Indigenous women[3]. More than 52 out of 100 Indigenous women are 24 years or younger when they have their babies, compared with less than 18 out of 100 non-Indigenous women. More than 21 in 100 Indigenous mothers are teenagers, compared with less than 4 in 100 non-Indigenous mothers.

On average, babies born to Indigenous women in recent years have weighed around 200 grams less than those born to non-Indigenous women[4]. Babies born to Indigenous women are more than twice as likely to be of low birth weight (less than 2500 grams) than are those born to non-Indigenous women[4]. (Low birth weight can increase the risk of health problems.)

DEATHS

Indigenous people are much more likely to die before they are old than people in the rest of the Australian population[5]. Estimates from the Australian Bureau of Statistics (ABS) indicate that at birth an Indigenous male born in the period 1996–2001 could be expected to live to 59 years, which is around 17 years less than a male in the total population at that time (who had a life expectancy of 76.5 years). In the same period, an Indigenous female could be expected to live to 65 years, which is around 17 years less than a woman in the total population (82 years).

In 2003, there were 2079 people who died and were identified as Indigenous[5]. Many Indigenous deaths are incorrectly identified as non-Indigenous – the actual number of Indigenous deaths is likely to be around 3600.

Death rates relate the numbers of deaths to the total numbers of people. After taking account of the facts that the Indigenous population is much younger overall than the non-Indigenous population and that many Indigenous deaths are not identified as such, the death rates for Indigenous males and females are likely to be around four times higher than those of their non-Indigenous counterparts[6].

Indigenous babies are more likely to die in their first year than non-Indigenous babies[5]. In 2001–03, the infant mortality rate for Indigenous babies was highest in Western Australia (16 babies died out of 1000 births) and the Northern Territory (16 babies died out of 1000 births) and lowest in New South Wales (nine babies died out of 1000 births). (The rate for the total Australian population is around five deaths per 1000 births.)

In 2000–02 the leading causes of death for Indigenous people living in Queensland,

3 Australian Bureau of Statistics (2004) *Births, Australia 2003.* (cat no. 3301.0), Canberra: Australian Bureau of Statistics.

4 Laws PJ, Sullivan EA (2004) *Australia's mothers and babies 2001.* (AIHW cat. no. PER 25) Sydney: AIHW National Perinatal Statistics Unit.

5 Australian Bureau of Statistics (2004) *Deaths Australia 2003.* (Cat. no. 3302.0), Canberra: Australian Bureau of Statistics.

6 Thomson N, Ali M (2003) Births, deaths, and hospitalisation. In: Thomson N, ed. *The health of Indigenous Australians.* South Melbourne: Oxford University Press: 44–74.

Western Australia, South Australia and the Northern Territory were: cardiovascular disease (including heart disease and strokes); injuries (including transport accidents, self-harm and assault); cancer; respiratory diseases; and diabetes[7]. (More information about these causes of death is provided below).

SPECIFIC HEALTH CONDITIONS

CARDIOVASCULAR DISEASE

More than one in four deaths registered as Indigenous in recent years were caused by cardiovascular disease[7, 8]. Indigenous people are much more likely to die from cardiovascular disease than other Australians at any age, and particularly in younger age groups. The cardiovascular disease death rate among Indigenous people aged between 25 and 54 years is at least eight to ten times, and possibly as high as 15 times, that of other Australians[9]. In the 2001 National Health Survey (NHS), about one in ten Indigenous people reported having a long-term cardiovascular condition, particularly in older age groups[10]. The most commonly reported condition was hypertension (high blood pressure).

CANCER

It is not known just how many Indigenous people develop cancer, but notification rates for new cases have been lower for Indigenous people than for non-Indigenous people in recent years[9]. On the other hand, death rates for people living in Queensland, Western Australia and the Northern Territory are generally higher for Indigenous people than for non-Indigenous people (these rates take account of the fact that the Indigenous population is much younger overall than the non-Indigenous population)[9, 11].

The leading causes of Indigenous cancer deaths include cancers of the digestive organs and lung cancer [8, 12]. Indigenous people have higher rates of smoking-related cancers than non-Indigenous people[9, 11, 12]. Indigenous women have higher rates of cervical cancer than non-Indigenous women, but lower rates of breast cancer.*

The fact that Indigenous people are more likely than non-Indigenous people to die

---

7 Australian Institute of Health and Welfare (2004) *Australia's health 2004: the ninth biennial report of the Australian Institute of Health and Welfare*. Canberra: Australian Institute of Health and Welfare.

8 Australian Bureau of Statistics (2003) *Causes of Death 2002*. (Cat no. 3303.0) Canberra: Australian Bureau of Statistics.

9 Australian Bureau of Statistics, Australian Institute of Health and Welfare (2003) *The health and welfare of Australia's Aboriginal and Torres Strait Islander peoples 2003*. (ABS Cat no.4704.0, AIHW Cat no. IHW11) Canberra: Australian Bureau of Statistics

10 Australian Bureau of Statistics (2002) *National Health Survey: Aboriginal and Torres Strait Islander results, Australia 2001*. (Cat. no. 4715.0) Canberra: Australian Bureau of Statistics.

11 Kirov E, Francis J, Thomson N (2003) Cancer. In: Thomson N, ed. *The health of Indigenous Australians*. South Melbourne: Oxford University Press: 207–23.

12 Condon JR, Barnes T, Cunningham J, Armstrong BK (2004) Long-term trends in cancer mortality for Indigenous Australians in the Northern Territory. *Medical Journal of Australia*;180(10): 504–511.

* © Australian Indigenous HealthInfoNet 3 www.healthinfonet.ecu.edu.au

from cancer could be because the cancers they develop (such as cancers of the lung and liver) are more likely to be fatal, or that the stage of cancer may be more advanced by the time it is recognised[9, 11].

DIABETES

Diabetes is a major health problem among Indigenous people, but it is difficult to know just how many Indigenous people have the disease. The best evidence suggests that diabetes is between two and four times more common among Indigenous people than among non-Indigenous people[13]. Indigenous people are likely to be diagnosed with diabetes at a much lower age than non-Indigenous people[14].

Deaths from diabetes are much more common for Indigenous people than for non-Indigenous people[8]. In recent years in Queensland, Western Australia and the Northern Territory, diabetes accounted for 11 times as many deaths as expected for Indigenous males and 18 times as many deaths as expected for Indigenous females (based on total Australian male and female rates, but, as with other estimated death rates, the actual difference is likely to be up to 30 per cent greater)[9].

In the 2001 National Health Survey, five out of every 100 Indigenous people reported that they had diabetes as a 'long-term health condition'[10]. Indigenous people living in remote areas were more likely to report having diabetes than Indigenous people in other areas. (It should be noted that for every person who reports in surveys that they have diabetes it is likely that there is another person who doesn't know they have the disease[15].)

RENAL DISEASE

Renal disease, which affects the kidneys, has only recently been fully recognised as a serious public health threat to Indigenous people. End-stage renal disease (ESRD) occurs when the kidneys are no longer able to function. Rates of ESRD are much higher for Indigenous people than they are for non-Indigenous people across most of the country, and particularly in remote areas where they are up to 30 times higher[16]. Death rates from chronic kidney disease for people living in Queensland, Western Australia, South Australia and the

---

13 de Courten M, Hodge A, Dowse G, King I, Vickery J, Zimmet P (1998) Review of the epidemiology, aetiology, pathogenesis and preventability of diabetes in Aboriginal and Torres Strait Islander populations. Canberra: Commonwealth Department of Health and Family Services © Australian Indigenous HealthInfoNet 7 <www.healthinfonet.ecu.edu.au>

14 Couzos S, Metcalf S, Murray R, O'Rourke S (1998) *Systematic review of existing evidence and primary care guidelines on the management of non insulin dependent diabetes in Aboriginal and Torres Strait Islander populations.* Canberra: Office for Aboriginal and Torres Strait Islander Health Services, Commonwealth Department of Health and Family Services.

15 Dunstan D, Zimmet P, Welborn T, et al. (2001) *Diabesity and associated disorders in Australia, 2000: the accelerating epidemic.* Melbourne: International Diabetes Institute.

16 Cass A, Cunningham J, Wang Z, Hoy W (2001) Regional variation in the incidence of end-stage renal disease in Indigenous Australians. *Medical Journal of Australia;*175:24–27.

17 Australian Institute of Health and Welfare (2004) *Australian hospital statistics 2002–03.* (AIHW cat. no. HSE 32) Canberra: Australian Institute of Health and Welfare

Northern Territory in 1999–2001 were 8 times higher for Indigenous people than for non-Indigenous people[9].

Dialysis (the usual treatment for ESRD – where the work of the kidneys is done artificially) accounted for more than one-third of all hospital admissions among Indigenous people in 2002–03 (many of these involved repeat admissions for the same people, some on an almost daily basis)[17]. Indigenous people were 7.5 times more likely to be hospitalised for dialysis than non-Indigenous people. In recent years, almost half of all Indigenous ESRD patients have come from regions without dialysis or transplant facilities, and around one in six from regions with only satellite dialysis facilities.

INJURY
Indigenous people are more likely to die from transport accidents, intentional self-harm and assault than other Australians[8]. Injury was the second most common cause of death for Indigenous males living in Queensland, Western Australia, South Australia and the Northern Territory in 2000–02, and the fourth most common cause of death for Indigenous females – rates were around three times those of the total Australian populations (the actual difference is likely to be up to 30 per cent greater)[7].

Across Australia in 2002–03, Indigenous people were around twice as likely as other Australians to be admitted to hospital for injuries[17]. Assault was the leading cause of hospitalisation as a result of injury for both Indigenous males and females, followed by accidental falls. Other common causes of hospitalisation for injury were transport accidents (particularly for Indigenous males), complications of medical and surgical care and intentional self-harm. Hospitalisation rates for injury among Indigenous people were higher than those among non-Indigenous people in nearly every age group.*

RESPIRATORY DISEASE
About 1 in 11 of all deaths registered as Indigenous in recent years was due to a respiratory disorder[7, 8]. For Indigenous people living in Queensland, Western Australia, South Australia and the Northern Territory in 2000–02, deaths from these disorders were around four times more common than for non-Indigenous people (the actual difference is likely to be up to 30 per cent greater)[7]. In the 35 to 44-years age group, the death rates for Indigenous people were around 20 times higher for males and ten times higher for females than for other Australian males and females. In recent years, Indigenous people were more likely to be hospitalised for respiratory disease than non-Indigenous people, particularly in infancy and early childhood[17].

COMMUNICABLE DISEASES
It is compulsory for some communicable diseases to be notified. The state and territories collect the information which is then collated and published by the National Notifiable Disease Surveillance System. Indigenous status is often not reported in notifications and only the information from Western Australia, South Australia and the Northern Territory is believed to be complete enough for publication by Indigenous status[9]. Information for

---

Australian HIV/AIDS cases relates to all states and territories and is collated and published by the National Centre in HIV Epidemiology and Clinical Research[18].

Recent information about communicable diseases includes:

- tuberculosis: the rate of newly diagnosed cases for Indigenous people in 2003 was ten times the rate for Australian-born non-Indigenous people[19]
- Haemophilus influenzae type B: the notification rate in 2000–02 for Indigenous children aged less than five years was 14 times that for the total Australian population in that age group[20]
- meningococcal infection: the notification rate for Indigenous people living in New South Wales, Western Australia, South Australia and the Northern Territory in 2000–02 was around twice that of the total population of those states[20]
- syphilis and gonorrhoea: notification rates for Indigenous people living in Western Australia, South Australia and the Northern Territory in 2003 were between 50 and 100 times higher than those for the total Australian population[18]
- HIV/AIDS: notification rates for HIV infection and AIDS are similar for the Indigenous population and the non-Indigenous population[18].

EYE HEALTH

Eye conditions that affect the Indigenous population include refractive error (requiring glasses for correction), cataract (clouding of the lens), trachoma (a bacterial infection that can lead to blindness if untreated) and diabetic retinopathy (damage to the retina, at the back of the eye, caused by diabetes). There has been progress in the eye health of Indigenous people, but many Indigenous people are still more likely than non-Indigenous people to suffer from preventable conditions[21]. The frequency and severity of trachoma, for example, has decreased generally, but the infection is still quite common among Indigenous children living in some remote parts of the country.

The eye health of many Indigenous people is limited also by their difficulty in accessing specialised ophthalmological or optometrist services (because they are not available where they live, or are not culturally appropriate, or they are too expensive).

EAR CONDITIONS

According to the 2001 National Health Survey, almost one in five Indigenous people has some degree of hearing loss, compared with around one in seven non-Indigenous people[10].*

---

18 National Centre in HIV Epidemiology and Clinical Research (2004) *2004 annual surveillance report: HIV/AIDS, viral hepatitis and sexually transmissible infections in Australia.* Sydney: National Centre in HIV Epidemiology and Clinical Research

19 Li J, Roche P, Spencer J, and the National Tuberculosis Advisory Committee (2004) *Tuberculosis notifications in Australia, 2003.* Communicable Diseases Intelligence; 28(4): 464–73.

20 Menzies, R, McIntyre P, Beard F (2004) *Vaccine preventable diseases and vaccination coverage in Aboriginal and Torres Strait Islander people, Australia, 1999 to 2002.* Communicable Diseases Intelligence;28(2): 127–59.

21 Taylor HR (1997) *Eye health in Aboriginal and Torres Strait Islander communities: the report of a review commissioned by the Commonwealth Minister for Health and Family Services, the Hon. Michael Wooldridge, MP.* Canberra: Commonwealth Department of Health and Family Services.

* © Australian Indigenous HealthInfoNet 5 <www.healthinfonet.ecu.edu.au>

This higher frequency of hearing loss, reported for all age groups except people aged 55 years or older, reflects mainly the much higher levels of otitis media (middle ear disease) that Indigenous people experience in their childhood years. The actual levels vary considerably – geographically and over time – but it was estimated that in the mid-1990s around one in seven Indigenous children under ten years of age had a perforated eardrum[22]. This level puts Indigenous children within the World Health Organization's 'extremely high risk' category. Disease of the middle ear can cause permanent hearing loss that limits life opportunities, particularly in education and in employment[23, 24].

ORAL HEALTH

The oral health of Indigenous people generally is not as good as that of other Australians. In contrast to the situation for young non-Indigenous children, whose oral health has improved in recent years, that of young Indigenous children has generally declined[25]. (There may be differences across the country, however, as Indigenous children in remote areas appear to have better oral health than those in urban areas.) Partly because the overall level of dental care is lower for Indigenous people than for non-Indigenous people, their oral health deteriorates with age, contributing to higher frequencies of periodontal (gum) disease and tooth loss.

SKIN INFECTIONS AND INFESTATIONS

Skin infections, which are more common for Indigenous people than for non-Indigenous people, are often the result of poor living conditions. The most common skin infections affecting Indigenous people are scabies (caused by a mite) and streptococcal pyoderma (a bacterial infection)[26]. Scabies, in particular, is a problem in many remote Indigenous communities where up to half the children may be infected.

Skin diseases cause very few deaths directly, but they can be linked with serious complications. They did, however, account for around one of every 40 hospital separations in 2002–03 for patients identified as Indigenous, at a rate around 2.5 times that of non-Indigenous people[17].

FACTORS CONTRIBUTING TO ILL-HEALTH

Indigenous people generally experience more risk factors for ill-health than do other Australians. Contributing generally to the poor health status of many Indigenous people

22 Morris P (1998) A systematic review of clinical research addressing the prevalence, aetiology, diagnosis, prognosis and therapy of otitis media in Australian Aboriginal children [review]. *Journal of Paediatrics and Child Health*, 34(6): 487–97.

23 Couzos S, Metcalf S, Murray R (2003) Ear health. In: Couzos S, Murray R, eds. *Aboriginal primary health care: an evidence-based approach*. 2nd ed. South Melbourne: Oxford University Press: 193–250.

24 Burrow S, Thomson N (2003) Ear disease and hearing loss. In: Thomson N, ed. *The health of Indigenous Australians*. South Melbourne: Oxford University Press: 247–72.

25 Harford J, Spencer J, Roberts-Thomson K (2003) Oral health. In: Thomson N, ed. *The health of Indigenous Australians*. South Melbourne: Oxford University Press: 313–38.

26 Currie BJ, Carapetis, JR (2000) Skin infections and infestations in Aboriginal communities in northern Australia. *Australasian Journal of Dermatology*, 41(3): 139–45.

are: social factors such as dispossession, dislocation and discrimination; disadvantages in education, housing, income and employment; and physical environmental factors. These social, economic and environmental disadvantages underlie specific health risk factors (such as smoking, obesity, physical inactivity and high blood pressure) and often contribute to lack of access to good quality health care.

Given the importance of these factors, substantial improvements in Indigenous health status are unlikely to be achieved without improvements in the overall circumstances of Indigenous people.

SUMMARY

Indigenous people remain the least healthy sub-population in Australia, and there is evidence that the difference between Indigenous and non-Indigenous health, at least measured by mortality, has widened in recent years[27].

The reasons why the health status of Indigenous people remains much worse than that of non-Indigenous people are complex, but represent a combination of general factors – such as education, employment, income and status – and factors more specific to the health sector. As the Australian health ministers noted in their introduction to the 2003 National Strategic Framework for Aboriginal and Torres Strait Islander Health, achievement of substantial improvements in Indigenous health will depend on long-term collaborative approaches involving Indigenous leaders and communities, the health and non-health sectors, and all levels of government[28]. Within the health sector, there is a need for further improvement in: health advancement programs; identification of health conditions before they become serious; and expansion of primary health care services. To achieve long-term health benefits, funding needs to be directed to a wide range of preventive and clinical services. Funding should take account of the fact that mainstream services may not be accessible for many Indigenous people who may also have difficulty in accessing Medicare and pharmaceutical benefits. However, without substantial reductions in the overall disadvantages experienced by many Indigenous people, even fully committed approaches within the health sector will have a limited impact on achieving major improvements in Indigenous health status.*

---

27 Ring IT, Firman, D (1998) Reducing Indigenous mortality in Australia: lessons from overseas. *Medical Journal of Australia*;169: 528–33.

28 National Aboriginal and Torres Strait Islander Health Council (2003) *National Strategic Framework for Aboriginal and Torres Strait Islander Health: framework for action by governments*. Canberra: National Aboriginal and Torres Strait Islander Health Council.

Registrar General's Occupational Class Categories, as used in the *Black Report*

1. Professional (for example, accountant, doctor, lawyer) (5 per cent)[1]

11. Intermediate (for example, manager, nurse, school teacher) (18 per cent)

111N. Skilled non-manual (for example, clerical worker, secretary, shop assistant) (12 per cent)

111M. Skilled manual (for example, bus driver, butcher, carpenter, coalface worker (38 per cent)

1V. Partly skilled (for example, agricultural worker, bus conductor, postman) (18 per cent)

V. Unskilled (for example, cleaner, dock worker, labourer) (9 per cent)[2]

---

1 The percentages are of the total number of economically active and retired males.

2 Townsend, Davidson and Whitehead, *Inequalities in Health*, p.4

The Effectiveness of Mission Work:
a missionary's view

I am working as a missionary on the Kopperamanna Mission Station and have been living amongst the aboriginals of this colony for the past eleven years, so I was able by knowing their language to study their habits in different directions. At first I have to mention that I have been wondering to find nothing in the Bill about the missions which has [sic] worked now for thirty six years amongst the aboriginals to civilise and christianise them. It is not only my opinion when I say that the mission has protected the aboriginals well, it can be seen by everyone who visits the mission station that this affords the best protection for them, because, not only do we teach the aboriginals Christianity, but we also give them instructions so they may live a human life. Of course it is not a work that can be done in a few weeks; it takes years to make these wandering people settle down perfectly, but, as can be seen, the results of the mission work are great. Many of them started a new life altogether, and I only wish this honorable Committee would pay us a visit to see the progress of the mission work. It would not be necessary then to impress upon this honorable Committee to invite their attention beyond this – the interests of the mission. We keep the children separate, the girls being in one house and the boys in the other, like they would be in an institute. They are under the protection of one missionary when they are in their apartments. They have to rise at a certain time in the morning to learn cooking, prepare themselves for school and to do any handy work that will prove useful to them. The mission also appoints one English teacher to teach them writing, reading, arithmetic, singing, history, etc. I wish you gentlemen could see how happy these children are living. The married couples have their own cottages each of which consists of two rooms. The natives are washed and combed in a way they never experienced in their natural life. The lubras are cooking their meals, mending their clothes, as you will see in the picture, baking their bread, and looking after their children etc. The husband is employed in station work, just in the way that his ability or talent suits him. The old, sick and infirm aborigines, who are mostly unable to do anything, are kept on the station to enjoy a human life in their old age. It has often been told me by strange people who visited the station that they are glad to see how nicely the aboriginals have improved with us. It must not be forgotten that £80 000 has been spent by the mission for the promotion of the welfare of the blacks. They have also sent out the missionaries to civilise, christianise and educate the poor aboriginals, in order that they may have a better outlook for their future lives. Now, in looking over the bill, I found nothing about the mission station, and I do not know whether the Government will exclude it from its operations or not. We are subject to the same instructions as any other stations although we have protected the abo-riginals for many years, and stations which employ blacks for their own benefit only do not act fairly. Remembering the Australians are the inhabitants of the country of the blacks, the Government should do what the mission is doing today for the blacks. In my opinion the government should grant to the mission stations the powers of protectors to enable them to fully protect the aboriginals. The mission station of Kopperamanna is well known by all the blacks up to the Queensland border and as far down as any blacks are living. The Finke River Mission Station is also well known on this side of the MacDonnell Ranges. So I am sure if the Government would allow each mission station to have a pro-tector, the results would be more favourable to the blacks than is the case now. What an unpleasant thing it would be for the mission station if the missionaries were compelled to abide by the provisions of clause 9, and go to a protector every twelve months to get a new agreement for every blackfellow. If the terms of clause 9 were enforced it would be impossible for the mission to do its duty. I doubt if any other stations are able to protect the blacks as they are compelled to do, there being no way to educate them in reading and writing, so that they may be able to understand an agreement. The aforesaid stations only employ well-bodied, strong blacks, but do not look to the old and infirm inhabitants. And I ask is it not the duty of the Government to protect the old and infirm as well as the young ones? If the government intends to protect the blacks, they should look to their education, but who does give them this education? Again, the mission only. I know that many of the white people do not pay much regard to the education of the blacks; they do not want to see a blackfellow educated, because were his mind trained at all it would not be so easy to cheat him. Not so long ago a blackfellow came to me with a piece of paper which had been given to him as a cheque for the payment of dog scalps. It turned out to be a ticket for horse racing. While the mission is the only place in the North where the aboriginals can be educated and protected as well as it is possible for them to be, the Government should go hand and hand with the mission, thereby promoting the welfare of the blacks. The provisions of this Bill are only practicable where educated aboriginals or half-castes – such as we have on our station – are concerned. What does a wild black-fellow know of an agreement, a period of twelve months, or of money given to him by means of a cheque? As he cannot read or write, he can neither understand an agreement, nor can he sign any certificate.[1]

---

1 Rev. John George Reuther, Lutheran missionary, Kopperamanna Mission Station on the effectiveness of mission work.
   Evidence before 1899 Select Committee inquiry on the Aborigines Bill, in Report of Protector of Aborigines, 30 June 1908,
   SAPP, no. 30 of 1910.

Appendix 4

Taplin's 1874 Advice
to Government

1. I do not see any decrease in the numbers of the aborigines since 1867; there was then a great muster of them and I do not think the tribes have grown less since then. This matter will soon be put to the test with the valuable help of my coadjutor, James Unaipon. I am going to make a register of every native in the Narrinyeri nation.

2. The health of the natives is better than it used to be. I attribute this to the more prompt medical assistance which they receive now. Those who now suffer most are those who now frequent the townships and the public-houses. Those who hang about Adelaide always return here in a low state of health. I have known of several deaths in past years which resulted from drunken exposure on the Adelaide Park Lands. It would be a work of mercy if the Government would direct the police to order the natives out of Adelaide. They have no right there; it is not their territory; and if the white man had not come here they would probably never have seen the ground on which the city stands.

3. Our great difficulty at present is the obtaining employment for the natives. Our location here would afford more employment if we had funds to expend in providing food and clothes for the workers, but unless we receive greater assistance from the government than we have done that is impossible.

   I hope the Government will benevolently grant us the means of making this station a better source of employment for the aborigines. At shearing time the natives are pretty well employed; they eagerly get all the shearing they can and are good and careful shearers; but the shearing time only lasts two months or so, and then they are not needed, except for a week or so, for dogging, and one or two men as boundary riders. At harvest time about half the natives are employed for about six weeks; at seed time a few get work at grubbing and clearing. These are the sources of employment outside this station.

   In proof of their eagerness for employment I may state that a lot of them are now dogging sheep for six shillings a week and rations. This job will last a fortnight perhaps.

   If we did not assist the unemployed natives I do not know what would be the result; I fear their starvation. Game around the Lakes has greatly decreased in number and are more difficult to get. Fish are much scarcer than they used to be, strange to say.

The land is all enclosed in sheep paddocks, and hunting almost impossible.

Nevertheless, if the natives are fraternally cared for and provided with employ-ment I do not think they need become an extinct race. I foresee that if employment is provided for them and homes, they may yet become a useful class of the community.

4. We very much need houses for them. Those we have are crowded. There are at least a dozen couples who require dwellings. One native is now having a house built for himself and another has built himself one; but only a few are able to do this. We have twelve cottages at present all fully occupied.

I have been informed that there is a probability of the Government introducing some special legislation for the aborigines. May I be allowed to make a few suggestions relative to this matter, which have occurred to me from my experience?

I. Might not something be done to give the natives a clear right to some portions of the land? As settlement increases they gradually get pushed off their country until they have not a place to build a hut upon. This was the case with these natives here until the Reserves were declared by the Government.

    The aboriginal reserves which are let are often in unsuitable places for native occupation. A well-wooded situation where there is game would always be the best. There are some pieces of land on the Coorong well adapted for this purpose. If ever surveys are carried on there while natives survive this might be borne in mind.

II. Some law ought to be enacted to forbid the giving or selling of poison to the natives. Our natives tell us that the Lacepede Bay natives get strychnine from the boundary riders and use it where they wish to gratify their desire for revenge upon other natives who may have offended them.

III. It will be remembered that some time ago the law officers of the Crown declared that the occupation licences under which some of the natives held certain sections of land were invalid, because illegal. Might not some measure be devised by which the Government could give a legal tenure to aboriginal natives, so that they might occupy their land of right and not merely by sufferance.

IV. It is exceedingly desirable that the aborigines should be compelled to send their children to school to be educated. Of course this could only be done where there are native schools. Natives do not see the good of education – that is, old natives – but they would respect a government measure. Such compulsory education would prevent interested white people from persuading natives not to send their children to school, because they want them as cheap servants. Of course, the more employment natives get the better, but yet it is desirable their employment should be preceded by sufficient schooling to teach them to read and write.

V. A law to facilitate the adoption of half-caste and quadroon children by benevo-lent white people would do much good. I mean a law which would render valid the conveyance of the child to the person adopting it and secure the child against going back to the tribe.

VI. The present law with reference to intoxicating drinks is very inadequate. The punishment for supplying the natives ought to be made more severe, and drunkenness of natives ought to be punished.

VII. Native customs which are injurious and a nuisance to either natives or whites ought to be prohibited, especially in settled districts. Of course every custom complained of must be taken on its own merits, but yet the general principle should be laid down.

VIII. Provision should be made that where an aboriginal native is brought before a Magistrate or a Court of Justice, an interpreter should be provided if possible. I know that in some cases mistakes have arisen from want of one. This will occur in the Northern Territory to a certainty if some one does not learn the language and customs of the aborigines there.

IX. Some means of summarily trying and convicting on the spot natives in the far interior who may commit crimes are necessary, but yet great care will be necessary lest their accusers be their judges. Prejudice against them is often very strong on distant stations.

X. It is very desirable that the aborigines should be forbidden to frequent Adelaide; it is a fruitful source of evil to them.

XI. The law with reference to their dogs should be altered; they are at present an awful nuisance; they destroy many sheep and lambs. I would suggest that the officers in charge of the aborigines should have a certain number of dog licences given them to issue gratis to the aborigines, and also collars, and that only those dogs which have the collars be allowed, and all others destroyed. This would moderate the nuisance and would really do no harm to the aborigines.[1]

---

1 Rev. George Taplin, Superintendent, Point McLeay Mission, Report for half-year ended 30 June 1874, *SAGG*, 20 August 1874, pp.1667–68

Minutes of Special Meeting of Aborigines Protection Board, 18 May 1956

Present: Professor JB Cleland, Deputy Chairman
Mrs W Ternent Cooke
Mrs Harvey Johnston
Rev. Gordon Rowe
Mr CE Bartlett
Apology received from Mr AJK Walker

Minutes: The minutes of the meeting held on 16 May 1956 were not confirmed as members had not had the opportunity of perusing them.

Definition of Aborigines Protection Board Policy: A.D 11/56
A statement of Policy of the Aborigines protection board was considered. The secretary reported that during 1941 a Policy Statement was issued and accepted as being in accord with overall Government Policy. Since that time certain modifications have been made and as monies have been provided by the Government it was presumed that these modifications received Government approval. The policy of the Board is the promotion of the welfare of aborigines to a standard whereat they are considered capable of complete assimilation into the white community. This is necessarily a wide range policy, brought about by the wide diversity existing between the unsophisticated primitive full-blood through a wide range of degrees to the highly sophisticated part aborigine. It is recognised that there is a rate of change beyond which a backward people cannot be pushed without great risk. It must be understood that such a task demands an adequate staff of great ability, suitably educated and experienced. After discussion the Board agreed that in order to achieve the objective of total assimilation the following policy would be adopted: –
1. The provision of vocational training facilities which will carry the children from the close of their primary school years up to the time when they have become fitted to obtain their livelihood in the community in various fields of employment. These fields include station and farm work, carpentry, joinery, plumbing and sheet metal work, motor mechanics or similar trades, domestic training, nursing, shorthand typists, physical culture, masseurs etc. In planning such training, the advice, assistance and co-operation of the Departments of Education and Agriculture will be necessary.

2. The provision of assistance to gain suitable employment for all aborigines, including those living at Point Pearce and Point McLeay reserves. Natives going out to employment require special consideration to enable them to be established in a white community.
3. The erection by the South Australian Housing Trust of twelve Trust homes, or more, each year in suitable country towns where there is available a continuity of employment, for allocation to selected aboriginal families.
4. Erection by the Aborigines Department of improved accommodation to replace unhygienic and unsanitary tin shacks and primitive encampments on Aboriginal Reserves, for allocation to selected aboriginal families.
5. Where necessary, the acquisition of suitable blocks of land and the development of Aboriginal Reserves as poultry farms, market gardens, small unit farms and fishing reaches, to be ultimately conducted by selected aboriginal families after suitable training in their efficient management.
6. The establishment of Campbell House as a training institution for aboriginal youths who will be trained in agriculture and pastoral pursuits to fit them for employment in country areas or for further agricultural training in such institutions as Roseworthy Agricultural College.
7. The depopulation of Point Pearce and Point McLeay, leading to the eventual establishment of havens for the aged and infirm aborigines and farms of suitable areas for selected natives.
8. The development of Point Pearce, sections of Point McLeay and Aboriginal Reserves operated by Missions on a share-farming basis with aborigines, leading to the ultimate establishment of unit farms operated by aborigines.
9. a. The provision of grants in aid to missions for improvement of living conditions and physical welfare of aborigines, where in the opinion of the Board such Missions are able to satisfactorily care for the aborigines.
9. b. Where in the opinion of the Board the living conditions, physical welfare, health, and advancement of the aborigines ar4e not provided for to the satisfaction of the Board by a Mission, such Mission or institution to be taken over by the Board, and, if necessary, maintained and controlled by the Department.
10. Medical supervision of health of aborigines of South Australia.
11. Provision of supplementary ration scales consistent with local needs of each group of aborigines and the issue of relief to necessitous aborigines where deemed necessary by the Department.

    The Board further agreed to this policy statement to be forwarded to the Honourable the minister for approval of the Government, and recommended the appointment of two male Welfare Officers (or Patrol Officers) and other staff as a beginning to implement the policy outlined.

Control of Neglected and Destitute Aboriginal Children. A.D. 19/56

At a meeting of the Board held on 3 February 1956 the Board agreed:-
1. Primarily the Aborigines Protection Board must accept the responsibility of control, welfare, maintenance and education of aboriginal children.

2. Should a child be neglected etc. the Aborigines Protection Board must make every endeavour to improve the situation.

3. If not successful:
   a. Full blooded aboriginal children to be committed to an institution under the control of the Children's Welfare and Public Relief Board (section 38 (1), Aborigines Act.
   b. Part aboriginal children to be charged as 'neglected' children through the Courts as are white children (Maintenance Act).

4. Where possible, aboriginal and white children to be placed in homes in approximately even numbers.

These recommendations were forwarded to the Children's Welfare and Public Relief Board and have now been returned. The Chairman of the Children's Welfare and Public Relief Board has now advised that his Board, after carefully considering the difficulties of adequately controlling and caring for aboriginal children, was of the opinion that these children should be provided for in the following manner:-

a. The part aboriginal, whether exempted or not, who is living a fairly independent life, earning and paying rates and taxes, should be accepted into our community life. Neglected or destitute children from this group should be subject to the same court orders as other children and should continue to be placed, when necessary, in our departmental institutions with white children.

b. All other destitute or neglected aboriginal or part aboriginal children should continue to be the responsibility of the Aborigines Protection Board. In some cases, e.g. myall aborigines living in a tribal life, etc., it would be unthinkable to remove the children from their parents. In others it seems hardly right to expect this Department to admit these children into departmental institutions when it has no power or authority in the matter of improving their usual living conditions.

The Children's Welfare and Public Relief Board, in addition, suggested and preferred that the Aborigines Protection Board endeavour to establish institutions and seek any legislative authority deemed necessary to adequately control and care for destitute aboriginal children. The Board are aware that throughout the State there are native children who are neglected, and that with the limited staff at the disposal of the Department little can at present be done. Further that the Aborigines Protection Board has no authority to remove such children from their parents other than that provided under Section 38(i) of the Aborigines Act, which is not acceptable to the Children's Welfare and Public Relief Board. As the Aborigines Act charges this Board with the duty of controlling and promoting the welfare of aborigines and in providing that the board shall be the legal guardian of every aboriginal child, it would appear that primarily the Board should provide for the control, welfare, maintenance and education of aboriginal children. The present position is that where a child is destitute or neglected, this Board has no authority to correct the situation. Board members realise that these conditions have existed for many yeas with neither the Children's Welfare nor the Aborigines Protection Board accepting responsibility. This Board is charged with certain duties which it cannot carry out without the necessary legal authority, or with the limited staff available to the department. In the meantime these children remain neglected and, to a large extent, uncared for. Should this Board eventually agree to accept the responsibility of promoting the welfare and control of this type of child, the following action would be necessary:-

1. The Aborigines Act to be amended and additional legislation would be needed to give this Board all the necessary powers to care for, protect, maintain and educate aboriginal children, as is at present vested in the Children's Welfare and Public Relief Board in regard to neglected white children.

2. Additional staff would be required as welfare officers, probation officers, a prosecuting officer, etc.

3. Institutions established and staffed, at least one for girls, one for boys, and a home for infants.

After consideration it was agreed that the whole mater is one for consideration by the Honourable the Minister as, to a large extent, it is a question of Government policy. The Honourable the Minister may wish to discuss these matters with the Minister in control of the Children's Welfare and Public Relief Board and/or submit this matter to Cabinet for expression of Government Policy.[1]

---

1 Minutes of the Special Meeting of the Aborigines Protection Board held in the Secretary's Office, Kintore Avenue, Adelaide, on Friday 18 May 1956, at 11a.m.

Summary of Aboriginal Reserves and Missions, 1972

Reserve or Mission	Area	Total Population at 30th June, 1972	Staff (Departmental and Mission)		Number of School Pupils		Employed as at 30th June, 1972	Number of Aboriginal Houses
			Established Positions	Positions Filled	Primary	Secondary		
Coober Pedy Aboriginal Reserve[1]	1 sq. mile	275	3	3	50	10	8[2]	10
Davenport Aboriginal Reserve[3]	200 acres	206	9	9	46	9	45	32
Gerard Aboriginal Reserve[4]	4,833 acres	96	5	5	17	6	19	24
Indulkana Aboriginal Reserve[5]	9,000 acres	293	7	7	38	-	32	2
Koonibba Aboriginal Reserve[6]	2,200 acres[7]	190	8	8	64	9	26	36
North-west Aboriginal Reserve[8]	27,620 sq. miles	319	11	9	83	-	47	8
Point McLeay Aboriginal Reserve[9]	2,716 acres	140	4	4	49	15	20	25
Point Pearce Aboriginal Reserve[10]	13,591 acres	275	9	7	81	37	43	58
Yalata Mission[11]	1,761 sq. miles	419	15	15	90	-	36	7
Ernabella Mission[12]	2,400 sq. miles	550	22	22	91	-	99	4
Nepabunna Mission[13]	31.5 sq. miles	84	5	5	21	-	18	13

1 Adjoins Eastern boundary of township

2 Excludes persons self-employed in mining or noodling for opal.

3 Two miles from Port Augusta

4 Five miles from Winkie

5 160 miles North-West of Oodnadatta

6 25 miles west of Ceduna

7 With 18,000 acres on lease

8 North-west corner of State; major centre – Amata

9 28 miles from Meningie

10 13 miles South-west of Maitland

11 126 North-West of Ceduna

12 80 miles East of Amata

13 40 miles East of Leigh Creek

SOURCE: Appendix to the Report of the Director-General of Community Welfare, for the year ended 30 June 1972, *SAPP*, 1972, vol.2, no.23, p.48

Distribution of Estimated Aboriginal Population in South Australia, 1972

Area	Totals
Metropolitan Area –	
Adelaide*	3,400
Far North –	
Coober Pedy	278
Ernabella Mission	550
Indulkana	293
North-West	319
Oodnadatta and Stations	187
Others*	220
Area Totals	1,847
Mid-North –	
Davenport	208
Nepabunna Mission	84
Umeewarra Mission	39
Port Augusta Area*	1,300
Leigh Creek Area	426
Others*	260
Area Totals	2,317
Yorke Peninsula –	
Point Pearce	274
Others*	100
Area Totals	374
West Coast –	
Ceduna Area	193
Koonibba	190
Port Lincoln Area	360
Yalata Mission	419
Area Totals	1,162
Murray Valley and South-East –	
Berri Area	184
Gerard	96
Point McLeay	140
Others*	260
Area Totals	680
State Totals*	9,780

* Estimates have been made where exact figures are not available

SOURCE: Appendix to the Report of the Director-General of Community Welfare,

for the year ended 30 June 1972, *SAPP*, 1972, vol.2, no.23, p.47

Bibliography

PUBLISHED

OFFICIAL PUBLICATIONS

SOUTH AUSTRALIAN

Aboriginal Affairs Board, Annual Reports: *SAPP*, 1962–1971

Aborigines Protection Board, Annual Reports: *SAPP*, 1940–1962

Good Health for South Australia (also published as *Public Health Notes, Health Notes, Health Notes for South Australia, Good Health*), Department of Public Health, South Australia, 1932–1977

Protector of Aborigines, Reports:

    Fifth Annual Report of the Colonization Commissioners for South Australia, British Parliamentary Papers relating to Australia 1842–1844, 1839–1841

    SAGG, 1841–1901

    South Australian Aborigines Department Reports, 1902–3 – 1936–7, 1902–1937

    SAPP, 1908–1940

Reports of Department of Social Welfare and Aboriginal Affairs, Department of Community Welfare: *SAPP*, 1971–1973

Report of the Select Committee of the Legislative Council upon 'the Aborigines', together with minutes of evidence and appendix, 16 October 1860: *SAPP*, no.165, 1860

Report of the Select committee of the Legislative Council on the Aborigines Bill, together with minutes of proceedings, *SAPP*, no.77A, 1899

Report of the Royal Commission on the Aborigines, together with minutes of proceedings, evidence and appendices, 1912

    Progress Report, 7 October 1913: *SAPP*, no.26, 1913

    Final Report, 3 October 1916: *SAPP*, no.21, 1916

Report of the Committee of Enquiry into Health Services in South Australia (CH Bright, Chairman), Government Printer, Adelaide, 1973

OTHER

Acheson, Sir Donald. *Independent Inquiry into Inequalities in Health Report*, The Stationery Office, London, 1999 [1998]

Bleakley, JW. *Report, 1928: The Aboriginals and Half-Castes of Central Australia and North Australia*, Government Printer, Victoria, 1929

Gale, Fay and Binnion, Joan. *Poverty among Aboriginal Families in Adelaide*, research report prepared for the Commission of Inquiry into Poverty, Australian Government Publishing Service, Canberra, 1975

Commonwealth Bureau of Census and Statistics. *The Aboriginal Population of Australia: a summary of characteristics*, Census of the Commonwealth of Australia, 30 June 1966, Canberra, 1969

Commonwealth Bureau of Census and Statistics. *Official Year Book of the Commonwealth of Australia*: 1908–2004, Melbourne/Canberra

House of Representatives Standing Committee on Aboriginal Affairs. 'Aboriginal Health', *Commonwealth of Australia Parliamentary Paper*, no.60, 1979

Human Rights and Equal Opportunity Commission. *Bringing Them Home: report of the National Inquiry into the Separation of Aboriginal and Torres Strait Islander children from their families*, Commonwealth of Australia, Canberra, 1997

Senate Community Affairs Committee. *Forgotten Australians: a report on Australians who experienced institutional or out-of-home care as children*, Commonwealth of Australia, Canberra, 2004

Smith, LR. *Aboriginal Vital Statistics: an analysis of trends*, Commonwealth Department of Health Aboriginal Health Bulletin, no.1, Australian Government Publishing Service, Canberra, 1980

ABORIGINAL HEALTH POLICY DOCUMENTS

Aboriginal Health Council of South Australia Inc. and South Australian Health Commission. *Dreaming Beyond 2000: our future is in our history. South Australian Aboriginal health policy and strategic framework*, Aboriginal Health Council of South Australia Inc. and South Australian Health Commission, Adelaide, 1994

National Aboriginal Health Strategy Working Party. *A National Aboriginal Health Strategy*, Australian Government Publishing Service, Canberra, 1989

National Aboriginal Health Strategy Evaluation Committee. *The National Aboriginal Health Strategy: an evaluation*, Australian Government Publishing Service, Canberra, 1994

National Aboriginal and Torres Strait Islander Health Council. *National Strategic Framework for Aboriginal and Torres Strait Islander Health: framework for action by governments*, Australian Government Publishing Service, Canberra, 2003

South Australian Aboriginal Health Partnership. *The First Step: South Australian Aboriginal health regional plans*, South Australian Aboriginal Health Partnership, Adelaide, 1998.

BOOKS/BOOK CHAPTERS

Anderson, Warwick. *The Cultivation of Whiteness: science, health and racial destiny in Australia*, Melbourne University Press, Melbourne, 2002

Attwood, Bain. *The Making of the Aborigines*. Allen and Unwin, Sydney, 1989

Attwood, Bain and Markus, Andrew, in collaboration with Dale Edwards and Kath Schilling. *The 1967 Referendum, or when Aborigines didn't get the vote*, Australian Institute of Aboriginal and Torres Strait Islander Studies, Canberra, 1997

Attwood, Bain and Foster SG (eds). *Frontier Conflict: the Australian experience*, National Museum of Australia, 2003

Attwood Bain and Foster SG. 'Introduction', in Attwood, Bain and Foster SG (eds). *Frontier Conflict: the Australian experience*, National Museum of Australia, 2003, pp.1–30

Barnes, Nancy. *Munyi's Daughter: a spirited Brumby*, Seaview Press, Adelaide, 2000

Basedow, Herbert. *The Australian Aboriginal*, FW Preece and Sons, Adelaide, 1929 [1925]

Bennett, MM. *The Australian Aboriginal as a Human Being*, Alston Rivers Ltd., London, 1930

Bennett, Scott. *Aborigines and Political Power*, Allen and Unwin, Sydney, 1992

Berndt, Catherine H. 'Out of the Frying Pan . . . or, back to square one?' in Berndt RM (ed.), *Aborigines and Change: Australia in the '70s*, Australian Institute of Aboriginal Studies, Canberra, 1977, pp.402–11

Berndt RM (ed.). *Aborigines and Change: Australia in the '70s*, Australian Institute of Aboriginal Studies, Canberra, 1977

Berndt, Ronald M. 'Aboriginal Identity: reality or mirage?' in Berndt RM (ed.), *Aborigines and Change: Australia in the '70s*, Australian Institute of Aboriginal Studies, Canberra, 1977, pp.1–12

Berndt, Ronald and Catherine. *From Black to White in South Australia*, FW Cheshire, Melbourne, 1951

Blacket, Rev. John. *History of South Australia: a romantic and successful experiment in colonization*, second edition, Hussey and Gillingham, Adelaide, 1911

Blainey, Geoffrey. *The Triumph of the Nomads: a history of ancient Australia*, Sun Books, Melbourne, 1976

Blane, David, Brunner, Eric and Wilkinson, Richard (eds). *Health and Social Organization: towards a health policy for the twenty-first century*, Routledge, London, 2000 [1996]

Blane, David, Brunner, Eric and Wilkinson, Richard. 'The Evolution of Public Health Policy: an anglocentric view of the last fifty years' in Blane, David, Brunner, Eric and Wilkinson, Richard (eds), *Health and Social Organization: towards a health policy for the twenty-first century*, Routledge, London, 2000 [1996], pp.1–17

Bourke, Colin, Bourke, Eleanor and Edwards, Bill (eds). *Aboriginal Australia: an introductory reader in Aboriginal studies*, (second edition), University of Queensland Press, St Lucia, Queensland, 1998

Briscoe, Gordon and Smith, Len. 'The Aboriginal Population in South Australia, 1921–1944', in Briscoe, Gordon and Smith, Len (eds), *The Aboriginal Population Revisited: 70 000 years to the present*, Aboriginal History Monograph 10, Aboriginal History Inc., Canberra, 2002, pp.16–40

Brock, Peggy. *Outback Ghettos: a history of Aboriginal institutionalisation and survival*, Cambridge University Press, Melbourne, 1993

Brodie, Veronica, as told to Mary-Anne Gale. *My Side of the Bridge*, Wakefield Press, Adelaide, 2002

Broome, Richard. *Aboriginal Australians: black response to white dominance, 1788–1994*, (second edition), Allen and Unwin, Sydney, 1994

Cockburn, Stewart, assisted by John Playford. *Playford: benevolent despot*, Axiom Publishing, Adelaide, 1991

Coghlan, TA. *Labour and Industry in Australia: from the first settlement in 1788 to the establishment of the Commonwealth in 1901*, vols I–IV, Oxford University Press, Melbourne, 1918

Cooke, Constance M Ternent. 'The Status of Aboriginal Women in Australia' [1930], in Jenkin, Graham (ed.), *Between the Wars: documents relating to Aboriginal affairs, 1919–1939*, South Australian College of Advanced Education, Magill, South Australia, 1989, pp.101–15

Couzos, Sarah and Murray, Richard, for the Kimberley Aboriginal Medical Services Council. *Aboriginal Primary Health Care: an evidence-based approach*, Oxford University Press, Melbourne, 1999

Cumpston, JHL. *Health and Disease in Australia: a history* [1928], introduced and edited by MJ Lewis, Australian Government Publishing Service, Canberra, 1989

Dagmar, Hans. 'Development and Politics in an Interethnic Field: Aboriginal interest associations', in Tonkinson, Robert and Howard, Michael (eds). *Going it Alone? Prospects for Aboriginal Autonomy:*

essays in honour of Ronald and Catherine Berndt, Aboriginal Studies Press, Canberra, 1990, pp.99–123

Dickey, Brian and Howell, Peter. *South Australia's Foundation: select documents*, Wakefield Press, Adelaide, 1986

Dugüid, Charles, *No Dying Race*, Rigby, Adelaide, 1963

Dugüid, Charles, *Doctor and the Aborigines*, Rigby, Adelaide, 1972

Elkin, AP. 'Introduction', in Berndt, Ronald and Catherine. *From Black to White in South Australia*, FW Cheshire, Melbourne, 1951, pp.11–17

Elmslie, Ronald G and Nance, Susan. 'Smith, William Ramsay (1859–1939), in Serle, Geoffrey (ed.), *Australian Dictionary of Biography*, vol.11, Melbourne University Press, Carlton, Victoria, 1988, pp.674–5

Foster, Robert, Hosking, Rick and Nettelbeck, Amanda. *Fatal Collisions: the South Australian frontier and the violence of memory*, Wakefield Press, Adelaide, 2001

Forte, Margaret. *Flight of an Eagle: the dreaming of Ruby Hammond*, Wakefield Press, Adelaide, 1995

Gale, Fay. 'Administration as Guided Assimilation (South Australia)', in Marie Reay (ed.). *Aborigines Now: new perspectives in the study of Aboriginal communities*, Angus and Robertson Ltd, Sydney, 1964, pp.101–14

Gale, Fay and Wundersitz Joy. *Adelaide Aborigines: a case study of urban life, 1966–1981*, Australian National University, Canberra, 1982

Greenway, John. *Bibliography of the Australian Aborigines and the Native Peoples of the Torres Strait*, Angus and Robertson, Sydney, 1963

Haebich, Anna. *For Their Own Good: Aborigines and government in the south west of Western Australia, 1900–1940* (third edition), University of Western Australia Press, Nedlands, 1998

Haebich, Anna. *Broken Circles: fragmenting indigenous families, 1800–2000*, Fremantle Arts Centre Press, Fremantle, 2000

Harmstorf, Ian. 'Basedow, Herbert (1881–1933)', in Nairn, Bede and Serle, Geoffrey (eds), *Australian Dictionary of Biography*, vol.7, Melbourne University Press, Carlton, Victoria, 1979, pp.202–3

Harris, John. *One Blood. 200 years of Aboriginal encounter with Christianity: a story of hope* (second edition), Albatross Books, Sutherland, New South Wales, 1994

Hicks, Neville. 'Cure and Prevention', in Curthoys, Ann, Martin AW and Rowse, Tim (eds), *Australians From 1939*, Fairfax, Syme and Weldon Associates, Sydney, 1987, pp.329–41

Hodder, Edwin. *The History of South Australia from its Foundation to the Year of its Jubilee with a Chronological Summary of all the Principal Events of Interest up to Date*, vol.11, Sampson Low, Marston and Company, London, 1893

Hunt, Arnold D. 'Blacket, John (1856–1935)', in Nairn, Bede and Serle, Geoffrey (eds), *Australian Dictionary of Biography*, vol.7, Melbourne University Press, Carlton, Victoria, 1979, pp.312–13

Hunter, Ernest. *Aboriginal Health and History: power and prejudice in remote Australia*, Cambridge University Press, Melbourne, 1993

Huxley, Julian S and Haddon, AC. *We Europeans: a survey of 'racial' problems*, Jonathan Cape, London, 1936

Inglis, Judy. 'Dispersal of Aboriginal families in South Australia (1860–1960)', in Marie Reay (ed.). *Aborigines Now: new perspectives in the study of Aboriginal communities*, Angus and Robertson Ltd, Sydney, 1964, pp.115–32

Jenkin, Graham. *Conquest of the Ngarrindjeri*, Raukkan Publishers, Point McLeay, South Australia, 1995 [1979]

Jones, Philip.'Unaipon, David (1872–1967)', in Ritchie, John (ed.), *Australian Dictionary of Biography*, vol.12, Melbourne University Press, Carlton, Victoria, 1990, pp.303–5

Kawachi, Ichiro, Kennedy, Bruce P and Wilkinson, Richard G (eds). *The Society and Population Health Reader, vol.1: Income Inequality and Health*, The New York Press, New York, 1999

Kawachi, Ichiro, Kennedy, Bruce P and Wilkinson, Richard G, 'Introduction', in Kawachi, Ichiro, Kennedy, Bruce P and Wilkinson, Richard G, (eds). *The Society and Population Health Reader, vol.1: Income Inequality and Health*, The New York Press, New York, 1999, pp.xi–xxiv

Kidd, Rosalind. *The Way We Civilise: Aboriginal affairs – the untold story*, University of Queensland Press, St Lucia, Queensland, 1997

Kritzman, Lawrence D (ed.). *Michel Foucault: politics, philosophy, culture. Interviews and other writings, 1977–1984*, Routledge, London, 1988

Kunitz, Stephen J. *Disease and Social Diversity: the European impact on the health of non-Europeans*, Oxford University Press, New York, 1994

Lewis, Milton J. *The People's Health: public health in Australia, 1788–1950* (vol.1) and *1950 to the present* (vol.2), Praeger, Connecticut, 2003

Lloyd, Moya and Thacker, Andrew (eds). *The Impact of Michel Foucault on the Social Sciences and Humanities*, Macmillan, Basingstoke, 1997

McGrath, Anne. *'Born in the Cattle': Aborigines in cattle country*, Allen and Unwin, Sydney, 1987

McGrath, Anne (ed.). *Contested Ground: Australian Aborigines under the British crown*, Allen and Unwin, Sydney, 1995

McGregor, Russell. *Imagined Destinies: Aboriginal Australians and the doomed race theory, 1880–1939*, Melbourne University Press, Carlton, Victoria, 1997

Marmot, Michael. 'The Social Pattern of Health and Disease', in Blane, David, Brunner, Eric and Wilkinson, Richard (eds). *Health and Social Organization: towards a health policy for the twenty-first century*, Routledge, London, 2000 [1996], pp.42–67

Marmot, Michael and Wilkinson, Richard G. *Social Determinants of Health*, Oxford University Press, Oxford, 1999

Mathers, Colin, assisted by Merton, Carolyn. *Health Differentials Among Adult Australians Aged 25–64 Years*, Australian Institute of Health and Welfare Monitoring Series, number 1, Australian Government Publishing Service, Canberra, 1994

Mellor, Doreen and Haebich, Anna, (eds). *Many Voices: reflections on experiences of indigenous child separation*, National Library of Australia, Canberra, 2002

No author. 'Moorhouse, Matthew (1813–1876)', in Pike, Douglas (ed.), *Australian Dictionary of Biography*, vol. 5, Melbourne University Press, Carlton, Victoria, 1984 [1974], pp.283–4

Mulvaney, DJ. 'Gillen, Francis James (1855–1912)', in Nairn, Bede and Serle, Geoffrey (eds), *Australian Dictionary of Biography*, vol.9, Melbourne University Press, Carlton, Victoria, 1983, pp.6–7

Mustard, J Fraser. 'Health and Social Capital', in Blane, David, Brunner, Eric and Wilkinson, Richard (eds). *Health and Social Organization: towards a health policy for the twenty-first century*, Routledge, London, 2000 [1996], pp.303–13

Palmer, Kingsley. 'Government Policy and Aboriginal Aspirations: self-management at Yalata', in Tonkinson, Robert and Howard, Michael (eds). *Going it Alone? Prospects for Aboriginal Autonomy: essays in honour of Ronald and Catherine Berndt*, Aboriginal Studies Press, Canberra, 1990, pp.165–83

Price, A Grenfell. *White Settlers and Native Peoples: an historical study of racial contacts between English-speaking whites and aboriginal peoples in the United States, Canada, Australia and New Zealand,* Georgian House, Melbourne, 1949

Quick, Allison and Wilkinson, Richard. *Income and Health,* Socialist Health Association, London, 1991

Raftery, Judith. 'The Social and Historical Context', in Baum, Fran (ed.), *Health for All: the South Australian Experience,* Wakefield Press, Adelaide, 1995, pp.19–37

Raftery, Judith. 'Health Policy Development in the 1980s and 1990s', in Fran Baum (ed.), *Health for All: the South Australian Experience,* Wakefield Press, Adelaide, 1995, pp.51–64

Raftery, Judith. 'Saving South Australia's Babies: the Mothers' and Babies' Health Association', in O'Neil, Bernard, Raftery, Judith and Round, Kerrie (eds), *Playford's South Australia: essays on the history of South Australia, 1933–1968,* Association of Professional Historians Inc., Adelaide, 1996, pp.275–94

Raynes, Cameron. *'A Little Flour and a Few Blankets': an administrative history of Aboriginal affairs in South Australia, 1834–2000,* State Records of South Australia, Adelaide, 2002

Reid, Janice and Trompf, Peggy. *The Health of Aboriginal Australia,* Harcourt, Brace, Jovanovich, Sydney, 1991

Reynolds, Henry. *This Whispering in Our Hearts,* Allen and Unwin, Melbourne, 1998

Rowley, CD. *The Destruction of Aboriginal Society. Aboriginal Policy and Practice – volume 1,* Australian National University Press, Canberra, 1970

Rowley, CD. *Outcasts in White Australia. Aboriginal Policy and Practice – volume 11,* Australian National University Press, Canberra, 1971

Rowley, CD. *The Remote Aborigines. Aboriginal Policy and Practice – volume 111,* Australian National University Press, Canberra, 1971

Rowse, Tim. 'Assimilation and after', in Curthoys, Ann, Martin AW and Rowse, Tim (eds). *Australians From 1939,* Fairfax, Syme and Weldon Associates, Sydney,1987, pp.133–49

Rowse, Tim. 'The Centre: a limited colonisation', in Curthoys, Ann, Martin AW and Rowse, Tim (eds). *Australians From 1939,* Fairfax, Syme and Weldon Associates, Sydney, 1987, pp.151–65

Rowse, Tim. *Traditions for Health: studies in Aboriginal reconstruction,* North Australia Research Unit, Australian National University, Casuarina, Northern Territory, 1996

Rowse, Tim. *White Flour, White Power: from rations to citizenship in Central Australia,* Cambridge University Press, Melbourne, 1998

Rowse, Tim. *Indigenous Futures: choice and development for Aboriginal and Islander Australia,* University of New South Wales Press, Sydney, 2002

Royal Geographical Society of Australasia, South Australian Branch. *Centenary History of South Australia,* supplementary to vol.xxxvi of the proceedings of the society, Adelaide, 1936

Rushbrook, Philippa and Radford, Anthony. *An Annotated Bibliography related to Aboriginal health in South Australia from 1965 to 1984,* Monograph 8, Unit of Primary Care and Community Medicine, Flinders University of South Australia, 1985

Smith, LR. *The Aboriginal Population of Australia,* Australian National University Press, Canberra, 1980

Stanner, WEH. *After the Dreaming: black and white Australians – an anthropologist's view* (Boyer lectures, 1968), Australian Broadcasting Commission, Sydney, 1969

Stevens, Christine. *White Man's Dreaming: Killalpaninna Mission, 1866–1915,* Oxford University Press, Melbourne, 1994

Swain, Tony and Rose, Deborah Bird. *Aboriginal Australians and Christian Missions: ethnographic and historical studies,* Australian Association for the Study of Religions, Bedford Park, South Australia, 1988

Syme, S Leonard. 'To Prevent Disease: the need for a new approach', in Blane, David, Brunner, Eric and Wilkinson, Richard (eds), *Health and Social Organization: towards a health policy for the twenty-first century*, Routledge, London, 2000 [1996], pp.21–31

Taffe, Susan. *Black and White Together FCAATSI: the Federal Council for the Advancement of Aborigines and Torres Strait Islanders, 1958–1973*, University of Queensland Press, St Lucia, Queensland, 2005

Taplin, the Rev. George. *The Narrinyeri: an account of the Tribes of South Australian Aborigines inhabiting the country around the Lakes Alexandrina, Albert and the Coorong, and the lower part of the River Murray: their names and customs. Also an Account of the Mission at Point Macleay*, TJ Shawyer, Printer, Adelaide, 1874

Tatz, Colin. 'Aborigines: political options and strategies', in Berndt RM (ed.), *Aborigines and Change: Australia in the '70s*, Australian Institute of Aboriginal Studies, Canberra, 1977, pp.384–401

Thacker, Andrew. 'Foucault and the writing of history', in Lloyd, Moya and Thacker, Andrew (eds), *The Impact of Michel Foucault on the Social Sciences and Humanities*, Macmillan, Basingstoke, 1997, pp.29–53

Thomson, Neil. 'The Health of Australian Aborigines and Torres Strait Islanders: a socio-cultural perspective', in Lupton GM and Najman JM (eds), *Sociology of Health and Illness: Australian readings*, (second edition), Macmillan Education Australia, Melbourne 1995, pp.113–42

Tindale, Norman B and Lindsay HA. *Aboriginal Australians*, Jacaranda Press, Brisbane 1963

Titmuss, Richard. *Essays on the Welfare State*, Unwin, London, 1958

Tonkinson, Robert and Howard, Michael (eds). *Going it Alone? Prospects for Aboriginal Autonomy: essays in honour of Ronald and Catherine Berndt*, Aboriginal Studies Press, Canberra, 1990

Tonkinson, Robert and Howard, Michael. 'Aboriginal autonomy in Policy and Practice: an introduction', in Tonkinson, Robert and Howard, Michael (eds), *Going it Alone? Prospects for Aboriginal Autonomy: essays in honour of Ronald and Catherine Berndt*, Aboriginal Studies Press, Canberra, 1990, pp.67–81

Townsend, Peter and Davidson, Nick (eds) and Whitehead, Margaret. *Inequalities in Health* (comprising *The Black Report* [1982] and *The Health Divide* [1988]), Penguin Books, London, 1988

Trigger, David. *Whitefella Comin': Aboriginal responses to colonialism in Northern Australia*. Cambridge University Press, Cambridge, 1992

Trudgen, Richard. *Why Warriors Lie Down and Die: towards an understanding of why the Aboriginal people of Arnhem Land face the greatest crisis in health and education since European contact*, Aboriginal Resource and Development Services Inc., Darwin, 2000

Turner, VE. *Pearls from the Deep: the story of Colebrook Home for Aboriginal children, Quorn, South Australia*, United Aborigines' Mission, Adelaide, n.d.[1936]

Turrell, Gavin. 'Social Class and Health: a summary of the overseas and Australian evidence', in Lupton, Gillian M and Najman, Jake M, (eds), *Sociology of Health and Illness: Australian readings*, (second edition), Macmillan Education Australia, Melbourne, 1995, pp.113–42

Vivienne, May. *Sunny South Australia: its city-towns, seaports, beauty-spots, fruit, vineyards, and flowers; its wheat, wool, wine, sheep, dairying, copper, iron, phosphates, and other progressive industries from 1837 to 1908 with map; 4000 miles of travel*, Hussey and Gillingham, Adelaide, 1908

Walker, Peter. 'Maori War', in Fraser, Morag (ed.), *Seams of Light: best antipodean essays*, Allen and Unwin, Sydney, 1988, pp.19–49

Woods, JD (ed.). *The Native Tribes of South Australia*, ES Wigg and Son, Adelaide, 1879

Wilkinson, Richard. *Unhealthy Societies: the afflictions of inequality*, Routledge, London, 1996

Wilkinson, Richard G. 'The Epidemiological Transition', in Kawachi, Ichiro, Kennedy, Bruce P and
    Wilkinson, Richard G (eds), *The Society and Population Health Reader, vol.1: Income Inequality and
    Health*, The New York Press, New York, 1999, pp.36–46
Wilkinson, Richard G. 'The Culture of Inequality', in Kawachi, Ichiro, Kennedy, Bruce P and
    Wilkinson, Richard G (eds), *The Society and Population Health Reader, vol.1: Income Inequality and
    Health*, The New York Press, New York, 1999, pp.492–498
Wilkinson, Richard and Marmot, Michael. *The Social Determinants of Health: the solid facts*, World
    Health Organization, Geneva, 1998

ARTICLES AND PUBLISHED PAPERS

Altman, JC and Sanders, W. *From Exclusion to Dependence: Aborigines and the welfare state in Australia*,
    Centre for Aboriginal Policy Research Discussion Paper, no.1, 1991, Australian National
    University, Canberra, 1991
Anderson, Christopher, Keen, Ian *et al.* 'On the Notion of Aboriginality: a discussion', *Mankind*,
    vol.15, no.1, April 1985, pp.41–55
Anderson, Warwick. 'Geography, Race and Nation: remapping 'tropical' Australia, 1890–1930',
    Historical Records of Australian Science, vol.11, no.4, December 1997, pp.457–468
Attwood, B and Arnold, J (eds). *Power, Knowledge and Aborigines.* (Special edition of the *Journal of
    Australian Studies*), La Trobe University Press, Bundoora, Victoria, in association with the National
    Centre for Australian Studies, Monash University, 1992
Attwood, Bain. 'Introduction', in Attwood B and Arnold, J (eds), *Power, Knowledge and Aborigines.*
    (Special edition of the *Journal of Australian Studies*) La Trobe University Press, Bundoora, Victoria,
    in association with the National Centre for Australian Studies, Monash University, 1992, pp.i–xvi
Bacchi, CL. 'The Nature-Nurture Debate in Australia, 1900–1914', *Historical Studies (Australia and
    New Zealand)*, vol.19, no.75, October 1980, pp.199–212
Berndt, Ronald M (ed.). *A Question of Choice: an Australian Aboriginal dilemma. A collection of papers
    presented at the Australian and New Zealand Association for the Advancement of Science Congress,
    Adelaide, 1969*, University of Western Australia Press, Perth, 1971
Berndt, Ronald M. 'Introduction', in Berndt, Ronald M (ed.), *A Question of Choice: an Australian Aboriginal
    dilemma. A collection of papers presented at the Australian and New Zealand Association for the Advancement
    of Science Congress, Adelaide, 1969*, University of Western Australia Press, Perth, 1971, pp.vii–xx
Berndt, Ronald M. 'The Concept of Protest within an Australian Aboriginal Context', in Berndt,
    Ronald M (ed.), *A Question of Choice: an Australian Aboriginal dilemma. A collection of papers
    presented at the Australian and New Zealand Association for the Advancement of Science Congress,
    Adelaide, 1969*, University of Western Australia Press, Perth, 1971, pp.25–43
Brady, Maggie. 'Leaving the Spinifex; the impact of rations, missions and the atomic tests on the
    southern Pitjantjatjara', *Records of the South Australian Museum*, vol.20, May 1987, pp.35–45
Cleland, J Burton. 'Disease amongst the Australian Aborigines', Parts 1–V, *Journal of Tropical
    Medicine and Hygiene*, vol.XXX1, no.5, 1 March 1928, pp.53–9; no.6, 15 March 1928, pp.65–70;
    no.11, 1 June 1928, pp.125–30; no.12, 15 June 1928, pp.141–5; no.13, 2 July 1928, pp.157–60;
    no.14, 16 July 1928, pp.173–7; no.17, 1 September 1928, pp.216–20; no.18, 15 September 1928,
    pp.232–4; no.20, 15 October 1928, pp.262–6; no.21, 1 November 1928, pp.281–2; no.22, 15
    November 1928, pp.290–4; no.23, 1 December 1928, pp.307–13; no.24, 15 December 1928,
    pp.326–30.

Cleland, JB. 'The Value of a Travelling Medical Service', in Aborigines' Friends' Association, *Aboriginal Problems; articles by various writers*, Aborigines' Friends' Association, Adelaide, nd, [c.1937], p.12

Clyne, Robert. 'At war with the natives: from the Coorong to the Rufus, 1841', *Journal of the Historical Society of South Australia*, no.9, 1981, pp.91–110

Cochrane, Peter. 'Hunting Not Travelling', *Eureka Street*, vol. 8, no.8, October 1998, pp.32–40

Cook, CE. 'The Native in Relation to the Public Health', *Medical Journal of Australia*, vol.1, 1949, pp.569–51

Cook, CEA. 'The Native Problem – why it is unsolved', *Australian Quarterly*, vol. XX11, no.4, December 1950, pp.11–24

Cowlishaw, Gillian. 'Studying Aborigines: changing canons in anthropology and history', in Attwood, B and Arnold, J (eds), *Power, Knowledge and Aborigines* (Special edition of the *Journal of Australian Studies*), La Trobe University Press, Bundoora, Victoria, in association with the National Centre for Australian Studies, Monash University, 1992, pp.20–31

De Maria, William. ' 'White Welfare: Black Entitlement'. The social security access controversy, 1939–59', *Aboriginal History*, vol.10, 1986, pp.25–39

Elkin, AP. 'Three Ways of Helping the Aborigines', Aborigines' Friends' Association. *Aboriginal Problems; articles by various writers*, Aborigines' Friends' Association, Adelaide, nd, [c.1937], p.11

Elkin, AP. 'Culture and Racial Clash in Australia', *Morpeth Review*, vol.2, no.21, September 1932, pp.35–45

Elkin, AP, 'Reaction and Interaction; a food gathering people and European settlement in Australia', *American Anthropologist*, vol.53, no.2, 1951, pp.164–86

Foster, Robert. 'Feasts of the Full-Moon: the distribution of rations to Aborigines in South Australia: 1836–1961', *Aboriginal History*, vol.13, nos.1–2, 1989, pp.63–78

Foster, Robert. 'The Aborigines Location in Adelaide: South Australia's first 'mission' to the Aborigines', *Journal of the Anthropological Society of South Australia*, vol.28, nos.1–2, December 1990, pp.11–37

Foster, Robert. 'Two Early Reports on the Aborigines of South Australia', with an introduction by Robert Foster, *Journal of the Anthropological Society of South Australia*, vol.28, nos.1–2, December 1990, pp.38–63

Haebich, Anna. *Stolen Wages and Consequential Indigenous Poverty: a national issue*. Occasional paper no.17, History Department, University of Melbourne, Melbourne, 2004

Glastonbury, AA. 'Aborigines', *Good Health*, no.138, 1972, pp.45–50

Inglis, Judy. 'One Hundred Years at Point Mcleay, South Australia', *Mankind*, vol.5, no.12, November 1962, pp.503–7

James, W Philip T, Nelson, Michael, Ralph, Ann and Leather, Suzi. 'The Contribution of Nutrition and Inequalities in Health', *British Medical Journal*, vol.314, 24 May 1997, pp.1545–9

Jones PG. 'South Australian Anthropological History: the Board for Anthropological Research and its early expeditions', *Records of the South Australian Museum*, vol.20, May 1987, pp.71–92

Kawachi, Ichiro and Kennedy Bruce P. 'Health and Social Cohesion: why care about income inequality', *British Medical Journal*, vol.314, 5 April 1997, pp.1037–40

Lawrie, WT. 'The Education of Half-caste Children', in Aborigines' Friends' Association, *Aboriginal Problems; articles by various writers*, Aborigines' Friends' Association, Adelaide, nd, [c.1937], pp.15–16

Lendon, AA. 'Dr Richard Penney (1840–1844)', *Proceedings of the Royal Geographical Society of Australasia, South Australian Branch*, vol.xxxi, 1929–30, pp.20–33

Marmot, Michael. 'Social Determinants of Health: from observation to policy', *Medical Journal of Australia*, vol.172, 17 April 2000, pp.379–82

Marmot, MG, Syme SL, Kagan A, Kato H, Cohen JB and Belsky J. 'Epidemiological Studies of
    Coronary Heart Disease and Stroke in Japanese Men Living in Japan, Hawaii and California:
    prevalence of coronary and hypertensive heart disease and associated risk factors', *American Journal
    of Epidemiology*, vol.102, no.6, December 1975, pp.514–25

Marmot, Michael and Theorell, Tores. 'Social Class and Cardiovascular Disease: the contribution of
    work', *International Journal of Health Sciences*, vol.18, no.4, 1988, pp.659–74

Mathews, John D. 'Health Research with Aboriginal Australians: perceptions and realities', the Ian
    Prior Oration for the Australasian Epidemiology Association Annual Scientific Meeting 1999,
    Australasian Epidemiologist, vol.6, no.4, December 1999, pp.2–7.

McGregor, Russell. 'Protest and Progress: Aboriginal activism in the 1930s', *Australian Historical
    Studies*, vol.25, no.101, October 1993, pp.555–68

McGregor, Russell. ' 'Breed out the Colour' or the Importance of Being White', *Australian Historical
    Studies*, vol.33, no.120, October 2002, pp.286–302

Millar, CJ. 'Aboriginal Affairs in South Australia', in Department of Adult Education, *The Aborigines
    of South Australia: their background and future prospects. Proceedings of a conference held at the
    University of Adelaide, 13–16 June 1969*, publication no.19, Department of Adult Education,
    University of Adelaide, 1969, pp.13–18

Millar CJ and Leung, JMS. 'Aboriginal Alcohol Consumption in South Australia', in Berndt, Ronald
    M (ed.), *A Question of Choice: an Australian Aboriginal dilemma. A collection of papers presented at
    the Australian and New Zealand Association for the Advancement of Science Congress, Adelaide, 1969*,
    University of Western Australia Press, Perth, 1971, pp.91–5

Morris, Barry. 'From Underemployment to Unemployment: the changing role of Aborigines in a rural
    economy', *Mankind*, vol.13, no.6, April 1983, pp.499–516

Mulvaney, DJ. 'The Australian Aborigines 1606–1929: opinion and fieldwork. Part 1: 1606–1859',
    Historical Studies Australia and New Zealand, vol. 8, November 1957–May 1959, pp.131–51

Mulvaney, DJ. 'The Australian Aborigines 1606–1929: opinion and fieldwork. Part 11: 1859–1929',
    Historical Studies Australia and New Zealand, vol. 8, November 1957–May 1959, pp.297–314

Navarro, Vicente. 'A Historical Review (1965–1997) of Studies on Class, Health, and Quality of Life:
    a personal account', *International Journal of Health Services*, vol.28, no.3, 1998, pp.389–406

Navarro, Vicente and Shi, Leiyu. 'The Political Context of Social Inequalities and Health', *Social
    Science and Medicine*, 52, 2001, pp.481–91

Pearson, Noel. 'On the Human Right to Misery, Incarceration and Early Death', *Quadrant*,
    December 2001, pp.9–20

Pettman, Jan. 'Gendered Knowledges: Aboriginal women and the politics of feminism', in Attwood B.
    and Arnold, J. (eds), *Power, Knowledge and Aborigines*. (Special edition of the *Journal of Australian
    Studies*) La Trobe University Press, Bundoora, Victoria, in association with the National Centre for
    Australian Studies, Monash University, 1992, pp.120–31

Pope, Alan. 'From Feast to Famine: the food factor in European–Aboriginal relations: South Australia
    1836–1845', *Forum*, Journal of the History Teachers Association of South Australia, vol.10, no1,
    July 1988, pp.47–54

Pope, Allan. 'Aboriginal Adaptation to Early Colonial Labour Markets: the South Australian
    experience', *Labour History*, no.54, May 1988, pp.1–15

Price, A Grenfell. 'Preserving the Aboriginal Race', in Aborigines' Friends' Association, *Aboriginal Problems;
    articles by various writers*, Aborigines' Friends' Association, Adelaide, nd, [c.1937], pp.14–15

Raftery, Judith. ' 'Mainly a Question of Motherhood': professional advice-giving and infant welfare', *Journal of Australian Studies*, no.45, June 1995, pp.66–78

Raftery, Judith. 'Aboriginal Health and 'Black Armband History', *Migration to Mining: medicine and health in Australian history. Collected papers of the fifth biennial conference of the Australian Society of the History of Medicine*, Historical Society of the Northern Territory, Casuarina, Northern Territory, 1998, pp.106–15

Raftery, Judith. 'Keeping Healthy in Nineteenth Century Australia', *Health and History*, vol.1, no.4, 1999, pp.274–97

Roe, Michael. 'A Model Aboriginal State', *Aboriginal History*, vol.10, 1986, pp.40–4

Stretton, Pat and Finnimore, Christine. 'Black Fellow Citizens: Aborigines and the Commonwealth franchise', *Australian Historical Studies*, vol.25, no.101, October 1993, pp.521–35

Sutton, Peter. 'The Politics of Suffering: Indigenous policy in Australia since the 1970s', *Anthropological Forum*, vol.11, no.2, 2001, pp.125–73

Szreter, Simon. 'Rapid Economic Growth and 'the Four Ds' of Disruption, Deprivation, Disease and Death: public health lessons from nineteenth century Britain for twenty-first century China?', *Tropical Medicine and International Health*, vol.4, issue 2, February 1999, pp.146–52

Szreter, Simon. 'The Population Health Approach in Historical Perspective', *American Journal of Public Health*, vol.93, no.3, March 2003, pp.421–31

Thomas, David. 'What Professor Cleland did in his Holidays: collecting expeditions to Central Australia as indigenous health research, 1925–39', *Health and History*, vol.4, no.2, 2002, pp.57–79

Tindale Norman B. 'Survey of the Half-caste Problem in South Australia', *Proceedings of the Royal Geographical Society of Australasia, South Australian Branch*, vol.xlii, November 1941, pp.66–161

Turrell, Gavin and Mathers Colin D. 'Socioeconomic Status and Health in Australia', *Medical Journal of Australia*, vol.172, 1 May 2000, pp.434–8

Unaipon, David. 'An Aboriginal Pleads for his Race', in Aborigines' Friends' Association, *Aboriginal Problems; articles by various writers*, Aborigines' Friends' Association, Adelaide, nd, [c.1937], p.16

Wallace, Rodrick and Wallace Deborah. 'Community Marginalisation and the Diffusion of Disease and Disorder in the United States, *British Medical Journal*, vol.314, 3 May 1997, pp.1341–5

Wilkinson, RG. 'Income Distribution and Life Expectancy', *British Medical Journal*, vol.304, 18 January 1992, pp.165–8

Wilkinson, Richard G. 'Health Inequalities: relative or absolute material standards?', *British Medical Journal*, vol.314, 22 February 1997, pp.591–5

Winter, JM. 'Public Health and the Extension of Life Expectancy in England and Wales, 1901–1960', in Keynes, M, Coleman, DA and Dimsale, NH (eds), *The Political Economy of Health and Welfare. Twenty Second Annual Symposium of the Eugenics Society 1985, Studies in Biology, Economy and Society*, Macmillan, London, 1988, pp.184–203

Woolmington, Jean. 'The Civilisation/Christianisation Debate and the Australian Aborigines', *Aboriginal History*, vol.10, 1986, pp.90–8

Wooton, Hal. 'Imprisoned by the Old Ways: what matters most', *Australian*, 19 April 2001, p.15

MISCELLANEOUS BOOKLETS, REPORTS, PAMPHLETS

Aborigines' Friends' Association Inc. *Aboriginal Problems; articles by various writers*, Aborigines' Friends' Association Inc., Adelaide, nd [c.1934]

Aborigines' Friends' Association Inc. *The Aborigines: a commonwealth problem and responsibility*,

Aborigines' Friends' Association Inc., Adelaide, 1934

Aborigines' Protection League. *Australian Aboriginals: a statement by the Aborigines' Protection League explaining its basic principles and proposals and discussing statements in the Public Press and recent reports and recommendations*, Aborigines' Protection League, Adelaide, 1929

Adler, Elizabeth, Barkat, Anwar, Bena-Silu, Duncan, Quince and Webb, Pauline. *Justice for Aboriginal Australians: report of the World Council of Churches team visit to the Aborigines, 15 June to 3 July 1981*, Australian Council of Churches, Sydney, 1981

Australian National Missionary Conference 1937: Report, Conference Continuation Committee in association with the National Missionary Council of Australia, Sydney, 1937

Evangelical Lutheran Synod in Australia, South Australian District Inc. *Koonibba Jubilee Booklet 1901–1926*, Lutheran Publishing Company, Adelaide, 1926, pp.11–17

Genders, JC. *The Aborigines' Protection League*, (report on conference convened by the Commonwealth Minister of State for Home Affairs to discuss the Bleakley Report, 1928, Melbourne, 12 April 1929), Aborigines' Protection League, Adelaide, 1929

Harms E and Hoff C (eds). *Koonibba: a record of fifty years work among the Australian Aboriginals by the Evangelical Lutheran Church of Australia,1901–1951*, Lutheran Publishing Company, Adelaide, 1951

Lewis, Milton J and Leeder, Stephen R. *Where To From Here? The need to construct a comprehensive national health policy*, Australian Health Policy Institute, University of Sydney, 2001

Report of the Proceedings of the Synodical Convention of the Evangelical Lutheran Synod in Australia, South Australian District, Inc., 1921–1925

Sexton, JH. *A Plea for the Aborigines*, Aborigines' Friends' Association Inc., Adelaide, nd [c. 1935]

Sexton, JH. *Legislation Governing the Australian Aborigines*, second edition, Aborigines' Friends' Association Inc. Adelaide, 1935

Sexton, JH. *An Extensive Survey of Australian Aboriginal Problems*, Aborigines' Friends' Association Inc., Adelaide, nd [c.1937]

Smith, W. Ramsay. *On Race-culture and the Conditions that Influence it in South Australia*, Government Printer, Adelaide, 1912

NEWSPAPERS

Adelaide Examiner
Advertiser
Australian
Australian Lutheran
Christian Colonist
News
Observer
Presbyterian Banner
South Australian Gazette and Colonial Register
South Australian
South Australian Register

UNPUBLISHED

ARCHIVAL MATERIAL

AT STATE RECORDS, SOUTH AUSTRALIA: Government Records
GRG 8 – Public Health Department
Central Board of Health
Correspondence received, 1877, 1898–1968: GRG 8/1
Minutes, 1876–1949: GRG 8/19

GRG 23 – Minister of Public Works
Office of the Commissioner of Public Works
Correspondence received, 1857–1967: GRG 23/1
Petition of the Aboriginals Inhabitants of South Australia to His Majesty's Government, 1935:
  GRG23/1/317

GRG 24 – Colonial (later Chief) Secretary's Office
Correspondence
received by Colonial Secretary, Governor etc,1836–1851: GRG 24/1
received by Colonial (later Chief) Secretary's Office,1842–1984: GRG 24/6
Reports of Protector of Aborigines
1837–1838: GRG 24/1
1842–43: GRG 24/6

GRG 35 – Department of Lands
Crown Lands and Immigration/Crown Lands Office
Correspondence received, 1856–1917: GRG 35/1
Reports of Protector of Aborigines, 1862–63: GRG 35/1

GRG 52 – Aborigines Office and successor agencies
Aborigines Office: GRG 52/1
Correspondence received, 1866–1968: GRG 52/1
George Taplin to Aborigines Office, together with paper 'The Diseases of the Aborigines of South
  Australia', 5 April 1870: GRG 52/1/73/1870

Advisory Council of Aborigines: GRG 52/10 – 52/15
Correspondence, 1921–1939: GRG 52/10
An historical review, 1939: GRG 52/10/5A/1939
Minutes, 1918–1939: GRG 52/12
Research Committee Minutes, 1937–1938: GRG 52/13
Cleland, JB. Some aspects of the problem of the Australian Aboriginal and his descendants in South
  Australia, typescript, [1938]: GRG 52/10/3/1938

Aborigines Protection Board: GRG 52/16 – 52/17
Minutes, 1940–1963: GRG 52/16

Miscellaneous Reports: GRG 52/18
Native (later Aboriginal) Welfare Conferences of Commonwealth and State Authorities, Proceedings
    and Decisions, 1961–1967: GRG 52/18/6 – 52/18/11

Certificates of Exemption: GRG 52/19 – 52/20
Certificates of Unconditional Exemption, 1941–1954: GRG 52/19
Certificates of Limited Exemption, 1941–1954: GRG 52/20

CJ Millar Papers: GRG 52/22
A Brief Outline of Aboriginal Affairs in South Australia since Colonisation, 1963: GRG 52/22/2

Miscellaneous Papers: GRG 52/37
Cleland, JB and Tindale, Norman B. Published papers, (includes unpublished items): GRG 52/37

GRS 4343 – Department of Aboriginal Affairs (1963–1971)
Aboriginal Affairs Board
Minutes, 1963–1971: GRS 4343/1/P

AT STATE LIBRARY OF SOUTH AUSTRALIA: Society Records and Personal Papers
Aboriginal Education Foundation, miscellaneous reports and papers, 1965–84: SRG 102
Aborigines' Friends' Association, Inc. miscellaneous records, Annual Reports: SRG 139;
    PRG 186/7/14
Daisy Bates Papers: PRG 878
Papers of Laurie Bryan: PRG 448
Duguid Papers: PRG 387
Lendon, AA. Short Biographical Sketches. Typescript, with hand written annotations, no date
    [circa 1933]: PRG 128/12/11

NON-ARCHIVAL MATERIAL

THESES AND UNPUBLISHED PAPERS
Bury, Warren R. The Foundation of the Point Macleay Aboriginal Mission, BA (Hons), University of
    Adelaide, 1964
Clark, Alan. 'For Their Own Good': the Aborigines Act 1911, BA (Hons), University of Adelaide, 1992
de Lawyer, Antonia. Davenport and Umeewarra since 1937, BA (Hons), University of Adelaide, 1972
Elton, Jude. Comrades or Competition? Factors affecting union relations with Aboriginal workers in
    the South Australian and Northern Territory pastoral industries, 1878–1958, PhD 2006,
    University of South Australia
Fitzgerald, Paul A. A Study of the Gerard Aboriginal Reserve Community, BA (Hons), University of
    Adelaide, 1971
Gale, Fay. A Study of Assimilation: part-Aborigines in South Australia, PhD, University of Adelaide, 1960

Gibbs, RM. Humanitarian Theories and the Aboriginal Inhabitants of South Australia to 1860, BA (Hons), University of Adelaide, 1959

Hart, Arthur Maxwell. A History of the Education of Full-Blood Aborigines in South Australia, MEd, University of Adelaide, 1970

Hunt, Jennifer M. Schools for Aboriginal Children in the Adelaide District, 1836–1852, BA (Hons), University of Adelaide, 1971

Jennings, Reece. The Medical Profession and the State in South Australia, 1836–1975, MD, University of Adelaide, 1997

Kidd, Rosalind. Regulating Bodies: administrations and Aborigines in Queensland, 1840–1988, PhD, Griffith University, 1994

Macilwain, Margaret. 'South Australian Aborigines Protection Board (1939–1962): tensions between expertise and the idea of representative government', Paper presented at Australian Political Science Association Conference, September 2004

Macilwain, Margaret. South Australian Aborigines Protection Board (1939–1962) and governance through 'scientific' expertise: a genealogy of protection and assimilation, PhD, University of Adelaide, 2005

Milich, Corinne. Official attitudes to the SA Aborigines in the 1930s, BA (Hons), University of Adelaide, 1967

INTERVIEWS (TAPES AND TRANSCRIPTS IN POSSESSION OF AUTHOR)

Rex Orr. Adelaide, 26 February 1999

Geoffrey Pope. Adelaide, 11 March 1999

Ian Cox. Goolwa, 9 December 2002

PRESENTATIONS

O'Donoghue, Lowitja. Address to Foreign Correspondents' Press Conference, 25 May 1999, Canberra; broadcast on ABC Radio National

O'Donoghue, Lowitja. Duguid Memorial Lecture, 13 August 2003, University of South Australia, Adelaide

O'Donoghue, Lowitja. Friday Forum, 8 April 2005, Flinders Street Baptist Church, Adelaide

Index

Wirangu, 109, 274
Women's Community Health Centres, 29
Wood, Peter, 147
Woodruff, Dr Philip, 191
Woodward, Justice AE, 259
Working Group on Inequalities in Health report *see Black Report*
World Council of Churches, 262–263
World Health Organization, 31, 36, 264, 285
'wurley natives', 102, 107, 117, 146
Wyatt, Dr William, 51, 52, 53, 61

Y

Yalata, 20, 109, 203, 231–232
  Aboriginal Reserve Council, 251; data, 299; population, 301; school, 232
Yorke Peninsula, 70, 81, 94, 144, 177, 229
  population, 301
Yorke's Peninsula Aboriginal Mission, 81, 94 *see also* Point Pierce *and* Point Pearce